DNA
Systematics

Volume II:
Plants

Editor

S. K. Dutta, Ph.D.

Professor
Departments of Botany,
Genetics and Human Genetics,
and Oncology
Howard University
Washington, D.C.

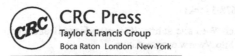

CRC Press
Taylor & Francis Group
Boca Raton London New York

CRC Press is an imprint of the
Taylor & Francis Group, an **informa** business

CRC Press
Taylor & Francis Group
6000 Broken Sound Parkway NW, Suite 300
Boca Raton, FL 33487-2742

Reissued 2019 by CRC Press

A Library of Congress record exists under LC control number:

Publisher's Note
The publisher has gone to great lengths to ensure the quality of this reprint but points out that some imperfections in the original copies may be apparent.

Disclaimer
The publisher has made every effort to trace copyright holders and welcomes correspondence from those they have been unable to contact.

ISBN 13: 978-0-367-25137-6 (hbk)
ISBN 13: 978-0-367-25138-3 (pbk)
ISBN 13: 978-0-429-28628-5 (ebk)

Visit the Taylor & Francis Web site at http://www.taylorandfrancis.com and the
CRC Press Web site at http://www.crcpress.com

FOREWORD

In the early 1960s in the now defunct Biophysics Section of the Carnegie Institution of Washington, Department of Terrestrial Magnetism, Ellis Bolton, Brian McCarthy and I were amazed that we could readily compare the reassociation of mammalian DNA-RNA and DNA-DNA; this, especially, since current dicta said that, because of great complexity, meaningful reassociation did not take place. Our examinations of unfractionated, sheared eukaryotic nucleic acids were mostly made possible by the presence of repeated families of sequences. These families were soon recognized and analyzed by Roy Britten, David Kohne and Michael Waring. Ultimately, Britten and Eric Davidson produced a theory in which the repeated DNA sequences were used as part of control mechanisms governing transcription functions; testing of this theory is still ongoing. At the same period of time, and before, another Carnegie Institution of Washington Staff Member, Barbara McClintock, was performing genetic experiments with maize which indicated "jumping genes". These experiments, finally recognized by a Nobel Prize, have stimulated a resurgence of interest in DNA control elements which are treated herein along with other forms of transcription translation controls such as the tRNAs and rRNAs. In this book series, an international mix of authors has been assembled to address current progress in control and genome comparison. The next 20 years should provide a very great increase in knowledge of these systems. What will the next related volume in this series contain?

Bill Hoyer

INTRODUCTION

In recent years, numerous studies have been performed that use various characteristics of DNA to estimate the diversity or relatedness between both closely and distantly related species. Some of these studies have been concerned with experimental microevolution dealing with the accumulation of relatively small changes within a species, and some with macroevolution involving taxonomic categories and measurements taken over long periods of time or on a geological scale. Most of this explosion of knowledge has been due to the utilization of the powerful methods of recombinant-DNA technology, and a new interdisciplinary science has evolved spontaneously which may be called "DNA Systematics". Included in this science are the characterization of DNA in nuclear and cytoplasmic genomes; DNA:DNA reassociation kinetics of repeated and nonrepeated DNA sequences; thermal stability measurements of heteroduplexes; restriction enzyme patterns analysis of specific nuclear and non-nuclear DNA segments, rDNAs, and mitochondrial and chloroplast DNAs; the rate of evolution of cell organelle genomes vs. nuclear genomes; the implication of gene duplication and gene fusion in evolution and the evolutionary history of specific genes like rRNA genes and hemoglobin genes; evolutionary trends in regulation; and species specificity and DNA sequencing of processing sites of introns and different RNA maturation sites.

Historically, DNA systematics studies were initiated more than 20 years ago by Ellis Bolton, Roy Britten, Bill Hoyer, David Kohne, Brian McCarthy, and others at the Carnegie Institution of Washington, Washington, D.C., and a few other scientists of England, France, and of U.S.S.R. whose work has been reviewed by Belozersky and Antonov during 1972 and 1980 at Moscow University Press, U.S.S.R. Their techniques were mostly based on DNA:DNA hybridization, which is now claimed as the "most favorable of all" methods for revealing family trees, as discussed by Lewin.* Based on these techniques Charles Sibley and Jon Ahlquist (see footnote) have proposed a "DNA clock" to construct phylogenetic trees. Antonov and his associates from the U.S.S.R proposed similar DNA clocks earlier. These molecular clock(s) are becoming very popular. So much so, that they are "now in danger of becoming the dogma that the fossils once were".* Unfortunately, there is no available comprehensive treatise of this vast amount of new knowledge particularly on microevolution based on studies in DNA systematics using new tools of recombinant-DNA technology. In the present work we attempt the first comprehensive review of new information on DNA systematics.

The enormous amount of accumulated information has been reviewed by authors who are active in their respective areas and then organized into three volumes. Volume I is devoted to general topics of DNA systematics with respect to general evolution. Hobish reviews the present state-of-the-art use of computers for storage and retrieval of DNA research data. The role of movable elements in evolution and species formation is reviewed by Georgiev and his associates. It is well established now that mobile DNA sequences provide variability for natural selection and for evolutionary jumps. It makes genomes flexible, and mobile sequences are widespread in living creatures. Studies have been performed on the evolutionary significance of various control mechanisms which regulate speciation and evolution. Studies dealing with the regulation of ribosomal RNA processing sites, regulation of transcription, and analysis of various small RNAs along with their phylogenetic significance are reviewed by Crouch and Bachellerie; Huang; and Beljanski and Le Goff, respectively. The examination of mitochondrial genomes from mammals, *Drosophila,* and fungi has produced models of mt-DNA variation and offers a comparative treatment of evolution with nuclear genomes; these investigations are reviewed by Birley and Croft. Two of the most important gene sets were selected for discussion in this volume. One is the histone gene set, most genes of which do not have introns, and the other is the hemoglobin gene set,

* Lewin, R., DNA reveals surprises in human family tree: the application of DNA-DNA hybridization, *Science,* 226, 1179, 1984.

which does have introns. Enormous amounts of information on these gene sets on the evolution of *Xenopus,* avians, rodents, and higher primates including humans are reviewed by Marzluff; and Winter, respectively.

The second volume is devoted primarily to the DNA systematics of plants, although, where necessary, reference species other than plants have been included to present a complete story. This volume starts with the classical approach to plant systematics using knowledge obtained from the contents of plant nuclear DNAs; this material is reviewed by Ohri and Khoshoo. Plant species, particularly higher green plants, show polyploidy and have 70 to 75% repeated DNA sequences. Studies made on these repeated and single copy DNA sequences of monocot and dicot plants are reviewed by Mitra and Bhatia; and Antonov, respectively. Appels and Honeycutt; and Troitsky and Bobrova have reviewed extensive studies done on ribosomal RNA genes of plants along with information obtained from other species and have given extensive analysis of phylogenetic significance of these studies. The DNA systematics of some fungal species are reviewed by Ojha and Dutta. The chloroplast genomes of green plants have provided excellent information on plant systematics; this information is reviewed by Palmer, whose group has done extensive work with chloroplast genomes of various plants. A critical glossary of different terminologies used in plant DNA systematics is given by A. K. Sharma.

The third volume, now in preparation in collaboration with Dr. William P. Winter as Co-Editor, is devoted primarily to the DNA systematics and evolution of *Homo sapiens* and related higher primate species. This volume will treat some of the newer insights into relationships within the higher primates and the origin of modern man from anthropoid ancestors. Also included will be discussions of the relationships between the races of man as determined by DNA analysis. In addition, several genes which are of vital concern to humans like neuron-specific genes, lipoprotein genes, HLA genes and others will be discussed. Dr. Ronald L. Nagel of Albert Einstein College of Medicine, New York; Dr. C. G. Sibley of Yale University; Drs. M. G. George, R. M. Millis, Mukesh Verma and S. K. Dutta, and William P. Winter of Howard University; Drs. T. B. Rajaveshisth, A. J. Lusis and others of the University of California at Los Angeles; Dr. I. A. Levedevan of Vavilov Institute of Human Genetics, Moscow, U.S.S.R.; Dr. R. L. Honeycutt of Harvard University; and Dr. R. D. Schmickel of the University of Pennsylvania will be writing chapters for this third volume.

These three volumes are expected to be valuable references, not only to students of evolution but also to others interested in efficient germ plasm resource maintenance and utilization, and fields which are vital for planning plant and animal breeding programs. Knowledge of DNA markers correlating the geographic distribution of genes responsible for heritable diseases such as human sickle cell anemia should be of profound importance to physicians and epidemiologists.

In addition to contributing authors, who have also helped in reviewing several chapters, several other authors have helped in organizing and improving various chapters. I would like to acknowledge particularly Fransciso Ayala of the University of California, Davis; Igor Dawid, H. Westphal and A. Schecter of the National Institutes of Health, Bethesda, Md; Professor A. K. Sharma of Calcutta University, Calcutta, India; R. L. Peterson, George Mathew and D. R. Maglott of Howard University, Washington, D.C.; H. James Price, Texas A&M University, College Station, Texas; H. R. Chen, National Biomedical Research Foundation, Georgetown University Medical Center, Washington, D.C.; Bill Hoyer of Georgetown University; E. S. Weinberg of the University of Pennsylvania, Philadelphia; and G. N. Wilson, Pediatric Genetics, The University of Michigan, Ann Arbor.

S. K. Dutta
Editor

THE EDITOR

Sisir K. Dutta, Ph.D., is Professor of Molecular Genetics in the Department of Botany; and Adjunct Professor in the Departments of Genetics and Human Genetics; and in the Department of Oncology at Howard University, Washington, D.C.

Dr. Dutta obtained his B.S. degree from Dacca University, Bangladesh in 1949, and thereafter, served for 6 years as Research Assistant in Genetics and Plant Breeding for the government of West Bengal, India. He received his M.S. and Ph.D. degrees in genetics from Kansas State University, Manhattan, Kansas in 1958 and 1960, respectively. He was a research associate and/or visiting scientist at the University of Chicago, Columbia and Rockefeller Universities in New York, the Pasteur Institute in Paris, the National Institutes of Health in Bethesda, Maryland, and Rice University in Houston, Texas. He was Chief Research Officer-*cum*-Director of the National Pineapple Research Institute of Malaysia from 1960 to 1964, Chairman of the Division of Natural Sciences, and Chairman of the Biology Department of the Christian University Affiliated College at Hawkins, at Texas Southern University from 1964 to 1967. In 1967 he assumed his present duties at Howard University.

He has been the organizer, chairman, and speaker of several national and international symposia held in the U.S., U.S.S.R., Europe, and Asia. He has been a member of the editorial board of the *East Pakistan Agricultural Journal,* a reviewer and panelist of several government and private agencies. He has been inducted as a personality in America's Hall of Fame for his contribution in molecular genetics, has appeared in *Who's Who in the World, Who's Who in America,* and *Who's Who in Frontier Sciences and Technology.* He is a member of several national and international professional societies, author or coauthor of more than 100 papers including monographs, and book chapters and editor of four books. He has been a recipient of several research awards for the U.S. National Science Foundation, National Institutes of Health, Department of Energy, Environmental Protection Agency, Research Corporation, Anna Fuller Fund, and several other agencies including the United Nations Development Projects.

His current research interest is in the areas of regulation of ribosomal RNA transcription and processing, molecular genetics of neuron-specific genes, and molecular evolution.

CONTRIBUTORS

Volume I

Jean-Pierre Bachellerie
Charge de Recherche
Centre Recherche Biochemie and
  Genetique Cellulaire
Centre National de la Recherche
  Scientifique
Toulouse, France

Mirko Beljanski
Master in Scientific Research
Department of Pharmacodynamie
Faculté des Sciences Biologiques et
  Pharmaceutiques
Chatenay-Malabry, France

A. J. Birley
Lecturer
Department of Genetics
University of Birmingham
Birmingham, England

J. H. Croft
Lecturer
Department of Genetics
University of Birmingham
Birmingham, England

Robert J. Crouch
Research Chemist
Laboratory of Molecular Genetics
National Institutes of Health
Bethesda, Maryland

Georgii P. Georgiev
Professor, Head
Department of Nucleic Acid Biosynthesis
Institute of Molecular Biology
U.S.S.R. Academy of Sciences
Moscow, U.S.S.R.

Tatiana I. Gerasimova
Chief
Group of Mobile Elements
Institute of General Genetics
U.S.S.R. Academy Sciences
Moscow, U.S.S.R.

Mitchell K. Hobish
Assistant Research Scientist
Laboratory of Chemical Evolution
Department of Chemistry
University of Maryland
College Park, Maryland

Pien Chien Huang
Professor of Biochemistry
Johns Hopkins University School of
  Hygiene and Public Health
Baltimore, Maryland

Yurii V. Ilyin
Doctor of Biological Science
Head, Department of Genome Mobility
Institute of Molecular Biology
U.S.S.R. Academy of Sciences
Moscow, U.S.S.R.

Liliane Le Goff
Docteur de Sciences
Department of Pharmacodynamie
Faculté des Sciences Biologiques et
  Pharmaceutique
Chatenay-Malabry, France

William F. Marzluff
Professor of Chemistry
Florida State University
Tallahassee, Florida

Alexei P. Ryskov
Senior Researcher
Department of Nucleic Acids
  Biosynthesis
U.S.S.R. Academy of Science
Moscow, U.S.S.R.

William P. Winter
Senior Biochemist
Center for Sickle Cell Disease
Associate Professor of Genetics and
  Human Genetics and Medicine
Howard University
Washington, D.C.

Volume II

Andrew S. Antonov
Professor
A. N. Belozersky Laboratory of
  Molecular Biology
Department of Evolutionary Biochemistry
Moscow State University
Moscow, U.S.S.R.

R. Appels
Principal Research Scientist
Division of Plant Industry
CSIRO
Canberra, ACT, Australia

Chittranjan R. Bhatia
Head
Nuclear Agriculture Division
Bhabha Atomic Research Centre
Trombay, Bombay, India

V. K. Bobrova
Department of Evolutionary Biochemistry
A. N. Belozersky Laboratory of
Molecular Biology and Bioorganic
  Chemistry
Moscow State University
Moscow, U.S.S.R.

Sisir K. Dutta
Professor in Molecular Genetics
Department of Botany
Howard University
Washington, D.C.

Rodney L. Honeycutt
Assistant Professor of Biology
Department of Organismic and
  Evolutionary Biology
Harvard University
Cambridge, Massachusetts

T. N. Khoshoo
Distinguished Scientist
CSIRO
New Delhi, India

Ranjit K. Mitra
Scientific Officer
Nuclear Agriculture Division
Bhabha Atomic Research Centre
Trombay, Bombay, India

Deepak Ohri
Scientist
Cytogenetics Laboratory
National Botanical Research Institute
Lucknow, India

Mukti Ojha
Maitre d'Enseignement et de Recherche
Biologie Vegetale
Universite de Geneve
Geneva, Switzerland

Jeffrey D. Palmer
Arthur F. Thurnau Assistant Professor of
  Molecular Genetics
Division of Biological Sciences
University of Michigan
Ann Arbor, Michigan

Arun Kumar Sharma
Indian National Academy of Science
Professor and Programme Coordinator
Centre of Advanced Study
Department of Botany
University of Calcutta
Calcutta, India

A. V. Troitsky
Department of Evolutionary Biochemistry
A. N. Belozersky Laboratory of
  Molecular Biology and Bioorganic
  Chemistry
Moscow State University
Moscow, U.S.S.R.

TABLE OF CONTENTS

Volume I

Volume II

Chapter 1

PLANT DNA: CONTENTS AND SYSTEMATICS

D. Ohri and T. N. Khoshoo

TABLE OF CONTENTS

I. INTRODUCTION

Quantitative estimation of nuclear DNA content, either chemically or by microdensito-metry, has added a new dimension in the study of evolutionary relationships. DNA being the genetic material, it is natural to presume a trend toward increasing contents during evolution. Quite expectedly, with advancing organismal complexity, the minimum DNA values of various major taxa do increase in a more or less regular way.[1-3] However, within major groups, particularly among eukaryotes, the DNA amounts show extremes of variation. Within angiosperms there is 600-fold variation with C-values ranging from 0.2 pg in *Arabidopsis thaliana* to 127.4 pg in *Fritillaria assyriaca*.[4] Besides, 40-fold difference occurs even within such families as Ranunculaceae[5] and Droseraceae.[6] Furthermore as earlier suggested on the basis of chromosome number, size, and nuclear volume,[7-9] even closely related species may show massive variation in DNA content. Over five-fold differences occur in genera including *Vicia,*[10] *Ranunculus,*[11] and *Crepis.*[12] Above all, gymnosperms, though possessing a narrow range of variation, have much larger mean genome size than that of the angiosperms, and particularly the woody dicots.[13] The situation among ferns is rather obscured by high polyploidy.[14]

This incongruency of organismal complexity or evolutionary status and DNA content has been termed C-value paradox,[15] where C stands for constant and refers to the DNA content of unreplicated haploid genome of a species.[16] Evidently, this paradox also implies that gain and/or loss of DNA has taken place many times during evolution. The marked differences even among closely related species indicate that C-value is under strong selection pressure and is a "character of fundamental biological significance",[4] and many studies have shown that this value is fairly constant within the limits of a species. Indeed, DNA content per genome has been correlated with various important characters such as mitotic and meiotic cell cycle duration,[17,18] minimum generation time and life cycle type,[11,19] latitudinal distribution of crop and noncrop species,[20,21] radiosensitivity,[22] and radiation-induced mutation rates.[23]

Thus, being an adaptive character, a comparison of C-values of related species may provide a natural way to elucidate evolutionary relationships. Therefore, our purpose presently is to consider the role of species DNA content in solving cytotaxonomical and evolutionary problems of narrow taxonomic groups.

II. VARIATION IN DNA CONTENT

A. Diploid Level

The role of DNA alterations at the diploid level will be discussed first as they are quite distinct from those caused by polyploidy which will be dealt with in the next section.

1. Intraspecific Variation

The presence of significant differences in nuclear DNA content within narrow taxonomic groups among higher plants is now well recognized. On the basis of the present data the role of relative DNA content in systematics and evolution at the genus or maybe at the family level can be assessed; however, before going into the feasibility of this approach, the nuclear DNA variation at subspecific level has to be given due consideration. The question arises, what is, if any, the extent of subspecific nuclear DNA alterations? The answer to this question will help in explaining the basic mechanism by which DNA is increased or decreased during species divergence.

Many workers have reported on the intraspecific differences. Up to now, the most thorough studies in this respect have been done in North American conifers. The DNA amount has been shown to vary from the lowest to highest by a factor of 1.5, 1.6, 1.7, and 1.9, respectively among the provenances of *Pinus banksiana, Picea glauca,*[24] *Picea sitchensis,*[25] and *Pseudotsuga menziesii.*[26] Furthermore, the increase in DNA shows a clinal pattern from south to north in the geographic range of the species. The maximum variation by a factor of 2.2, without clinal pattern was detected in 20 seed sources of *Pinus resinosa*[27] over a relatively small geographical distribution. Teoh and Rees,[28] however, failed to repeat Miksche's observations in *Picea glauca,* collected from the same range. A constancy in DNA amount was observed, except for some differences between provenances due to a variable number of B-chromosomes. Similar uniformity in DNA values was also observed in *Pinus contorta* and *Picea engelmanni.*[28] Ohri and Khoshoo[13] also observed a constancy of DNA values in different seed sources of *Pinus taeda, P. mugo,* and *Cupressus sempervirens.* A rather notable uniformity in DNA content was observed in two provenances of *Pinus wallichiana,* one from an extremely dry area of the northwestern Himalayas with annual precipitation of 10 to 20 in. and the other from a wet eastern region (Bhutan) with annual precipitation of up to 200 in.[13]

Similarly, Chooi[10] reported subspecific variation by a factor of 2.0 in *Vicia sativa* and 1.6 in *V. villosa.* However, in *Lathyrus sativus* 13 cultivars showed complete uniformity of DNA values despite significant differences in total chromosome volume which depended on the stage of fixation.[29] Similar constancy was observed in ten cultivars of *Lathyrus odoratus.*[30]

In several *Allium* species Zakirowa and Vakhtina[31] reported considerable intraspecific variation as also intravarietal variation in IC DNA of up to 77% in *Allium cepa* cv. Dungansky. Bennett and Smith[32] attributed it to faulty technique adopted by the authors. *Allium cepa* is not known to show intraspecific DNA variation,[33] and after independent investigation Ohri and Khoshoo[30] found uniformity of DNA values in five different seed sources of *Allium cepa.* This is significant because of the importance of *Allium cepa* as standard material in Feulgen densitometry.

Various crop species known to have undergone intense selection pressure show intraspecific constancy such as *Hordeum vulgare,*[34] *Triticum aestivum,*[35] and *Triticum monococcum.*[36] The case is similar in different cultivars of three elemental species of *Bougainvillea* (cultivars of a species show similar DNA) and their natural hybrids even though they have been under cultivation for several hundred years.[37] On the contrary, Bennett et al.,[38] have reported significant intraspecific variation in *Secale cereale, S. vavilovi,* and *S. silvestre.* Among *Aegilops* species a uniformity is observed in *Ae. speltoides* and *Ae. bicornis,*[39] however considerable intraspecific variation was observed in *Ae. sharonensis.*[39] This led Furuta et al.,[36] to remark that "it seems not feasible to formulate the general rule of intraspecific variability of nuclear DNA content even in a single genus".

Recently, Price et al.,[40] after analyzing 222 plants representing 24 geographically, ecologically, and morphologically diverse populations of *Microseris douglasii* in California, reported 14% interpopulation differences. The higher DNA content has been correlated with mesic sites and well-developed soil and lower DNA content with conditions of water stress. Similar results have also been obtained in four populations of *Microseris bigelovii.*[41] Such studies need to be extended further in more species.

While it may not be possible to assess the extent of intraspecific variation among higher plants from the examples cited above, some conclusions may nevertheless be drawn. It is evident that with some exceptions no detailed analysis has been made on a wider scale in any species. While it may be true that the same standards of intraspecific constancy cannot be applied to all the species, it is also true that the instances of intraspecific constancy are overwhelmingly more than those of intraspecific variation. This is despite the fact that many cases of intraspecific uniformity have not been reported in literature.[32] Moreover, many reports of intraspecific variation have not been confirmed by subsequent studies.[32] Even the same worker has sometimes reported different values for the same species as a result of faulty technique as in *Scilla bifolia* of which six distant provenances were later conclusively shown to be uniform with respect to nuclear DNA amount.[42,43]

Furthermore, it may be mentioned that significant differences in DNA content caused by aneuploidy, presence of variable number of B-chromosomes, and loss or duplication of chromosome segments are not the genuine instances of intraspecific variability. Bennett and Smith[32] have mentioned the sources of true intraspecific variation. First, such variation as caused by ribosomal DNA genes noticed in *Zea mays*, wheat, rice, and peas is so small as to be undetected by densitometry or chemically. Second, the differences as shown by megachromosomes in *Nicotiana* hybrids, or by various genotrophs of flax may just be the rare exceptions.

The point is not to prove or to altogether reject the intraspecific DNA variation, but such variation has not been conclusively shown in an unbiased manner. Much more information is required to settle this point.

2. Interspecific Variation

The presence of remarkable differences even among closely related species shows that C-value is one of the salient characters of a species having been selected because of its adaptive value. Moreover, instead of being random, the alterations in DNA content indeed follow some evolutionary pattern. Tables 1 and 2 give ample idea of both increase and decrease in DNA having occurred many times during the evolution of higher plants.

Table 1 shows the instances in which alterations in DNA content can be correlated with relative evolutionary advancement. A study of 21 diploid (2n = 14) species of *Lathyrus* depicts a four-fold difference in DNA content, which is less in inbreeding annual species and more in outbreeding perennial species.[44,45] The evidence from breeding system and life form together with taxonomic considerations led the authors to conclude that a phylogenetic diminution in DNA has taken place. Stebbins,[46] however, recognizes evolutionary trends even among perennial species in which specialization has been accompanied by increase in DNA.

A similar trend has been indicated in *Crepis*[12] and *Ranunculus*.[11] In *Ranunculus* a 5-fold difference is found in 9 diploid species (from 7.88 pg in *R. laterifolius* to 38.4 pg in *R. ficaria*) and 8 tetraploid species (from 16.5 pg in *R. scleratus* to 78.5 pg in *R. ficaria*.) The annual and perennial species in both diploids and tetraploids, taken separately, are so well defined that DNA values of perennials are more than twice that of annuals. In *Crepis* there is threefold difference in the 8-chromosome group and a tenfold difference in the 10-chromosome group, the overall difference being ninefold, which is equivalent to a ploidy range of 2 to 18 times. Another notable observation is that with the reduction in nuclear DNA there has been a reduction of mean arm ratio. That means a trend from asymmetrical to symmetrical karyotypes.

The *Scilla bifolia* group shows another instance in which DNA diminution has been correlated with advanced characters. A progressive decrease of DNA by a factor of 0.5 has been shown to occur during evolution from primitive yellow seeded (*S. kladnii* IC, 8.6 pg) to advanced black seeded species (e.g., *S. luciliae* IC = 4.3 pg), while brown and gray seeded species, supposed to be intermediary evolutionary stages, also show intermediate DNA amounts.[43] Thus, the grouping based on seed color and the distribution of DNA amounts indicates natural relationships.

The subtribe Microseridinae illustrates rather clearly the presence of opposing trends, i.e., increasing and decreasing DNA contents with species divergence, in a narrow taxonomic group.[47] The DNA varies by a difference of 7.7-fold, the highest being depicted by *Phalacroseris bolanderi* (124.5 units) and the lowest by *Agoseris heterophylla* (16.2 units). The perennial *Microseris laciniata* (48.1 units), occupying the mesic woodlands and open meadows along the Pacific Coast of North America, is considered to be the most primitive on

Table 1
INTERSPECIFIC VARIATION IN DNA CONTENTS WITH PHYLOGENETIC TRENDS

Genus	Direction of change	Least specialized species	More specialized species	Specialized characters	Ref.
Anemone	Increase	Anemone spp. (0.66—1.522)[a]			5
Hepatica			Hepatica spp. (1.85—1.86)	Calyx-like bracts derived karyotype	138, 139
Pulsatilla	Decrease		Pulsatilla spp. (0.487—0.581)	Elongate styles derived karyotype	5, 139
Lolium	Increase	L. perenne (4.16)[b]	L. persicum (6.35)	Annual, inbreeding	49, 50
Lathyrus	Decrease	L. vistitis (29.22)	L. miniatus (6.86)	Annual, inbreeding	44, 45
Chrysanthemum	Increase	C. parthenium (15.6)[a]	C. viscosum (55.7)[a]	Annual	52
Anacyclus	Increase	A. depressus (12.42)[b]	A. radiatus (16.92)	Annual	53, 54
	Decrease		A. clavatus (10.48)	Annual	—
Anthemis	Increase	A. tinctoria (7.46)[b]	A. cota (15.78)	Annual	53, 54
Artemisia	Decrease	A. absinthium (7.28)[b]	A. annua (4.05)	Annual	—
Phalaris (2n = 14)	Increase	P. caerulescens (100.0)[a]	P. angusta (145.9)	Annual	51
Phalaris (2n = 12)	Increase	P. truncata (226.1)[a]	P. canariensis (277.3)[a]	Annual	—
Ranunculus (2x)	Decrease	R. ficaria (19.20)[b]	R. laterifolius (3.94)	Annual	11
Ranunculus (4x)	Decrease	R. ficaria (39.25)[b]	R. scleratus (8.25)	Annual	—
Microseris	Increase	M. laciniata (48.1)[a]	M. borealis (55.7)	Specialized Achenes	47
			Phalacroseris bolanderi (124.5)		
	Decrease		M. elegans (19.6)	Annual	—
Agoseris	Decrease	A. glauca (50.3)[a]	A. heterophylla (16.2)	Annual, ephemeral	—
Crepis	Decrease	C. sibirica (40.25)[a]	C. bulbosa (4.90)	Annual	12
Scilla hohenackeri group	Increase	S. vvedenskyi (20.18)[b]	S. bisotunensis (45.42)	Derived DNA content	140
Scilla bifolia group	Decrease	S. vindobonensis (18.4)[b]	S. nivalis (7.8)	Black seeded	43
Arachis	Decrease	A. villosa var. villosa (5.98)[b]	A. duranensis (4.92)	Annual	141

[a]   The figures in arbitrary units used by the authors of the references cited.
[b]   The figures representing 2C DNA content in picograms.

the basis of morphological characters and is similar to some such ancestral species from which three lines of adaptive radiation have emerged.[48] One line led to such specialized perennial species as *Microseris borealis* and *Phalacroseris bolanderi* adapted to swampy or boggy montane habitats. Clearly, the adaptation to cooler moisture habitats has been ac-

Table 2
RANGE OF INTERSPECIFIC VARIATION IN DNA CONTENT:
PHYLOGENETIC TRENDS UNKNOWN

Genus	Species with lowest DNA content	Species with highest DNA content	Ref.
Allium(x = 9)	*A. zebdanense* (25.3)[a]	*A. karataviense* (45.4)	89
Allium (x = 8)	*A. sibiricum* (15.2)[a]	*A. cepa* (33.5)	—
Alliium (x = 7)	*A. fuscum* (18.4)[a]	*A. hirsutum* (35.9)	—
Drosera	*D. intermedia* (30.2)[a]		
Drosophyllum		*Drosophyllum lusitanicum* (521.0)	6
Vicia	*V. villosa* ssp. *eriocarpa* (15.7)[a]	*V. faba* (100.0)	10
Hordeum	*H. vulgare* var. *Algerie*[48] (13.05)[b]	*H. murinum* (13.55)	34
Avena	*A. nudi-brevis* (10.6)[b]	*A. wiestii* (12.4)	91
Sorghum	*S. roxburghii* (6.83)[b]	*S. durra* (11.42)	142
Lotus	*L. coimbrensis* (1.75)[a]	*L. pedunculatus* (2.12)	143
Gossypium	Species having D genome (10.95)[a]	Species having C genome (20.30)	144
Aegilops	*Ae. squarrosa* ssp. *eusquarrosa* var. *typica* (139.0)[a]	*Ae. bicornis* (255.0)	145
Machaeranthera	*M. brevilingulata* (10.1)[a]	*M. parviflora* (27.2)	55
Aster	*A. hydrophilus* (19.4)[a]	*A. riparius* (36.4)	—
Nicotiana	*N. tomentosiformis* (7.39)[b]	*N. paniculata* (9.64)	98
Phaseolus	*P. lathyroides* (2.3)[b]	*P. dumosus* (3.8)	61
Brassica	*B. nigra* (1.56)[b]	*B. oleracea* (1.81)	97
Crotalaria	*C. grahamiana* (1.91)[b]	*C. incana* (3.43)	146
Oryza	*O. barthii* (1.03)[b]	*O. officinalis* (3.43)	147
Secale	*S. silvestre* PBI R52 (14.42)[b]	*S. vavilovii* UM 2D49 (17.29)	38
Secale	*S. cereale* ssp. *dighoricum* PBI R40 (15.76)[b]	*S. cereale* ssp. *afghanicum* PBI R8 (16.61)	—
Secale	*S. vavilovii* PBI R11 (16.47)[b]	*S. vavilovii* UM 2D49 (17.29)	—
Amaranthus	*A. edulis* (2.40)[b]	*A. hypochondriacus* (2.47)	56
Bougainvillea	*B. peruviana* (7.00)[b]	*B. spectabilis* (8.91)	37
Ficus	*F. mysorensis* (1.37)[b]	*F. benghalensis* (1.45)	57
Cycas	*C. revoluta* (25.54)[b]	*C. circinalis* (29.51)	13
Araucaria	*A. cookii* (19.14)[b]	*A. cunninghamii* (21.77)	—
Picea	*P. mariana* (31.61)[b]	*P. glauca* (40.41)	—

Table 2 (continued)
RANGE OF INTERSPECIFIC VARIATION IN DNA CONTENT:
PHYLOGENETIC TRENDS UNKNOWN

Genus	Species with lowest DNA content	Species with highest DNA content	Ref.
Larix	*L. sibirica* (24.59)[b]	*L. eurolepis* (30.77)	—
Pinus	*P. banksiana* (34.35)[b]	*P. gerardiana* (57.35)	—
Callitris	*C. glauca* (16.53)[b]	*C. rhomboidea* (22.33)	—
Cupressus	*C. sempervirens* (22.62)[b]	*C. macrocarpa* (28.36)[b]	13
Chamaecyparis	*C. pisifera* (22.11)[b]	*C. lawsoniana* (30.10)[b]	13

[a] The figures in arbitrary units used by the authors of the references cited.
[b] The figures representing 2C DNA content in picograms.

companied by increases in DNA as *Microseris borealis* has the highest DNA content (55.7 units) of its genus and *Phalacroseris bolanderi* the highest (124.5 units) in the subtribe. Another line led, by reduction in DNA content, to the specialized inbreeding annual species adapted to warmer and drier regions of the western U.S. A third line of evolution from *M. laciniata* gave rise to a group of perennial *Microseris* species adapted to alpine habitats which subsequently evolved to the genus *Agoseris*. The most primitive perennial species of *Agoseris*, *A. glauca*, does not differ much in DNA content from perennial species of *Microseris*. The specialization and speciation within *Agoseris* have very clearly occurred by reduction in DNA content as highly specialized ephemeral annual *A. heterophylla* (16.2 units), growing in xeric habitats, has only one third the DNA content of *A. glauca* (50.3 units).

On the contrary, there are examples which depict more DNA content in annual species, which means that evolution from perennial to annual habit has been accompanied by the increase in DNA. The grouping of eight *Lolium* species on the basis of breeding system has shown that the inbreeders have 50% more DNA than the outbreeders.[49,50] The species are so well demarcated on the basis of breeding system and DNA content that they seem to form a natural grouping.

In the genus *Phalaris* the species with 2n = 12 have approximately double the DNA content as compared to those with 2n = 14 and seem to form a natural grouping in this respect. The perennial species in each chromosome number group have less DNA than the annual, the least DNA in both the groups is depicted by *P. coerulescens*, supposedly the most primitive perennial species.[51] Similar results have been reported in *Chrysanthemum*,[52] *Anacyclus* and *Anthemis*,[53,54] and *Aster*.[55] There are also genera in which speciation has occurred without any change in DNA, e.g., *Hordeum*,[34] *Amaranthus*,[56] and *Ficus*.[57]

The phylogenetic trends in the examples given in Table 2 are not clear; however, some of them require further explanation.

Thirteen species of a tropical hardwood genus *Ficus* show remarkable uniformity in DNA content. In other words, it may be stated that the speciation in this enormous genus (comprising 600 to 1500 species) is not concomitant with appreciable changes in DNA content.[57] This is despite striking differences in the habit as *F. pumila* studied is a climber in contrast to the other species characterized by large trees. It may be because *Ficus* spp. form climax vegetation in the stable and favorable habitats of tropical rain forests requiring adaptation to comparatively uniform climatic conditions.[48,58,59]

In *Bougainvillea* the DNA values of three elemental species support the crossability relationships among them. *B. peruviana* (BB), which is genetically different from *B. spec-*

tabilis (A_1,A_1) and *B. glabra* (AA) to the extent of forming sterile hybrids when crossed with them,[60] also differs significantly in DNA content from the latter two species.[37] In other words, the genetic differentiation and divergence in DNA content have been concomitant.

Similar observations have been made in *Phaseolus*, in which DNA values fall into two sharply defined groups with means of 2.6 pg (*P. angularis, P. geophilus, P. lathyroides,* and *P. lunatus*) and 3.6 pg (*P. coccineus, P. dumosus, P. leucanthus,* and *P. vulgari*). This natural grouping is supported by the fact that successful interspecific hybrids can be obtained within and not between the species of two groups.[61]

Many more such cases as the examples cited above may be presently uninvestigated. However, a word of caution may be added that genetic divergence and quantitative DNA alterations do not always go together, in view of the instances in which speciation has occurred without any appreciable alterations in DNA content as also massive DNA variation is present in species with close genetic relationship.

Quantitative determination of relative DNA amounts has also been applied to settle the problems of basic chromosome number in groups characterized by aneuploid series, as has been done in the tribe Astereae.[55] A study of three species each of *Aster* and *Machaeranthera* shows that those species with n = 9, e.g., *Aster hydrophilus* and *Machaeranthera brevilingulata*, have remarkably less nuclear DNA amounts than other closely related species with either n = 4 or 5. This evidence, along with data on meiotic pairing, suggests that n = 9 is not derived by polyploidy from the taxa with lower numbers and in fact is the base number from which the taxa with n = 4 and 5 have been derived by meroaneuploid reduction.[55]

Gymnosperms as a group apart show a much more narrow range of DNA content as compared with angiosperms. At the same time the DNA values are so consistently high that they are surpassed in angiosperms only by some monocots.[19,32] Price et al.[62] analyzed DNA contents from nuclear volume measurements of 236 gymnosperm species. The discrepancies in their technique and the low reliability of their results have been enumerated.[63] Subsequently, Ohri and Khoshoo[13] measured 2C values of 57 species belonging to 22 genera of gymnosperms. The range between minimum (*Gnetum ula*, 2C = 4.54 pg) and maximum (*Pinus gerardiana*, 2C = 57.35 pg) is 12-fold. A notable feature is that this variation has occurred primarily at diploid level because of rarity of polyploidy among gymnosperms;[64] this point will be discussed in a later section. Among Cycadales the maximum DNA content is depicted by *Encephalartos villosus* (42.17 pg). *Ginkgo biloba*, the only living species of Ginkgoales, has 19.86 pg. Among Coniferales the genera belonging to Pinaceae show higher mean DNA content than those of other families. Within the order Coniferales the DNA content shows 3.5-fold difference. Furthermore, the genus *Pinus* shows more mean DNA content than other genera of Pinaceae. Very remarkable interspecific differences are depicted in *Picea, Larix, Pinus, Callitris, Cupressus,* and *Chamaecyparis* (Table 2). In Ephedrales, *Ephedra tweediana* (17.75 pg) shows a lower DNA value than the members of Coniferales. *Gnetum ula* is quite distinct with the lowest DNA value (4.54 pg) among all gymnosperms.

To speculate on any overall phylogenetic trends on the basis of these DNA values would be an impossible task considering the antiquity and great divergence of the living gymnosperm families. A definite conclusion which can be drawn, however, is that both phylogenetic increase and decrease in DNA content have taken place many times during evolution. Even within different genera sizeable DNA content variation has taken place during species divergence, as exemplified by *Pinus* which shows as much as a twofold difference. Nothing, however, can be said about the direction of interspecific DNA alterations in different genera. In an ecological perspective of the reproductive cycle of *Pinus*, Francini-Corti[65] has mentioned that the genus originated in the tropics and later adapted itself to temperate conditions. The evidence is long-time (2 to 3 years taken by the seeds to mature), and as in temperate conditions the events in the reproductive cycle are so adjusted as to utilize the short growing season. If this is true, the direction of evolution within *Pinus* has been from lower to higher DNA content, as the tropical pine species presently under study show distinctly lower DNA content than the temperate ones. The highest value is depicted by *P. gerardiana*, a temperate species growing in highly xeric habitats. This point will be discussed in more detail in a later section. Similar phylogenetic considerations can also be deduced in other genera by correlating the trends in DNA content with a knowledge of their past history of ecogeographical distribution.

Finally, the DNA contents of *Ephedra* and especially *Gnetum* do substantiate what Ehrendorfer[66] remarked: "the deep evolutionary hiatus between Gnetatae and other gymnosperms . . .".

Taking an overall perspective, a question which ultimately arises is that if massive differences in DNA can arise even in closely related species, what is the genetic nature of this extra DNA, or in other words, its role in speciation? To put the question in a different way we can ask if there is any correspondence between any particular species characters and increase/decrease in "extra" DNA. Our research is still in a too preliminary stage to answer this question.

An attempt to genetically assay this "extra" DNA has been made in F_1 and F_2 progenies of *Lolium* species varying in DNA content by as much as 50%.[50,67,68] The results from both backcrosses and F_2 progeny depict a remarkable tolerance for "extra" DNA by both gametes and zygotes. In both cases we find a range from low to high DNA parent except for some crosses in which some selection against high nuclear DNA is indicated. Apparently this shows that the sequences comprising this "extra" DNA are inactive. An analogous situation is the disregard for chromosome balance shown by some polyploid taxa, e.g., *Gladiolus*.[69] Furthermore, a study of 19 phenotypic and other characters and this "extra" DNA as appearing in backcross and F_2 families showed no correlation in most of the cases.[50,68]

In contrast to this, no evidence of segregation of DNA content in F_2 progeny was found in an intraspecific cross between *Microseris douglasii* biotypes differing by 10% in 2C DNA content. In a second intraspecific cross the F_2 progeny from two sister hybrids differed significantly in DNA content. Furthermore, the F_1 progeny from an interspecific cross (*M. douglasii* x *M. bigelovii* differing by 10% in DNA content) did not cluster around the parental midpoint and instead depicted an entire range between the parents. Five families of F_2 progeny showed a mean DNA content corresponding to the particular F_1 from which they were obtained.[70] The authors have suggested that the DNA sequences accounting for the differences among plants are unstable and can undergo deletion or amplification in a hybrid.

Studies on almost similar lines have been done in *Microseris* species which show DNA diminution with specialization.[71] Along with the nucleotypic changes and the reduction in dimension of organs, qualitative changes concerning the increase in the degree of developmental canalization are also correlated with reduction in genome size. The latter changes have been found to be due to polygenic systems which are quite independent of the nuclear DNA content in different species. An hypothesis has been stated that these polygenically determined canalizations in development are influenced by different environments provided by different genome sizes in the species.[71] Other approaches to this problem will be discussed in a later section.

The present avaiable evidence leads to the assumption that a large proportion of eukaryotic DNA is superfluous; in other words, its sequences have no specific effect on the phenotype. Moreover, massive differences in closely related species must take place through very rapid changes in DNA on an evolutionary scale. Significant differences in satellite DNA and other very highly repeated sequences as also less repeated DNA have been found in closely related species.[72] This bulk of DNA of the eukaryotes has been termed "junk" and "selfish".[73,74] The multiplication of selfish DNA is suggested to take place by duplicative transposition,[74,75] a mechanism originally postulated to account for the increase in copy number of transposed elements. Moreover, the accumulation of such sequences takes place in such a way as to stimulate further accumulation of similar sequences. The amount of this added nonspecific DNA depends upon intragenomic spread of selfish sequences and phenotypic selection against excess DNA. In other words, the weaker the phenotypic selection against nonspecific DNA the larger the genome size. The authors propose that this selfish DNA may explain the C-value paradox. This concept has been criticized by Cavalier-Smith[76] and Dover[77] who pointed out that this extra DNA may have phenotypic effects independent of any biochemical or coding functions. Dover[77] termed this DNA as "ignorant" as it frequently gets out of hand and is quite capable of generating a multitude of sequence arrangements. Selection on these sequences acts by way of the phenotypic effects they cause due to the mere presence or position within a genome.[77] Subsequently, Orgel et al.[78] did distinguish between two kinds of repeated sequences — "parasitic", whose presence is determined mainly by the efficiency with which they spread intragenomically, and "symbiotic", which exist because of the adaptability they confer upon the individuals in a population. This topic will be discussed further in subsequent sections.

B. Polyploidy

Except for gymnosperms, polyploidy has been a widespread cytogenetic mechanism affecting higher plant evolution. Our purpose here is not to discuss the evolutionary role of polyploidy, a subject which has been much elaborated upon.[9,79-82] One of the most direct effects of polyploidy is the abrupt quantitative increase in chromosome number and nuclear DNA content. We shall therefore confine the subject here to DNA contents of polyploid taxa as related to that of their putative diploid ancestors.

A much-discussed problem has been the DNA diminution in polyploids. Some claims of polyploids having less DNA in proportion to their ploidy level as compared with the related diploids have been made. In *Tulipa* and *Chrysanthemum* some polyploid species contain less DNA when seen in light of their diploid parents,[52,83] while in *Betula* a reduction in DNA content is proposed to be associated with the establishment of highest ploidy level (12x).[84,85] Furthermore, many amphidiploids have been shown to contain less DNA than the expected values obtained on the basis of DNA contents of their presumed diploid ancestors.[86-88] The real problem in such cases is not of diminution of DNA contents in polyploids as such, but that of misinterpretation of results. First, one must be sure about the actual diploid ancestors which have given rise to the polyploids. It may be that the diploids with exactly half the DNA values existed in the past. To clarify, in *Allium* the DNA content of some diploid species exceeds, while that of others is just one half the DNA values of tetraploid species.[89] At the same time in *Ranunculus*, the tetraploid *R. ficaria*, which reproduces vegetatively by bulbils shows exactly double the DNA content of diploid *R. ficaria* which reproduces sexually.[11] The case is similar with the tetraploid race of *Briza media*, which has twice as much DNA as the diploid plants.[90] In *Chrysanthemum morifolium* complex a direct correlation between ploidy levels and DNA content was demonstrated, as it was in natural triploid cultivars of *Bougainvillea*.[37,56] Similarly, 2x, 4x, and 6x species of *Avena* and *Hordeum* maintain a ratio of 1:2:3 in DNA contents.[34,91]

Results such as those above may have been obtained because of faulty techniques as indicated by the initial claims of Pai et al.[87] and the subsequent papers by Upadhya and Swaminathan,[92] Rees and Walters,[93] Pegington and Rees,[94] and Nishikawa[95] which clearly demonstrated that no reduction has taken place during the evolution of allohexaploid *Triticum aestivum*. Furthermore, Furuta et al.[96] have shown that the sum of DNA contents of the AA and BB genomes in present-day allo-hexaploid wheat is not significantly different from that of the present-day allo-tetraploid emmer wheat (AA BB). Thus, we may conclude that no significant quantitative changes in DNA have occurred during the past 7000 years of cultivation, despite many genetic changes having been occurred. Pegington and Rees[94] also revealed that while chromosome volume, mass, or DNA remains constant, the chromosome length in hexaploid *Triticum aestivum* is shorter than that in its tetraploid and diploid ancestors, thus showing more compact chromosome organization. In the same way the earlier claims of DNA diminution in allotetraploid *Brassica* species[88] were refuted by Verma and Rees[97] who demonstrated that the denser nuclei of allotetraploid *B. napus*, *B. carinata*, and *B. juncea* resulted in the underestimation of their DNA contents by microdensitometry. However, after applying correction their DNA values were found to be equal to the sum of their respective diploid parents. Similar results were obtained in amphidiploids of *Nicotiana*; moreover, on the basis of DNA values, *N. sylvestris* and *N. tomentosiformis* were confirmed to be the diploid ancestors of *N. tabacum*[98]

Similarly, the induced colchiploids show an additive effect, i.e., the exact doubling of DNA content. After studying colchicine-induced 4n, 8n, and 16n nuclei in the root tip meristem cells of *Vicia faba*, Deka and Sen[99] showed that in polyploid nuclei while the chromosome numbers remained normal the DNA content showed a progressive decline at successive ploidy levels. Bennett and Jellings,[100] however, showed by a similar experiment that while progressive DNA diminution does take place, it was actually because of increasing frequency of micronuclei and higher nuclear density at higher ploidy levels, denying therefore any real decrease in DNA. In *Amaranthus*, the autotetraploids representing C-10 generation show an exact twofold increase in DNA over the diploids.[56] The case is similar in colchiploids of *Bougainvillea*.[37] This evidence proves the absence of DNA diminution in polyploids and once again demonstrates nuclear DNA constancy for a given set of chromosomes within a species.

C. Mechanism of Change

As the multinemic concept has been almost discarded, the discussion on the relative quantitative differences in nuclear DNA content will be based on uninemic structure of chromosomes.

For an unassailable structural proof of where exactly the increase in chromosomal DNA takes place, we have to relate the work on chironomids, *Chironomus thummi thummi*, *Ch. thummi piger*, and their F_1 hybrid. Phylogenetically, *Ch. th. thummi* is derived from *Ch. th. piger*.[101] The total amount of DNA in salivary gland nuclei of *Ch. th. thummi* is 27% higher than *Ch. th. piger*. This difference is demonstrated by unpaired regions of the salivary gland chromosomes of the hybrid where some bands of *Ch. th. thummi* contain 2, 4, 8, or 16 times the amount of DNA as compared with the corresponding bands of *Ch. th. piger*.[102,103] Hence, the difference in their chromosomes is caused by localized increase of DNA in *Ch. th. thummi*.

Equally convincing proof of lengthwise repetition or deletion has been obtained from the pachytene analysis of the F_1 hybrids between the species differing markedly in DNA content. In such cases loops and overlaps are expected where repetition or deletion of chromosome segments has taken place. Exactly this has been revealed in *Lolium temulentum* x *L. perenne*, *Festuca drymeja* x *F. scariosa*, and *Allium cepa* x *A. fistulosum* hybrids.[2,49,89,104,105]

Furthermore, among tribe Asterae, Stucky and Jackson[55] discovered unpaired loops in *Machaeranthera parviflora* (n = 5) x *Aster hydrophilus* (n = 9), *Machaeranthera boltoniae* x *M. tenuis* (n = 4), and *Machaeranthera parviflora* x *Aster riparius* hybrids. In *Crepis* hybrids the situation is obscured because of the presence of multiple translocations and inversions; however, the difference in sizes of parental chromosomes is revealed at metaphase I of *C. laciniata* x *C. aurea* (2n = 10) and *C. neglecta* x *C. capillaris* (2n = 6). Though the chromosomes of *C. laciniata* are larger by volume than those of *C. aurea* by 20%, the difference in size between homoeologs as found at metaphase I varies from 6 to 40%, which means that the differences in DNA amount are not equally distributed to all the chromosomes of the complement.[12] This case is similar to that of the *Allium cepa* x *A. fistulosum* hybrid in which the size differences between homoeologs at metaphase I vary from 10 to 60%, although the former has 27% more nuclear DNA than the latter.[89] In contrast to this, in *Lolium* and *Festuca* it has been conclusively shown that the increase in DNA was achieved by each chromosome of the complement sharing roughly equal amounts of DNA. Chromosome volume measurements at metaphase I of F_1 hybrids *Festuca drymeja* x *F. scariosa* and *Lolium temulentum* x *L. perenne* revealed that each chromosome of haploid complement of *F. drymeja* and *L. temulentum* is bigger than its homoeolog in *F. scariosa* and *L. perenne* by 0.17 and 0.15 pg of DNA, respectively.[105]

This obviously means that with increasing DNA content the karyotypes became more symmetrical, and as a result of this the smaller homoeologs showed incomplete pachytene pairing because of larger differences in DNA content as compared to the bigger homoeologs.[105] Much the same pattern was noticed by an analysis of the distribution of nuclear DNA in chromosome complements of four *Lathyrus* species showing twofold differences.[45,106] This kind of uniformity of relative chromosome sizes within complements despite marked differences in DNA content has also been noticed within diverse genera of both plants and animals, i.e., salamanders,[107] anguilloid fishes,[108] acridid grasshoppers,[109] *Blennius*,[110] conifers,[13,111-116] etc. In the genus *Pinus*, particularly, the interspecific differences in karyotype are hardly detectable, so much so that the karyotype of species with the highest DNA content appears to be only the larger version of that of the species with the least DNA content.[13] Such a remarkable uniformity provides compelling evidence for some sort of constraint upon the DNA increments in each of the chromosomes of the complements. This is indeed significant and may not be without any adaptive value.

Equally significant and much more surprising is the fact that the interspecific variation in DNA content, being far from random, shows a discontinuous pattern and in some cases even geometric progression. Plant genera showing this type of variation are *Anemone*,[5] *Vicia*,[117] several genera within graminae,[118] *Phaseolus*,[61] *Phalaris*,[51] *Lathyrus*, *Clarkia*, and *Nicotiana*.[45] Among these, the results on *Lathyrus* need to be explained in detail. On the basis of their nuclear DNA content 21 diploid species showing a range of 22.4 pg can be clustered into 7 DNA groups, with successive groups differing equally by 3.71 pg of DNA. Further detailed analysis on 12 species taking 12 nuclear characters revealed that the species can be grouped into 6 sharply defined clusters. There is marked similarity of species within clusters in contrast to large intercluster differences for most of the characters. The relatively larger divergence in one group, D, comprised of *L. hirsutus* and *L. tingitanus*, was due mainly to the difference in the amount of constitutive heterochromatin, which is 10.7% higher in the latter species. An additive influence of C-bands on the DNA amount has also been shown in *Scilla siberica* and *S. bifolia* subgroups.[43,119]

Similarly, in *Secale* the evidence is presented which shows that the addition of heterochromatin at telomeres is responsible for large increases in DNA amount.[38] Coming back to *Lathyrus*, it has been postulated that the divergence of species is accompanied by "discrete quantum jumps" and the groups represent "steady states" in genome evolution.

Finally, the question arises about the composition of DNA lost or gained, as the case may be, during evolution. It is worth pointing out here that the constraints seen at the cytological level are present at a biochemical level as well. A proportionate increase of repetitive DNA with the genome size has been indicated;[120] however, the studies on narrow taxonomic groups in both plants and animals have revealed that both repetitive and nonrepetitive fractions are involved in the evolutionary increase or reduction of genome size. In *Lathyrus* the ratio of repetitive to nonrepetitive DNA in "supplementary DNA" is constant throughout the genus, i.e., for every 3.9 pg increase in the former there is an addition of 1 pg in the latter fraction.[121] Similarly, in *Lolium* the increase in 5.5 pg of repetitive DNA is accompanied by a 1 pg addition of nonrepetitive DNA.[122] Such a regularity of ratios between the two fractions contributing to varying DNA amounts has been shown to be a consistent feature in many plant and animal genera.[122] The situation is indeed interesting. What these constraints signify will be discussed later, though our present knowledge is too meager to deal with it.

D. Temperate vs. Tropical

It has long been known from the observations primarily on Graminae of Avdulov[123] and Stebbins[9] that tropical species or those growing during warm periods in temperate regions possess small- to medium-sized chromosomes and nuclei in contrast to larger chromosomes of those growing in cool temperate regions. The same situation was later pointed out for Leguminosae and the order Liliales.[58] An hypothesis was also put forth which stated that high nuclear DNA content means each gene controlled metabolic process being controlled by many gene loci leading to slowing down of metabolic activity, which is an adaptation to limited supply of raw materials to growing cells at low temperatures.[58]

The presence of differences in genome size between tropical and temperate species has been largely corroborated by the later studies. In a literature survey of 368 tropical and 524 temperate herbaceous species, Levin and Funderburg[124] clearly showed that mean and total chromosome lengths and 4C DNA contents of temperate species are almost twice that of the tropical species. However, it may not be true for larger cosmopolitan families such as Leguminosae and Compositae in which no significant differences were detected. As mentioned earlier, a similar marked difference in DNA content has been detected in tropical vs. temperate species of *Pinus*.[13] This correlation, however, becomes modified at high latitudes as has been shown in the case of 23 angiosperm species from South Georgia or the Antarctic which have much smaller ranges of DNA amounts than that of angiosperms taken as a whole.[21] This suggestion by the authors is due to the selection of species with only the low DNA amounts at such altitudes because of the constraints applied by the duration of minimum generation time, which becomes inordinately long in species with high DNA amounts at low temperatures (0 to 5°C).

That the geographical ranges are determined by the amount of nuclear DNA content has also been comprehensively demonstrated in the case of crop plants. A DNA amount-latitude cline has been shown for cereal grain crops, cultivated pasture grasses, and pulses.[20] Furthermore, a clear correlation exists between the latitude of supposed sites of domestication, thereby implying the natural distribution of wild progenitors and DNA amount. This shows that the cline is a natural phenomenon and crop species with increasingly low DNA amounts were selected at successively lower latitudes. This cline has evidently been modified and exaggerated in agriculture later on.

E. Life Form

Bennett[19,125] introduced the term "nucleotype" to denote the role of nuclear DNA in controlling various developmental processes and phenotype in quantitative terms quite independent of its informational content. As the topic has been dealt with in much detail,[11,19,20,126] it will not be repeated here. Regardless, it may be mentioned that in the case of herbaceous plants a positive correlation of DNA content has been indicated with chromosome and nuclear volume, cell size, nucleolar and nuclear dry mass, seed dry mass, minimum cell cycle time, meiotic duration, pollen maturation time, and minimum generation time.[19]

F. Woody vs. Herbaceous

As compared with the herbaceous, woody angiosperms are known to possess small-sized chromosomes.[127,128] Thirteen species of a tropical hardwood genus *Ficus* show uniform and very low 2C DNA values ranging from 1.35 to 1.47 pg.[57] If chromosome size is taken as a good indicator of DNA content, it may be stated that the hardwoods have particularly low and uniform C-values. This may seem to support as Mehra[127] has remarked "Hutchinson's[129] broad division of angiosperms into Lignosae and Herbaceae, if considered in its proper perspective". Moreover, it raises another point that by being a constant feature the small genome size must be of a high adaptive value in woody angiosperms. An explanation most often considered is based upon proportionality between nuclear and cell size,[130] which means that a check is likely to be exercised by the smallest cells in the life of a plant. In woody dicots these are cambial cells which form wood fibers.[7,9,113] While the point certainly seems to be explained reasonably well, it may not be exclusively so, as Mehra and Bawa[131] have reported the presence of polyploid series in many woody taxa which seem to tolerate different cell/nucleus ratios. Also, the concept of positive correlation between minimum generation time and DNA content as seen in herbaceous angiosperms[19] is not true in their woody counterparts.

In sharp contrast to this the conifers depict very high DNA values showing a fourfold variation.[13] This is because the function of water conduction in conifers is performed by tracheids in contrast to woody angiosperms which have vessels. Therefore, the need for efficient water conduction has resulted in strong selection for bigger cell size as depicted by giant cambial cells in *Pinus strobus*,[132,133] and consequently in increased nuclear volume and DNA content.[126] In this context it is significant to note the association of very high DNA values, as in the case of *Pinus gerardiana* (2C = 57.35 pg), with a temperate and highly xeric habitat.[13] It would be worth studying tracheid dimensions vis a vis DNA content in conifer species in relation to ecological conditions. The rarity of polyploidy among gymnosperms may be because the selection for larger genome size has almost reached a saturation point and further increase through polyploidy cannot be tolerated. It is pertinent to remark here that endopolyploidy, which is so characteristic of angiosperms has not so far been found in gymnosperms.[134] This may mean that any increase in nuclear and cell size is not tolerated during ontogeny. Furthermore, as this increase in DNA content has taken place by tandem duplications, thereby implying much DNA redundancy, the more active and divergent evolution by (allo)polyploidy has been denied to gymnosperms.[66,135-137] Similarly, high DNA values and slow rate of development may have been responsible for the absence of annual habit among gymnosperms.[19,126]

III. CONCLUSIONS

The salient points which have emerged from this review are as follows:

1. On the basis of our present understanding it can reasonably be stated that the concept of intraspecific constancy of nuclear DNA amount is practically valid, and therefore C-value is one of the basic characteristics of a species.
2. Remarkable variation in DNA content can be found even among closely related species at the diploid level, and the direction of change may be correlated with specialized or primitive features. The grouping of taxa according to C-values may sometimes correspond with taxonomic affinities suggested by the morphological traits. Most often, evolutionary advancement or specialization is accompanied by a reduction in genome size, but the reverse is also true in some cases.
3. There is no correspondence between the level of genetic differentiation of species and their DNA amounts; in other words, the quantitative genome variation is not a prerequisite of species divergence. Furthermore, the "extra" DNA does not form a fertility barrier between the species which can be crossed to obtain F_1 hybrids, as it also shows a random distribution among backcrosses and F_2 progeny, depicting a remarkable tolerance by both gametes and zygotes.
4. Some groups such as gymnosperms and certain perennial monocots have particularly high DNA values. This may be because of large-scale accretion of DNA without any selection for reduction in genome size. The potential for the further evolution of such groups is quite different from those having a moderate genome size of 1 to 10 pg, as depicted by the absence of polyploidy in gymnosperms.

5.   In the large majority of the groups the increase or decrease in DNA is not random but shows a discontinuous pattern forming clusters of taxa or even geometric progression.
6.   The DNA alterations take place by tandem duplications or deletions as evidenced by unpaired loops at pachytene of F_1 hybrids. Furthermore, the DNA accretions are distributed equally among all the chromosomes of the complement, thus maintaining karyotypic uniformity. However, as smaller chromosomes gain proportionally more DNA, the karyotypes become more symmetrical with increasing DNA content.
7.   The constraints seen at the cytological level are also maintained at the biochemical level, where repetitive and nonrepetitive sequences increase in proportionally equal amounts, i.e., their ratios remain constant during evolution.
8.   The adaptive parameters which govern evolutionary gain or loss of DNA are nuclear and cell volume, chromosome size, minimum mitotic and meiotic duration, and minimum generation time.

REFERENCES

1. **Sparrow, A. H., Price, H. J., and Underbrink, A. G.,** A survey of DNA content per cell and per chromosome of prokaryotic and eukaryotic organisms. Some evolutionary considerations, *Brookhaven Symp. Biol.*, 23, 451, 1972.
2. **Rees, H. and Jones, R. N.,** The origin of the wide species variation in nuclear DNA content, *Int. Rev. Cytol.*, 32, 53, 1972.
3. **Price, H. J.,** Evolution of DNA content in higher plants, *Bot. Rev.*, 42, 27, 1976.
4. **Bennett, M. D., Smith, J. B., and Heslop-Harrison, J. S.,** Nuclear DNA amounts in angiosperms, *Proc. R. Soc. Lond. Ser. B:*, 216, 179, 1982.
5. **Rothfels, K., Sexsmith, E., Heimburger, M., and Krause, M. O.,** Chromosome size and DNA content of species of *Anemone* L. and related genera (Ranunculaceae), *Chromosoma*, 20, 54, 1966.
6. **Rothfels, K. and Heimberger, M.,** Chromosome size and DNA values in sundews (Droseraceae), *Chromosoma*, 25, 96, 1968.
7. **Darlington, C. D.,** *Recent Advances in Cytology*, 2nd ed., Churchill, Livingston, London, 1937.
8. **Stebbins, G. L.,** Cytological characteristics associated with the different growth habits in the dicotyledons, *Am. J. Bot.*, 25, 189, 1938.
9. **Stebbins, G. L.,** *Variation and Evolution in Plants*, Columbia University Press, New York, 1950.
10. **Chooi, W. Y.,** Variation in nuclear DNA content in the genus *Vicia*, *Genetics*, 68, 195, 1971.
11. **Smith, J. B. and Bennett, M. D.,** DNA variation in the genus *Ranunculus*, *Heredity*, 35, 231, 1975.
12. **Jones, R. N. and Brown, L. M.,** Chromosome evolution and DNA variation in *Crepis*, *Heredity*, 36, 91, 1976.
13. **Ohri, D. and Khoshoo, T. N.,** Genome size in gymnosperms, *Plant Syst. Evol.*, in press, 1985.
14. **Mehra, P. N.,** Cytological evolution of ferns with particular reference to Himalayan forms, in *Proc. 48th Indian Sci. Congr.*, II, 1, 1961.
15. **Thomas, C. A.,** The genetic organisation of chromosomes, *Ann. Rev. Genet.*, 5, 237, 1971.
16. **Swift, H.,** The constancy of deoxyribose nucleic acid in plant nuclei, *Proc. Natl. Acad. Sci. U.S.A.*, 36, 643, 1950.
17. **Van't Hof, J.,** The duration of chromosomal DNA synthesis, of the mitotic cycle, and of meiosis of higher plants, in *Handbook of Genetics*, Vol. 2, King, R. C., Ed., Plenum Press, New York, 1975, 363.
18. **Bennett, M. D.,** The time and duration of meiosis, *Philos. Trans. R. Soc. Lond.*, B277, 201, 1977.
19. **Bennett, M. D.,** Nuclear DNA content and minimum generation time in herbaceous plants, *Proc. R. Soc. Lond. Ser. B:*, 181, 109, 1972.
20. **Bennett, M. D.,** DNA amount, latitude and crop plant distribution, *Environ. Exp. Bot.*, 16, 93, 1976.
21. **Bennett, M. D., Smith, J. B., and Lewis-Smith, R. I.,** DNA amounts of angiosperms from the antarctic and South Georgia, *Environ. Exp. Bot.*, 22, 307, 1982.
22. **Underbrink, A. G., Sparrow, A. H., and Pond, V.,** Chromosomes and cellular sensitivity. II. Use of interrelationships among chromosome volume, nucleotide content and DO of 120 diverse organisms in predicting radiosensitivity, *Rad. Bot.*, 8, 205, 1968.
23. **Abrahamson, S., Bender, M. A., Conger, A. D., and Wolff, S.,** Uniformity of radiation-induced mutation rates among different species, *Nature (London)*, 245, 460, 1973.

24. **Miksche, J. P.,** Quantitative study of intraspecific variation of DNA per cell in *Picea glauca* and *Pinus banksiana*, *Can. J. Genet. Cytol.*, 10, 590, 1968.

25. **Miksche, J. P.,** Intraspecific variation of DNA per cell between *Picea sitchensis* (Bong) carr. provenances, *Chromosoma*, 32, 343, 1971.

26. **El-Lakany, M. H. and Sziklai, O.,** Intraspecific variation in nuclear characteristics of douglas-fir, *Adv. Frontiers Plant Sci.*, 28, 363, 1971.

27. **Dhir, N. K. and Miksche, J. P.,** Intraspecific variation of nuclear DNA content in *Pinus resinosa*, *Can. J. Genet. Cytol.*, 16, 77, 1974.

28. **Teoh, S. B. and Rees, H.,** Nuclear DNA amounts in populations of *Picea* and *Pinus* species, *Heredity*, 36, 123, 1976.

29. **Verma, S. C. and Ohri, D.,** Chromosome and nuclear phenotype in the legume *Lathyrus sativus* L., *Cytologia*, 44, 77, 1979.

30. **Ohri, D. and Khoshoo, T. N.,** Unpublished data, 1984.

31. **Zakirowa, R. O. and Vakhtina, L. I.,** Cytophotometrical and caryological investigation of some species of the genus *Allium*, subgenus *Melanocrommyum* (Webb et Berth.) Wedelbo, Sect. Melanocrommyum, *Bot. Zh. S.S.S.R.*, 12, 1819, 1974.

32. **Bennett, M. D. and Smith, J. B.,** Nuclear DNA amounts in angiosperms, *Philos. Trans. R. Soc. Lond.*, B274, 227, 1976.

33. **Rees, H.,** personal communication, 1982.

34. **Bennett, M. D. and Smith, J. B.,** The 4C DNA content of several *Hordeum* genotypes, *Can. J. Genet. Cytol.*, 13, 607, 1971.

35. **Nishikawa, K. and Furuta, Y.,** Comparison of DNA content per nucleus between Japanese and U.S. varieties of common wheat, *Jpn. J. Breeding*, 18, 30, 1967.

36. **Furuta, Y., Nishikawa, K., and Haji, T.,** Uniformity of nuclear DNA content in *Triticum monococcum* L., *Jpn. J. Genet.*, 58, 361, 1978.

37. **Ohri, D. and Khoshoo, T. N.,** Cytogenetics of cultivated bougainvilleas X. Nuclear DNA content, *Z. Pflanzenzucht.*, 88, 168, 1982.

38. **Bennett, M. D., Gustafson, J. P., and Smith, J. B.,** Variation in nuclear DNA in the genus *Secale*, *Chromosoma*, 61, 149, 1977.

39. **Furuta, Y., Nishikawa, K., and Kimizuka, T.,** Quantitative comparison of the nuclear DNA in section sitopsis of the genus *Aegilops*, *Jpn. J. Genet.*, 52, 107, 1977.

40. **Price, H. J., Chambers, K. L., and Bachmann, K.,** Geographical and ecological distribution of genomic DNA content variation in *Microseris douglasii* (Asteraceae), *Bot. Gaz.*, 142, 415, 1981.

41. **Price, H. J., Chambers, K. L., and Bachmann, K.,** Genome size variation in diploid *Microseris bigelovii* (Asteraceae), *Bot. Gaz.*, 142, 156, 1981.

42. **Greilhuber, J.,** DNA contents, Giemsa banding, and systematics in *Scilla bifolia, S. drunensis* and *S. vindobonensis* (Liliaceae), *Plant Syst. Evol.*, 130, 223, 1978.

43. **Greilhuber, J.,** Evolutionary changes of DNA and heterochromatin amounts in *Scilla bifolia* group (Liliaceae) *Plant Syst. Evol.*, 2(Suppl.), 263, 1979.

44. **Rees, H. and Hazarika, M. H.,** Chromosome evolution in *Lathyrus*, *Chromosomes Today*, 2, 158, 1969.

45. **Narayan, R. K. J.,** Discontinuous DNA variation in the evolution of plant species; the genus *Lathyrus*, *Evolution*, 36, 877, 1982.

46. **Stebbins, G. L.,** Chromosome, DNA and plant evolution, *Evol. Biol.*, 9, 1976.

47. **Price, H. J. and Bachmann, K.,** DNA content and evolution in the Microseridinae, *Am. J. Bot.*, 62, 262, 1975.

48. **Stebbins, G. L.,** *Flowering Plants: Evolution Above Species Level*, Belknap Press, Cambridge, Mass., 1974.

49. **Rees, H. and Jones, G. H.,** Chromosome evolution in *Lolium*, *Heredity*, 22, 1, 1967.

50. **Hutchinson, J., Rees, H., and Seal, A. G.,** An assay of supplementary DNA effects in *Lolium*, *Heredity*, 43, 411, 1979.

51. **Kadir, Z. B. A.,** DNA values in the genus *Phalaris* (Gramineae), *Chromosoma*, 45, 379, 1974.

52. **Dowrick, G. J. and El-Bayoumi, A. S.,** Nucleic acid content and chromosome morphology in *Chrysanthemum*, *Genet. Res.*, 13, 241, 1969.

53. **Nagl, W. and Ehrendorfer, F.,** DNA content, heterochromatin, meiotic index and growth in perennial and annual Anthemideae, *Plant Syst. Evol.*, 123, 35, 1974.

54. **Nagl, W.,** Role of heterochromatin in the control of cell cycle duration, *Nature (London)*, 249, 53, 1974.

55. **Stucky, J. and Jackson, R. C.,** DNA content of seven species of Astereae and its significance to theories of chromosome evolution in the tribe, *Am. J. Bot.*, 62, 509, 1975.

56. **Ohri, D., Nazeer, M. A., and Pal, M.,** Cytophotometric estimation of nuclear DNA in some ornamentals, *Nucleus*, 24, 39, 1981.

57. **Ohri, D. and Khoshoo, T. N.,** Nuclear DNA contents in the genus *Ficus* (Linn.) Tourn. (Moraceae), *Plant Syst. Evol.*, (communicated), 1984.

58. **Stebbins, G. L.,** Chromosome variation and evolution, *Science*, 152, 1463, 1966.
59. **Ashton, P. S.,** Speciation among tropical forest trees: some deductions in the light of recent evidence, *Biol. J. Linn. Soc.*, 1, 155, 1969.
60. **Zadoo, S. N., Roy, R. P., and Khoshoo, T. N.,** Cytogenetics of cultivated bougainvilleas. VI. Hybridization, *Z. Pflanzenzucht.*, 75, 114, 1975.
61. **Ayonoadu, U. W. U.,** Nuclear DNA variation in *Phaseolus*, *Chromosoma*, 48, 41, 1974.
62. **Price, H. J., Sparrow, A. H., and Nauman, A. F.,** Evolutionary and developmental considerations of the variability of nuclear parameters in higher plants. I. Genome volume, interphase chromosome volume, and estimated DNA content of 236 gymnosperms, *Brookhaven Symp. Biol.*, 25, 390, 1973.
63. **Hesemann, C. U.,** Cytophotometrical measurement of nuclear DNA content in some coniferous and deciduous trees, *Theor. Appl. Genet.*, 57, 187, 1980.
64. **Khoshoo, T. N.,** Polyploidy in gymnosperms, *Evolution*, 13, 24, 1959.
65. **Francini-Corti, E.,** Ecology of the haploid generation in *Pinus*, *Adv. Frontiers Plant Sci.*, 1, 35, 1962.
66. **Ehrendorfer, F.,** Evolutionary significance of chromosomal differentiation patterns in gymnosperms and primitive angiosperms, in *Origin and Early Evolution of Angiosperms*, Beck, C. B., Ed., Columbia University Press, New York, 1976, 220.
67. **Gupta, P. K. and Rees, H.,** Tolerance of *Lolium* hybrids to quantitative variation in nuclear DNA, *Nature (London)*, 257, 587, 1975.
68. **Gupta, P. K.,** Nuclear DNA and meiosis in parents, F_1 hybrids and F_2 segregates of a *Lolium temulentum* $\times$ *L. rigidum* cross, *Nucleus*, 22, 177, 1979.
69. **Ohri, D. and Khoshoo, T. N.,** Cytogenetics of garden gladiolus. III. Hybridization, *Z. Pflanzenzucht.*, 91, 46, 1983.
70. **Price, H. J., Chambers, K. L., Bachmann, K., and Riggs, J.,** Inheritance of nuclear 2C DNA content variation in intraspecific and interspecific hybrids of *Microseris* (Asteraceae), *Am. J. Bot.*, 70, 1133, 1983.
71. **Bachamann, K., Chambers, K. L., and Price, H. J.,** Genome size and phenotypic evolution in *Microseris* (Asteraceae, Cichorieae), *Plant Syst. Evol.*, 2(Suppl.), 41, 1979.
72. **Thompson, W. F. and Murray, M. G.,** The nuclear genome: structure and function, in *Biochemistry of Plants*, Vol. 6, Marcus, A., Ed., Academic Press, New York, 1981.
73. **Ohno, S.,** So much "junk" DNA in our genome, *Brookhaven Symp. Biol.*, 23, 366, 1972.
74. **Orgel, L. E. and Crick, F. H. C.,** Selfish DNA: the ultimate parasite, *Nature (London)*, 284, 604, 1980.
75. **Doolittle, W. F. and Sapienza, C.,** Selfish genes, the phenotype paradigm and genome evolution, *Nature (London)*, 284, 601, 1980.
76. **Cavalier-Smith, T.,** How selfish is DNA?, *Nature (London)*, 285, 617, 1980.
77. **Dover, G.,** Ignorant DNA, *Nature (London)*, 285, 618, 1980.
78. **Orgel, L. E., Crick, F. H. C., and Sapienza, C.,** Selfish DNA, *Nature (London)*, 288, 645, 1980.
79. **Stebbins, G. L.,** *Chromosome Evolution in Higher Plants*, Arnold, London, 1971.
80. **Jackson, R. C.,** Evolution and systematic significance of polyploidy, *Ann. Rev. Ecol. Syst.*, 7, 209, 1976.
81. **Lewis, W. H.,** *Polyploidy: Biological Relevance*, Plenum Press, New York, 1980.
82. **Nagl, W.,** Search for the molecular basis of diversification in phylogenesis and ontogenesis, *Plant Syst. Evol.*, 2(Suppl.), 3, 1979.
83. **Southern, D. I.,** Species relationships in the genus *Tulipa*, *Chromosoma*, 23, 80, 1967.
84. **Grant, W. F.,** Decreased DNA content of Birch (*Betula*) chromosomes at high ploidy level as determined by cytophotometry, *Chromosoma*, 26, 326, 1969.
85. **Taper, L. J. and Grant, W. F.,** The relationship between DNA content and chromosome size in birch (*Betula*) species, *Caryologia*, 26, 263, 1973.
86. **Pai, R. A. and Swaminathan, M. S.,** Differential radiosensitivity among the probable genome donors of bread wheat, *Evolution*, 14, 427, 1960.
87. **Pai, R. A., Upadhya, M. D., Bhaskaran, S., and Swaminathan, M. S.,** Chromosome diminution and evolution of polyploid species in *Triticum*, *Chromosoma*, 12, 398, 1961.
88. **Yamaguchi, Y. and Tsunoda, S.,** Nuclear volume, nuclear DNA content and radiosensitivity in *Brassica* and allied genera, *Jpn. J. Plant Breeding*, 19, 350, 1969.
89. **Jones, R. N. and Rees, H.,** Nuclear DNA variation in *Allium*, *Heredity*, 23, 591, 1968.
90. **Murray, B. G.,** The cytology of the genus *Briza L.* (Gramineae). I. Chromosome numbers, karyotypes and nuclear DNA variation, *Chromosoma*, 49, 299, 1975.
91. **Bullen, M. R. and Rees, H.,** Nuclear variation within avenae, *Chromosoma*, 39, 93, 1972.
92. **Upadhya, M. D. and Swaminathan, M. S.,** Deoxyribonucleic acid and the ancestry of wheat, *Nature (London)*, 200, 713, 1963.
93. **Rees, H. and Walters, M. R.,** Nuclear DNA and the evolution of wheat, *Heredity*, 20, 73, 1965.
94. **Pegington, C. and Rees, H.,** Chromosome weights and measures in Triticinae, *Heredity*, 25, 195, 1970.
95. **Nishikawa, K.,** DNA content of individual chromosomes and genomes in wheat and its relatives, *Seikan Ziho*, 22, 57, 1971.

96. **Furuta, Y., Nishikawa, K., and Tanino, T.,** Stability in DNA content of AB genome component of common wheat during the past seven thousand years, *Jpn. J. Genet.,* 49, 179, 1974.

97. **Verma, S. C. and Rees, H.,** Nuclear DNA and the evolution of allotetraploid Brassicae, *Heredity,* 33, 61, 1974.

98. **Narayan, R. K. J. and Rees, H.,** Nuclear DNA, heterochromatin and phylogeny of *Nicotiana* and amphidiploids, *Chromosoma,* 47, 75, 1974.

99. **Deka, P. C. and Sen, S. K.,** Decrease in chromosomal DNA content at a higher polyploidy level in *Vicia faba* root meristems, *Can. J. Genet. Cytol.,* 15, 863, 1973.

100. **Bennett, M. D. and Jellings, A. J.,** DNA content of colchicine-induced endopolyploid nuclei in *Vicia faba* L., *Heredity,* 35, 261, 1975.

101. **Keyl, H.-G.,** Chromosomenevolution bei *Chironomus.* II. Chromosomenumbauten and phylogenetische Beziehungan der Arten, *Chromosoma,* 13, 464, 1962.

102. **Keyl, H.-G.,** A demonstrable local and geometric increase in the chromosomal DNA of *Chironomus, Experientia,* 21, 191, 1965.

103. **Keyl, H.-G.,** Duplikationen von unterienheitan der chromosomalen DNS wahrend der evolution von *Chironomus thummi, Chromosoma,* 17, 139, 1965.

104. **Rees, H.,** DNA in higher plants, *Brookhaven Symp. Biol.,* 23, 394, 1972.

105. **Seal, A. G. and Rees, H.,** The distribution of quantitative DNA changes associated with the evolution of diploid festuceae, *Heredity,* 49, 179, 1982.

106. **Narayan, R. K. J. and Durrant, A.,** DNA distribution in chromosomes of *Lathyrus* species, *Genetica,* 61, 47, 1983.

107. **Mizuno, S. and Macgregor, H. C.,** Chromosomes, DNA sequences and evolution in salamanders of the genus *Plethodon, Chromosoma,* 48, 239, 1974.

108. **Park, E. H. and Keng, Y. S.,** Karyotype conservation and difference in DNA amount in anguilloid fishes, *Science,* 193, 64, 1976.

109. **Rees, H., Shaw, D. D., and Wilkinson, P.,** Nuclear DNA variation among acridid grass hoppers, *Proc. R. Soc. Lond. Ser. B:,* 202, 517, 1978.

110. **Cano, J., Alvarez, M. C., Thode, G., and Munoz, E.,** Phylogenetic interpretation of chromosomal and nuclear-DNA content data in the genus *Blennius* (Blenniidae: perciformes), *Genetica,* 58, 11, 1982.

111. **Mehra, P. N. and Khoshoo, T. N.,** Cytology of conifers. I., *J. Genet.,* 54, 165, 1956.

112. **Mehra, P. N. and Khoshoo, T. N.,** Cytology of conifers. II., *J. Genet.,* 54, 181, 1956.

113. **Khoshoo, T. N.,** Cytogenetical evolution in the gymnosperms — Karyotype, in Proc. Summer School, Darjeeling, Govt. of India, 1962, 119.

114. **Pederick, L. A.,** Chromosome relationships between *Pinus* species, *Silvae Genet.,* 19, 171, 1970.

115. **Saylar, L. C.,** Karyotype analysis of *Pinus* group Lariciones, *Silvae Genet.,* 13, 165, 1964.

116. **Saylar, L. C.,** Karyotype analysis of the genus *Pinus* — subgenus *Pinus, Silvae Genet.,* 21, 155, 1972.

117. **Martin, P. G. and Shank, R.,** Does *Vicia faba* have multistranded chromosome? *Nature (London),* 211, 658, 1966.

118. **Sparrow, A. H. and Nauman, A. F.,** Evolutionary changes in chromosome size and DNA content in grasses, *Brookhaven Symp. Biol.,* 25, 367, 1973.

119. **Greilhuber, J. and Speta, F.,** Quantitative analysis of C-banded karyotypes, and systematics in the cultivated species of the *Scilla siberica* group (Liliaceae), *Plant Syst. Evol.,* 129, 63, 1978.

120. **Flavell, R. B., Bennett, M. D., Smith, J. B., and Smith, D. B.,** Genome size and the proportion of repeated nucleotide sequence DNA in plants, *Biochem. Genet.,* 12, 257, 1974.

121. **Rees, H. and Narayan, R. K. J.,** Evolutionary DNA variation in *Lathyrus, Chromosomes Today,* 6, 131, 1977.

122. **Hutchinson, J., Narayan, R. K. J., and Rees, H.,** Constraints upon the composition of supplementary DNA, *Chromosoma,* 78, 137, 1980.

123. **Avdulov, N. P.,** Karyo-systematische Untersuchungen der Familie Gramineen, *Bull. Appl. Bot. Genet. Plant Breeding,* 44(Suppl. 4), 1, 1931.

124. **Levin, D. A. and Funderburg, S. W.,** Genome size in angiosperms: temperate versus tropical species, *Am. Nat.,* 114, 784, 1979.

125. **Bennett, M. D.,** The duration of meiosis, *Proc. R. Soc. Lond. Ser. B:,* 178, 277, 1971.

126. **Cavalier-Smith, T.,** Nuclear volume control by nucleoskeletal DNA selection for cell volume and cell growth rate and the solution of the DNA C-value paradox, *J. Cell. Sci.,* 34, 247, 1978.

127. **Mehra, P. N.,** Cytogenetical evolution of hardwoods, *Nucleus,* 15, 64, 1972.

128. **Mehra, P. N.,** *Cytology of Himalayan Hardwoods,* Sree Saraswaty Press, Calcutta, 1976.

129. **Hutchinson, J.,** *The Families of Flowering Plants,* Oxford University Press, London, 1973.

130. **Price, H. J., Sparrow, A. H., and Nauman, A. F.,** Correlations between nuclear volume, cell volume and DNA content in meristematic cells of herbaceous angiosperms, *Experientia,* 29, 1028, 1973.

131. **Mehra, P. N. and Bawa, K. S.,** Chromosomal evolution in tropical hardwoods, *Evolution,* 23, 466, 1969.

132. **Wilson, B. F.,** A model for cell production by the cambium of conifers, in *The Formation of Wood in Forest Trees,* Zimmermann, M. H., Ed., Academic Press, London, 1964, 19.
133. **Wilson, W. F.,** Mitotic activity in the cambial zone of *Pinus strobus, Am. J. Bot.,* 53, 364, 1966.
134. **Nagl, W.,** *Endopolyploidy and Polyteny in Differentiation and Evolution,* North-Holland, Amsterdam, 1978.
135. **Miksche, J. P. and Hotta, Y.,** DNA base composition and repetitious DNA in several conifers, *Chromosoma,* 41, 29, 1973.
136. **Grant, W. F.,** The evolution of karyotype and polyploidy in arboreal plants, *Taxon,* 25, 75, 1976.
137. **Ohno, S.,** *Evolution by Gene Duplication,* Springer-Verlag, Basel, 1970.
138. **Marks, G. E. and Schweizer, D.,** Giemsa banding: karyotype differences in some species of *Anemone* and in *Hepatica nobilis, Chromosoma,* 44, 405, 1974.
139. **Baumberger, H.,** Chromosomenzahlbestimmungen and Karyotypanalysen bei den gattungen *Anemone, Hepatica* and *Pulsatilla, Ber. Schweiz. Bot. Ges.,* 80, 17, 1970.
140. **Greilhuber, J.,** Nuclear DNA and heterochromatin contents in *Scilla hohenackeri* group, *Scilla persica* and *Puschkinia scilloides* (Liliaceae), *Plant Syst. Evol.,* 128, 243, 1977.
141. **Ressler, P. M., Stucky, J. M., and Miksche, J. P.,** Cytophotometric determination of the amount of DNA in *Arachis* L. sect. Arachis (Leguminosae), *Am. J. Bot.,* 68, 149, 1981.
142. **Paroda, R. S. and Rees, H.,** Nuclear DNA variation in Eu-Sorghums, *Chromosoma,* 32, 353, 1971.
143. **Cheng, R. I. J. and Grant, W. F.,** Species relationships in *Lotus corniculatus* group as determined by karyotype and cytophotometric analyses, *Can. J. Genet. Cytol.,* 15, 101, 1973.
144. **Edwards, G. A., Endrizii, J. E., and Stein, R.,** Genomic DNA content and chromosome organization in *Gossypium, Chromosoma,* 47, 309, 1974.
145. **Furuta, Y.,** Quantitative variation of nuclear DNA in the genus *Aegilops, Jpn. J. Genet.,* 50, 383, 1975.
146. **Gupta, P. K.,** Nuclear DNA, nuclear area and nuclear dry mass in thirteen species of *Crotalaria* (Angiospermae, Leguminosae), *Chromosoma,* 54, 155, 1976.
147. **Iyengar, G. A. S. and Sen, S. K.,** Nuclear DNA content of several wild and cultivated *Oryza, Environ. Exp. Bot.,* 18, 219, 1978.

Chapter 2

REPEATED DNA SEQUENCES AND POLYPLOIDY IN CEREAL CROPS

R. Mitra and C. R. Bhatia

TABLE OF CONTENTS

I. INTRODUCTION

Cereals are the most important group of plants as they are the principal source of food for humans and feed for domesticated animals. They belong to the grass family Gramineae. Polyploidy has played an important role in the evolution of this family. Stebbins[1] estimated that nearly 70% of the grass species are polyploids; this is twice the mean number of polyploid species among the flowering plants. With the beginning of argriculture approximately 10,000 years ago, some of the present-day cereal crops or their ancestral species were domesticated. Since then, this group of plants has evolved under strong human selection. Among the old world crops wheat and barley were domesticated earlier than oats and rye.[2] The earliest evidence for the domestication of maize in the new world goes back to 5000 B.C.[2] Thus, the total period of evolution under domestication ranges from 7000 years for maize to about 10,000 years for barley and wheat.

Contemporary techniques and knowledge have been applied at all times to understand the origin and evolution of these important food plants. As a result, the origin and evolutionary trends in the major cereal species were reasonably well investigated during the first half of this century; these investigations were based on the evidence from archaeology, morphology, cytology, and cytogenetics.

With the recognition of DNA as the hereditary material and the availability of techniques to estimate the amount of DNA per cell in the 1950s and early 1960s, such data were obtained in several laboratories. In the mid-1960s, the pioneering work of the Carnegie group established that most eukaryotes, including plants, have a large proportion of their DNA as repeated sequences.[3] This discovery has, since 1970, led to extensive investigations on the structure, function, organization, divergence, and evolutionary trends of repeated and nonrepeated sequences in plants. A substantial amount of information has been gathered on plant genomes. This information is available in several reviews.[4-8] Cereals in general and especially wheat and its related species have been well investigated. This chapter deals with the structure, organization, chromosomal location, divergence, and evolution of repeated DNA sequences in cereals. These aspects are discussed at greater length for the polyploid wheats.

II. COMPARATIVE EVOLUTIONARY ACCOUNTS OF DIFFERENT CEREALS

Extensive accounts of the origin and evolution of specific cereal crops are available (barley,[9] maize,[10] rice,[11] sorghum,[12] and wheat[13]). Harlan et al.[14] have examined the evolution and species relationships on the basis of gene pools because this method provides a better insight into genome organization. This approach is certainly more relevant in the present context of repeated DNA sequences. Levels of ploidy and primary and secondary gene pools as identified by Harlan et al.[14] are given in Table 1. Although polyploidy is very common in the family Gramineae, among the major cereal crops only wheat and oats are polyploid. The origin and evolution of polyploid wheats and triticale are shown in Figures 1 and 2. There are many features that are common to the evolution of all cereals. All of them have originated from wild grasses, and the wild and weedy relatives continue to occupy the same habitats permitting gene flow in both directions, i.e., from weeds and wild relatives to

Table 1
PRIMARY AND SECONDARY GENE POOLS OF THE MAJOR CEREALS

Cereal	Ploidy	Primary gene pool[a]			Secondary gene pool[b]
		Cultivated sp.	Wild races	Weed races	
Wheat					
Einkorn	2x	*Triticum monococcum*	*T. boeoticum*	*T. boeoticum*	*Triticum, Secale, Aegilops*
Emmer	4x	*T. dicoccum*	*T. dicoccocoides*	None	*Triticum, Secale, Aegilops*
Timopheevi	4x	*T. timopheevi*	*T. araraticum*	*T. timopheevi*	*Triticum, Secale, Aegilops*
Bread	6x	*T. aestivum*	None	None	*Triticum, Secale, Aegilops*
Rye	2x	*Secale cereale*	*S. cereale*	*S. cereale*	
Barley	2x	*Hordeum vulgare*	*H. spontaneum*	*H. spontaneum*	None
Oats	2x	*Avena strigosa*	*A. hirsuta*	*A. strigosa*	*Avena* spp.
	4x	*A. abyssinica* *A. vaviloviana*	*A. barbata*	*A. barbata*	*Avena* spp.
	6x	*A. sativa*	*A. sterilis* *A. fatua*	*A. sterilis*	*Avena* spp.
Rice	2x	*Oryza sativa*	*O. rufipogon*	*O. rufipogon*	*Oryza* spp.
African	2x	*O. glaberrima*	*O. barthii*	*O. stapfii*	*Oryza* spp.
Sorghum	2x	*Sorghum bicolor*	*S. bicolor*	*S. bicolor*	*S. halepense*
Pearl millet	2x	*Pennisetum americanum*	*P. violaceum*	*P. americanum*	*P. purpureum*
Maize	2x	*Zea mays*	*Z. mexicana*	*Z. mexicana*	*Tripsacum* spp. *Z. perennis*

[a] Primary gene pool corresponds to the concept of biological species. It includes those races that can be freely crossed with the cultivated species giving rise to fertile or nearly fertile hybrids. The hybrids show normal or nearly normal chromosome pairing. Genetic segregations are reasonably normal.

[b] The secondary gene pool includes the species that can be crossed with the cultivated species but the gene flow is restricted. Hybrids are weak, show poor chromosome pairing, and sterility.

cultivated species and vice versa. It is implied that in most cereals evolution has taken place almost entirely within the primary gene pools.[14] Wheat differs from the other cereals in that the secondary gene pool of *Aegilops* contributed to the evolution of tetraploid wheats and the D genome from *Aegilops squarrosa* was added in nature after domestication. Triticale, of course, is a new cereal developed and evolving under intense human manipulation and selection. Domestication has led to wide variation between the cultivated and the wild relatives. The main genetic traits that differentiate the cultivated forms from their progenitors are large seed size, improved seed retention, determinate growth, large or more number of inflorescences, lack of seed dormancy, and wider adaptation.

III. HAPLOID DNA CONTENT

The haploid DNA content shows extensive variation in the flowering plants. The values range between less than 1 to over 200 pg.[15] The annual monocots contain more DNA than the annual dicots (Table 2). Among the monocots, the polyploid species have more DNA per haploid cell than do the diploid species (Table 2). The haploid DNA content also varies considerably among the cereals (Table 3). In the diploid cereals rice has the lowest amount of DNA (0.6 pg), while rye has the highest (8.60 pg). In general, the polyploid cereals have a higher DNA content compared to the diploids; however, the DNA content in finger millet (1.60 pg) and hexaploid oats (4.30 pg) is lower in comparison to many diploid cereals. The

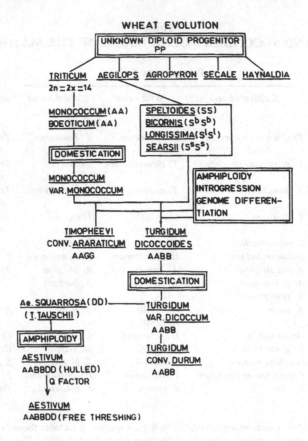

FIGURE 1. Evolutionary relationships of the wheats.

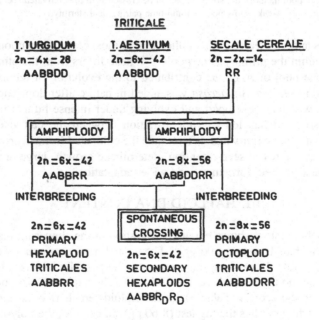

FIGURE 2. Evolution of triticale.

Table 2
THE MEAN AND RANGE OF HAPLOID
DNA CONTENT IN ANNUAL
MONOCOT AND DICOT SPECIES

Subclass	Ploidy	Haploid DNA content (pg)[a]	
		Mean	Range
Monocots	Diploids (29)	6.16	1.43—9.46
	Polyploids (30)	11.24	3.40—27.57
Dicots	Diploids (22)	5.82	0.27—14.67
	Polyploids (5)	1.10	0.70—1.73

Note: Values are recalculated from Table 3 of Bennett.[16]
Values in parentheses indicate number of species.

[a] The original 3C values are divided by 3.

nuclear DNA content has been shown to be positively correlated with chromosome volume, nuclear volume, cell size, nucleolar and nuclear dry mass, seed dry mass, minimum cell cycle time, meiotic duration, pollen maturation time, and mean generation time.[16] It was also observed in wheat species that the duration of meiosis decreased as the level of ploidy increased.[17]

Attempts have been made to estimate the proportion of nuclear DNA necessary to encode for the gene function (proteins) in higher plants. The estimates for expressed genes in plants vary between 10,000 to 15,000 and 25,000 to 35,000.[18,19] These numbers, however, can only be considered educated guesses at the moment. The average mRNA molecule contains about 1200 bases. If it is assumed that there are 20,000 genes per haploid genome of cereals each coding for a single mRNA, then 2.4×10^7 bp of DNA would be required. One picogram of DNA is equivalent to approximately 10^9 bp. Thus, 0.024 pg DNA would code for all the genes in a cereal. The mean haploid DNA content of 6 diploid cereals, barley, maize, pearl millet, rice, rye, and sorghum is 4.58 pg (Table 3). Hence, the fraction of the diploid cereal genome that codes for mRNA constitutes only 0.52% $[(2.4 \times 10^7 \div 4.58 \times 10^9) \times 100]$. On the other hand, 4x and 6x species of wheat have duplicate and triplicate genes for the same function, each contributed by one of the parental genomes. The precise number of single, duplicate, and triplicate loci in polyploid species is not known. However, if it is assumed that all the loci are duplicate and triplicate in 4x and 6x wheats, respectively, the fraction of DNA coding sequences in these two groups is estimated to be about 0.38% $[(4.8 \times 10^7 \div 12.63 \times 10^9) \times 100]$ and 0.40% $[(7.2 \times 10^7 \div 18.1 \times 10^9) \times 100]$. Flavell[6] reported that less than 1% of the cereal genome codes for proteins. It is thus interesting that all the genetic information we have for the cereals relates to less than 1% of the genomes.

IV. REPEATED DNA SEQUENCES

The reassociation of dissociated DNA essentially follows a biomolecular reaction. The rate of reassociation provides a measure of the concentration of complementary sequences. The fast reassociating fraction represents the nucleotide sequences which are present in multiple copies while the slow reassociating fraction comprises the sequences which are either present as single copies or are multiplied to a low degree. The former has been referred to as repeated DNA and the latter as nonrepeated, single copy, or low copy number DNA.

Table 3
HAPLOID DNA CONTENT AND PROPORTION OF REPEATED DNA SEQUENCE IN DIFFERENT CEREALS

Cereals	Ploidy	DNA content (pg)	Ref.	Repeated DNA (%)	Ref.	Experimental conditions: DNA fragment length, incubation temp., salt conc., and assay method
Barley	2x	5.40	15	70.0	62	300—400 bp: 60°C: 0.18 M Na$^+$; HAP
Maize	2x	5.50	82	68.4[a]	8	400—600 bp: Tm-25°C: 0.18 M Na$^+$; optical
Rye	2x	8.60	15	75.0	62	300—400 bp: 60°C: 0.18 M Na$^+$; HAP
Rice	2x	0.60	35	52.0	35	500—700 bp: 60°C: 0.18 M Na$^+$; HAP
Sorghum	2x	4.87	83	Not known	—	—
Pearl millet	2x	2.50	35	54.0	35	500—700 bp: 60°C: 0.18 M Na$^+$; HAP
Finger millet	4x	1.60	35	49.0	35	500—700 bp: 60°C: 0.18 M Na$^+$; HAP
Oats	6x	4.30	15	75.0	62	300—400 bp: 60°C: 0.18 M Na$^+$; HAP
Triticum monococcum	2x	7.00	84	67.0	45	450 bp: 60°C: 0.18 M Na$^+$; HAP
Ae. speltoides	2x	6.06	84	Not known	—	—
Ae. squarrosa	2x	5.03	84	Not known	—	—
T. durum	4x	12.63[b]	16	74.0	45	450 bp: 60°C: 0.18 M Na$^+$; HAP
T. aestivum	6x	18.10[b]	16	75.0	62	300—400 bp: 60°C: 0.18 M Na$^+$; HAP
Triticale	8x	27.57[b]	16	50.3	46	1 × 10^6 mol wt; 65°C: 0.18 M Na$^+$; optical

[a] Represents an average value pooled from 3 different DNAs isolated from 3 different tissues.

[b] Original 3C values are divided by 3; when corrected for ploidy the respective haploid DNA contents for 4, 6 and 8× wheat are 6.32, 6.03, and 6.89 pg.

However, in considering the repeated and nonrepeated sequences, it should be realized that these are operational definitions and should always be considered in relation to the criteria used for reassociation experiments, especially the size of DNA fragments, incubation temperature, and salt concentration.[7,20,21] Tissue- and age-dependent variation in the proportion of repeated DNA has also been reported in *Zea mays*.[8] The melting temperature (Tm) of the reassociated DNA provides a measure of the fidelity of reassociation and indicates divergence among the nucleotide sequences reassociated. Mismatch of bases decreases the Tm of the duplexes, and the greater the change in Tm (ΔTm) the higher the divergence.

A. Copies of Repeated Sequences

Eukaryotic DNA can be divided into three broad classes:[22] (1) unique or single or few copy, (2) moderately repeated, and (3) highly repeated. The unique sequences are present approximately as one copy per haploid genome. Some such sequences contain the genes that code for proteins, although other protein genes are in the repeated sequences. Genes coding for seed storage proteins[23] and wheat histone H4 gene[24] are present in multiple copies. The other gene sequences present in multiple copies are the ribosomal RNA, 5S RNA, and tRNA genes. They occur as tandemly repeated sequences.[25]

Nucleotide sequences present in 1000 to 100,000 are considered as moderately repeated. They can be further resolved into two types, long and short, depending upon their size. Both types are interspersed with single copy or few copy sequences and are transcribed.[22]

The highly repeated DNA consists of clustered repetitions of relatively short sequence units. They are not interspersed with other types of sequences and are considered to be the structural components of chromosomes. They are located mainly at centromeric and telomeric regions.[22]

B. Arrangement of Repeated DNA Sequences in Plant Chromosomes

Four different types of arrangements of repeated DNA sequences have been described as a result of the data compiled on sequence organization from several plant species.[4,6,7] They are shown schematically in Figure 3.

1. Length of Repeated and Interspersed Single or Few Copy Sequences

Repeated DNA sequences are short in species with larger genome sizes. Repeated sequences ranging in size from 200 to 600 bp are interspersed with short single copy sequences. On the other hand, in species with small genomes, the interspersed repeats are larger in size, around 1000 bp.[6] The lengths of the single copy sequences also vary among species with different genome size.[6] In species with genomes containing more than 2 pg DNA, 75 to 95% of the single copy DNA is in lengths shorter than 2000 bp. Further, about 66% of such DNA is in lengths shorter than 2000 bp. Species with genomes containing less than 2 pg DNA have a larger proportion of single copy DNA sequences that are longer than 4000 bp.

2. Reverse Repeats

Less than 5% of the plant genomes is composed of reverse repeats which after denaturation shows intrastrand reassociation in the form of duplex structure[6] (Figure 3). The length of such duplex structures varies between 50 to 900 bp. The number of reverse repeats in a genome is related to the DNA content. The large genomes show more copies of reverse repeats as compared to small genomes.[6] Over 1 million copies of reverse repeats occur per haploid genome of hexaploid wheat.[26] In chromosomes such reverse repeat sequences are located in clusters and are frequently separated by short sequences.[6]

3. Satellite DNA

In spite of the presence of an unusually large amount of repeated DNA sequences in the

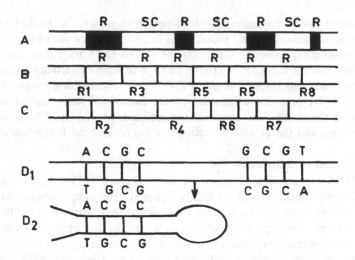

FIGURE 3.   General arrangements of repeated DNA in plant chromosomes. (A) Short pieces of repeated DNA (R) 50 to 2000 bp long are interspersed with single copy (SC) 200 to 4000 bp long sequences. (B) Essentially identical repeating units (R) in tandem arrays. (C) Unrelated short repeats (R1 to R8) are interspersed with each other in different permutations. (D1) Reverse repeats in their native configuration and (D2) after denaturation and intrastrand renaturation. The letters ACGT denote bases.[6,7,50]

monocots, no satellite DNA fraction has been found.[27,28] However, after ultracentrifugation of total DNA in heavy salt gradients (CsCl or Cs_2SO_4) containing actinomycin D, Ag^+, or HG^{++}, satellite fractions have been isolated from barley,[29,30] rye,[31] wheat,[29,30,32] and pearl millet.[33] The cryptic satellite fractions comprising highly repeated DNA sequences have also been isolated using the renaturation properties discussed earlier.

C. Repeated DNA From Different Cereals

The proportion of repeated DNA sequences in the genome of different cereals is given in Table 3. Important cereal species are discussed below.

1. Rice

The proportion of repeated DNA in eight rice species (*Oryza sativa* ssp. *indica*, *O. sativa* ssp. *japonica*, *O. rufipogon* — annual and perennial, *O. glaberrima*, *O. longistaminata*, *O. stapfii*, and *O. barthii*) varied from 56 to 66%.[34] It was reported that 52% of rice genome consists of repeated DNA.[35] The reassociation kinetic curves indicate an absence of sequence interspersion of both repeated as well as single copy sequences[36] at the DNA fragment length of 6500 bp. The size distribution of repeated DNA showed that about 35 to 40% of the S1 nuclease-resistant duplexes consisted of 6000 to 6400 bp and 60 to 65% had a fragment size of less than 150 bp. The implications of the absence of sequence interspersion under the experimental conditions in rice are not understood.

2. Pearl Millet

Repeated DNA in pearl millet varies from 54[35] to 69%.[33] About 80% of the repeated DNA is of at least 5000 bp in length. Nearly half of the single copy DNA is short (750 to 1400 bp) and interspersed with long repeated sequences. The other half of the single copy sequences varies in size from 1400 to 8600 bp. The moderately repeated fraction constitutes 46.6% of the genome and shows a reiteration frequency of 298.[33] When the total DNA was

Table 4
SEQUENCE ORGANIZATION PATTERN IN
DIFFERENT CEREALS EXPRESSED AS PERCENT OF
THE GENOME[50]

Type of sequences	Wheat	Rye	Barley	Oats
Short nonrepeats (single copy sequences) interspersed with short repeats	30—40	25—35	25—35	25—40
Interspersed repeats or tandem repeats	55—65	60—70	55—65	50—65
Long nonrepeats	2	5	9	9
In addition, 2—4% reverse repeats which are situated close to each other				

resolved in Cs_2SO_4-HG^{++} or Ag^+ gradients, a satellite fraction was detected.[33] Ten percent of the genome was made up of this fraction.

3. Finger Millet

Approximately 49% of the genome consists of repeated sequences.[37] The interspersed repeated sequences are in the size range of 150 to 200 and 4000 to 4200 bp. The two classes respectively constitute about 60 and 20% of the repeated sequences; 4000 to 4200 bp sequences are involved in a long range interspersion pattern, while 150 to 200 bp long sequences are involved in short period interspersion. Single copy DNA sequences are 1900 bp long.

4. Maize

Hake and Walbot[38] reported that 64% of the maize genome consists of repeated DNA. Nagl et al.[8] found that the proportion of repeated DNA varies depending upon the development stage and types of tissue from which the DNA is isolated. These findings are significant and if similar results are obtained in other species, the values summarized here from different sources may also vary. In maize they[8] reported that 68.5 and 78.0% of the genome is comprised of repeated sequences.

5. Barley, Rye, Oats, and Wheat

The most extensive investigations on genome analysis and interspecies comparisons of repeated DNA have been carried out in barley,[39-42] rye,[39,43,44] oats,[39,42] and wheat.[39,45-50] Different sequence organization patterns observed in these cereals are given in Table 4. Most of the single copy DNA in wheat and rye is dispersed in pieces shorter than 1200 bp. They reside between repeated DNA segments whose lengths range between 200 to 600 bp.[50]

6. Triticale

About 50% of the triticale genome consists of repeated DNA sequences.[46] The repeated DNA fraction was further resolved into three subfractions with high, intermediate, and low degrees of repetition. The highly repeated fraction contains two families having 3×10^7 and 5×10^6 order of repetitions of nucleotide sequences. They constitute 8.3 and 2.4% of the triticale genome, respectively. Compared with triticale, only one family of repeated DNA with 2 to 5×10^7 nucleotide frequency was observed in rye and wheat. The authors have emphasized that there could be selective deletion of repeated DNA sequences in triticale and polyploidization could be accompanied by selective loss of repeated DNA as was observed in *Drosophila*.[51] However, as yet, there is no experimental evidence for selective elimination of rye repeated sequences in triticale.

V. RESTRICTION ENDONUCLEASES IN THE ANALYSIS OF REPEATED DNA

Restriction endonucleases[52] cleave DNA at specific sites and thus produce a defined set of fragments which are separated by electrophoresis on agarose gels, stained with ethidium bromide, and observed under UV light. Such analyses of genomic DNA with different restriction endonucleases are extremely important for investigating repeated sequences. However, among the cereals, the studies so far are limited to rye and other species of *Secale*.[53-56] Their important findings are summarized in the following four sections.

When repeated sequences do not contain the sites for a restriction endonuclease, they are not cut and remain in high molecular form. After digestion of the total DNA, such undigested "spared" sequences are found at the top of the gel and have been referred to as "relic" DNA. Repeated digestion of DNA with restriction enzymes followed by steep, linear sucrose gradient centrifugation provides a method for enrichment of the spared, repeated sequences. Various restriction endonuclease spared fractions of rye were purified by velocity sedimentation. Each of the Hind III, Eco RI, Bam HI, and Bgl II digests of *Secale cereale* and *S. silvestre*, DNA showed a higher proportion of "relic" DNA in *S. cereale*. "Hind III relic" in the two species were 5 and 2.3% of the total DNA of *S. cereale* and *S. silvestre* respectively.

When repeated sequences include restriction sites, such families appear as distinct bands superimposed on the background smear of fluorescence. The limitation of the method, however, is that only a small percentage of the total DNA is represented as distinct bands. A higher proportion of *S. cereale* (1.24 of 8.3 pg = 11.4%) was found as bands compared to *S. silvestre* (0.72 of 7.2 pg = 75%) in Eco RI digests of nuclear DNA. The relative proportion for *S. cereale* and *S. silvestre* for the Bam H1 digestion was 10.1 and 6.9%, respectively, while for Hind III digestion it was 15.4 and 10%, respectively.

The size distribution of the DNA fragments produced after digestion with restriction endonucleases can be predicted on the basis of random fragmentation theory and the base composition of the genome. In rye DNA, the mean fragment size was higher after restriction with Sma I, Hpa II, and Pst I enzymes. When Eco RI and Bam HI were used, the mean fragment size was similar to that expected, but the fragments of higher and lower molecular weights were more than expected on the basis of random fragmentation. These deviations from expectations have been attributed to methylation of cytosine residues and the presence of repeated sequences. In this context, variation in the fragment lengths obtained after restriction among the seven inbreds of strains of maize is of interest and points to extensive variation among the different genotypes of the same species.[57] The authors[57] have named this heterogeneity "restriction fragment length polymorphism" (RFLP) and have discussed its possible applications in genetics and breeding.

The sensitivity of the restriction analysis is further enhanced by transferring the bands on agarose gels to nitrocellulose by the method of Southern[58] and hybridizing with the cloned, labeled complementary "probe" of repeated sequences. In the autoradiographs, DNA fragments having homology with the probe appear as a "ladder". This approach revealed the organization of a repeated sequence family in rye. These sequences are organized in two different repeating units of 120 and 2.2 k bp.

Mutations, deletions, translocations, and amplifications of the DNA sequences alter the sites cleaved by restriction enzymes. This is reflected by a change in the fragmentation pattern. This approach has been extremely useful in estimating divergence among the families of the repeated sequences.

VI. MOLECULAR CLONING OF REPEATED DNA SEQUENCES

The minimum number of clones required for the complete genomic library of cereal species was estimated to be 10^6 for most restriction endonucleases.[53] Extensive cloning of specific repeated DNA sequence families has been carried out in wheat and rye, and on a limited scale in maize and barley. The available information is summarized in Table 5.

VII. POLYPYRIMIDINE-POLYPURINE SATELLITE DNAs IN WHEAT, RYE, AND BARLEY

As mentioned earlier, satellite DNA can be isolated from wheat and barley using AG^+/Cs_2SO_4 gradients. It constitutes about 1.2 and 3.8% of the wheat and barley genomes, respectively.[30] These DNAs are highly repeated, each with a complexity of about 10 bp.

Reassociation kinetics, restriction enzyme analysis, and sequencing of complementary RNA transcripts of this DNA show that it is composed of tandem repeats of a simple sequence. Restriction endonuclease Mbo II digests of the cloned satellite fraction further suggests that it is composed of long tandem arrays of a single 12 bp repeating unit (CTT)n (CTC)n; i.e., one strand is a polypyrimidine sequence.[5,53] Polypurine satellite DNA was also reported in rye.[92]. The barley insert of 1.4 kb which was cloned shows the sequence of poly-CTT.[53]

VIII. REPEATED SEQUENCES IN pSC$_{7235}$

The rye genome contains about 2×10^5 copies of the pSC$_{7235}$ sequences, which is equivalent to about 1.5% of the rye genome.[56] The nucleotide sequence of the pSC$_{7235}$ was determined. The sequence contains 21 tracts of pyrimidines 5 to 10 residues long and the sequences

```
5'AACATTTTTTGAA3'        5'AAATTTGA3'
3'TTGTAAAAAACTT5'        3'TTTAAACT5'
```

are repeated twice and three times, respectively. When all possible reading frames were tested, it was determined that the sequences could not be translated into proteins longer than 70 amino acids.

IX. RIBOSOMAL RNA GENE (rDNA) REPEATING UNITS

Ribosomal genes are the DNA nucleotide sequences that specify the RNA components of the protein synthesizing machinery. They are composed of ribosomal RNAs (rRNA), 5S RNA, and tRNAs. Ribosomal genes of higher organisms are divided into four parts: 26-28S and 18S cistrons, a "nonconserved RNA" portion, and a spacer.[59] The spacer region separates one segment of ribosomal gene from the next.[25] They are organized in the form of tandemly repeated segments. The genes for 5S rRNA are separate and not linked to 18S and 26-28S rRNA genes. These genes also occur in tandemly arranged clusters interspersed with spacer region.[25]

In rye, wheat, and barley the repeating unit of rDNA is 9 to 10 kb in length.[60] A significant fraction of the rDNA in these species is located in the C-band proximal to the secondary constriction of mitotic chromosomes.[60] A diagrammatic representation of the rDNA repeating units is given in Figure 4. The two subclones (130.6 and 130.8) representing the tandemly repeating units of spacer region of rDNA have been sequenced.[61]

The estimated number of rRNA genes in different cereals is given in Table 6. The number per haploid genome varies from 2870 in diploid *Hordeum bulbosum* to 6350 in hexaploid wheat. The number of rRNA genes may have increased proportionately with ploidy level; in 6x wheat, it was genotype-dependent.

In situ hybridization has shown that in wheat cultivar Chinese Spring, 90% of the rRNA

Table 5
MOLECULAR CLONING OF REPEATED DNA IN CEREALS

Designation of chimeric plasmids and characterization	Restriction enzymes; vector and host	Ref.
Wheat		
61 inserts varying in size from 0.1 to 14 kb (mean 2.9 kb)	Eco RI digest of total nuclear DNA pACYC 184 E. coli HB 101	53
5200 bp highly repeated DNA, pTA8	Eco RI pACYC 184 E. coli	50
0.25 kb fragment, pCS(1)TC226	M13	69
4.70 kb fragment, pCS(1)40 repeated DNA	pACYC 184	
5S DNA pTA531, 410 bp pTA704, 410 bp pTA729, 410 bp	Isolation of 5S DNA fraction by actino-mycin-CSCl density gradient centrifugation	68
pTA794, 410 bp pTA665, 500 bp pTA630, 640 bp pTA710, 1190 bp	Bam HI pBR322 E. coli HB 101	
rDNA 9 kb repeating unit which consists of 18S, 5.8S, and 26S rRNA genes plus associated spacer DNAs	Eco RI pACYC 184	85
pTA71 (9 kb repeating unit)	E. coli HB101	53
pTA250 (shortest 9kb length variant) Sub-clones from pTA250 pTA250.1, 4.4 kb Bam HI/Eco RI fragment	Bam HI pBR322	61
pTA250.2, 3.6 kb Bam HI fragment containing coding sequences pTA250.4, 2.7 Taq fragment entirely within the spacer region pTA250.3, 0.9 kb Bam HI/Eco RI fragment from 26S RNA gene pTA250.10, 1 kb Taq fragment from 18S RNA gene pTA250.11, 0.5 kb Taq fragment for 26S RNA gene pTA250.15, 0.75 kb Hpa II fragment from the spacer region pTA250.16, 0.65 kb Hpa fragment from the spacer region pTA250.17, 0.65 kb Hinf fragment containing 0.3 kb of the 18S rRNA gene 130 bp Hha I repeated units from pTA250.4, 130.6, 130.8 (spacer region consists of a 130 bp tandemly repeating unit)	E. coli	

Table 5 (continued)
MOLECULAR CLONING OF REPEATED DNA IN CEREALS

Designation of chimeric plasmids and characterization	Restriction enzymes; vector and host	Ref.
Rye		53
Repeated DNA sequences from te-lomeric heterochromatin	pBR322 pACYC E. coli HB101	55
12 repeated DNA sequence bands obtained after Hae III digestion of restriction spared total DNA were purified, cloned, and characterized		70
pSC 210, 480 bp repeat from a family which constitutes about 6% of the rye genome		
pSC34, 610 bp repeat from a family which constitutes about 3% of the genomic DNA		
pSC119, 120 bp sequence from a family which constitutes about 2% of the genomic DNA		
pSC33, 630 bp repeat which consti-tutes 0.5% of the genomic DNA		56
pSC310, 2200 bp repeat unit		
pSC7235, 643 bp repeat	Hind III spared DNA Eco RI digested pBR 325 E. coli ED8624	
Barley		53
rDNA 9—10 kb	pACYC184 E. coli HB101	
Maize		86, 87
Corn insert (Cin1)	Eco RI	
Dispersed repetitive elements: size variation to approximately 700 bp NF-1 clone 5.7 kb genomic DNA fragment containing Cin1	λgtWES 14 Eco RI maize in-serts LC102—LC115 were isolated and sub-cloned into Eco RI sites of pACYC184 E. coli HB101	

genes are located on chromosomes 1B and 6B and the remaining repeating units on chromosome 5D.[5,60] Eco RI and Bam HI digests of rRNA repeating units of several diploid and polyploid wheat species showed variation in fragment lengths.[5]

X. LOCATION OF REPEATED DNA IN CEREAL CHROMOSOMES

The technique of *in situ* hybridization between a labeled nucleic acid probe and the homologous region on the fixed metaphase chromosomes offers an unique opportunity to locate chromosomal sites for specific DNA sequences. This technique has been extensively used for the location of repeated DNA sequences in cereals using cloned DNA probes. Chromosomal locations of repeated DNA sequences are summarized in Table 7.

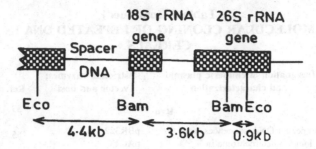

FIGURE 4.   Diagrammatic representation of the ribosomal RNA gene repeating unit from wheat. Sites for the restriction enzymes Bam H1 and Eco R1 are indicated. The fragment lengths obtained following simultaneous digestion with these two enzymes are marked.[5]

Table 6
NUMBER OF rRNA GENES IN DIFFERENT CEREALS

Species	No. of rRNA genes/haploid genome	Ref.
Hordeum bulbosum	2,870	25
H. parodii	4,830	
H. procerum	3,560	
H. vulgare	4,200	
Secale cereale	4,200	
Triticum aestivum	6,350	
Zea mays	3,100 or 8,500	
Triticum aestivum	2,300	60

	No. of rRNA genes/2C nucleus	
T. monococcum (AA)	5,700	88
T. tauschii (DD) *Aegilops squarrosa*	5,700	
T. speltoides (SS) *Ae. speltoides*	5,800	
T. dicoccoides (AABB)	10,800	
T. turgidum (AABB)	11,100	
T. durum (AABB)	12,400	
T. timopheevi (AAGG)	13,600	
T. aestivum cv. Atlas 66	18,400	
cv. Era	12,500	
cv. Chinese Spring	15,700	

XI. REPEATED DNA SEQUENCE DIVERGENCE IN CEREAL GENOME

A. Intra- and Interspecies Repeated DNA Sequence Divergence

These types of divergence have been investigated by reassociation kinetics involving homo- and heterologous sequences. In earlier studies on DNA-DNA hybridization between wheat, rye, barley, and oat DNA involving predominantly repeated sequences,[39,47] it emerged that:

1   Rye is more primitive among these cereals and shares a higher proportion of sequences with wheat, barley, and oats than any of these species do with each other.

2.   Maximum homology was found between rye and diploid as well as polyploid wheat sequences.

Table 7
LOCATION OF REPEATED DNA SEQUENCES IN CEREAL CHROMOSOMES AS REVEALED BY *IN SITU* HYBRIDIZATION

Species	Repeated DNA sequence	Probe used	Chromosomal location	Ref.
Wheat	Ag$^+$/Cs$_2$SO$_4$ satellite	^{3}H-c RNA transcript	All 7 B genome chromosomes, 4A, 7A; minor sites on chromosomes of A and D genomes	30
	pTA8, 5200 bp	^{3}H-c RNA transcript	Dispersed over most, if not all, chromosomes	50
	pCS(1)TC22b, 0.25 kb pCS(1)C40, 4.40 kb	^{3}H-c RNA transcript	Specific sites on the B genome chromosomes and 4A; a good correlation between the distribution of these sequences and heterochromatin as revealed by C-banding was observed	69
	Cot 10^{-2} DNA	^{3}H-c RNA transcript	All chromosomes of the B genome; other locations were visualized after heating the *in situ* hybridization reaction	89
	pTA71, rRNA gene repeating unit	^{3}H-c RNA transcript	1B, 6B, 1A, 5D	90
T. dicoccoides	"130" bp sequence subcloned from pTA 250.4 restricted with HhaI	^{3}H-c RNA	1B and/or 6B	61
	18S and 26S RNA	^{125}I RNAs	1B, 6B, 5D	5, 60
Rye	pCS(1)TC22b, 0.25 kb pCS(1)C40, 4.40 kb	^{3}H-c RNA transcripts	Telomeric and interstitial sites	69
Different rye species and triticale	pSC210, 480 bp pSC179, 120 bp pSC34, 610 bp pSC33, 630 bp	^{3}H-c RNA transcripts	Largely located on the heterochromatic region at the telomeres	70, 71
	pSC7235, 643 bp (and Class I sequence)	^{3}H-c RNA transcripts	Telomeric heterochromatic blocks, terminal heterochromatic blocks of 1R, 2R, DR and 5R	56, 91
Barley	Ag$^+$/Cs$_2$SO$_4$ satellite	^{3}H-c RNA transcript	All chromosomes pericentric location	30
	pCS(1)TC22b, 0.25 kb	^{3}H-c RNA transcript	Regions near the centromeres of all chromosomes	69

3.　Oats DNA was only distantly related to wheat, rye, and barley.
4.　Among the wheat species, divergence between A (*T. monococcum*) and D (*Ae. squarrosa*) was greater than between A and AB (4x wheat) or A and ABD (6x wheat) genomes.

Heterologous reassociation of repeated and nonrepeated fractions separated at an arbitrary Cot value of 100 showed considerably more divergence in the repeated sequences at both diploid and polyploid levels.[45] Nonrepeated sequences of wheat species showed greater homologies and appeared to be more conservative in composition.[45] Subsequent investigations using more refined experimental techniques have by and large confirmed these observations.[62-64]

Flavell and his group[62-64] further extended the reassociation studies of the repeated sequences of wheat, rye, barley, and oats. They have classified the repeated sequences into seven groups based upon their distribution among these species. Their distribution and relative proportions in the four cereals are given in Table 8. Sequences common to the four cereals are classified as group I. Closely related species have more groups of sequences in common,

Table 8
DISTRIBUTION AND RELATIVE
PROPORTION OF DIFFERENT
FAMILIES OF REPEATED
SEQUENCES IN WHEAT, RYE,
BARLEY, AND OATS GENOME[50]

Sequences	Wheat	Rye	Barley	Oats
Group I[a]	21	22	13	20
Group II	26	11		
Group III	5	6		
Group IV	16			
Group V		26		
Group VI			34	
Group VII				45

Note: Sequences of the group shared by different
cereals are shown by horizontal bars.

[a] Group I sequences are shorter than 600 bp and
interspersed with single copy sequences. Other
group sequences are shorter than 3000 bp or different repeats of similar length distribution.

Table 9
COPY NUMBERS OF SEQUENCES
RELATED TO pTA8 FRAGMENTS[50]

Fragments	*Triticum monococcum*	*Aegilops squarrosa*
B	33,000	27,000
C	1,500	650
D	800	<50
F	27,000	2,800

for example, wheat and rye share group I, II, and III sequences while only group I sequences
are common between wheat and oats. Species specific sequences in wheat (group IV), rye
(group V), barley (group VI), and oats group (VIII) respectively constitute 16, 24, 34, and
35% of the genome.

When a highly repeated DNA fraction renaturing at Cot 10^{-2} from *Ae. speltoides* was
used as the probe, diploid *Aegilops* species could be differentiated from diploid *Triticum*
species.[64] A higher proportion of DNA from *Aegilops* species reassociated with this fraction
than did that from diploid wheat species *T. monococcum*, *T. boeoticum*, and *T. urartu*.
Reassociation with 4x and 6x wheat species that respectively carry one and two genomes
from *Aegilops* species was similar to the homologous reassociation within the *Aegilops*
species.

As mentioned previously, a 5200 bp highly repeated sequence from wheat was cloned
(pTA8). Four fragments B, C, D, and F obtained from this fraction after restriction with
Hind III and Eco RI enzymes were used in hybridization experiments to estimate the copy
number of related sequences in *Triticum* and *Aegilops* species.[50] The sequences in the four
fragments were not related to each other. The estimated copy number of sequences related
to each fragment in *T. monococcum* and *Ae. squarrosa* is given in Table 9. The copy
numbers related to the four fragments were different in these two species.

A pTA8 sequence was hybridized with Eco RI restricted wheat DNA separated by agarose gel electrophoresis and transferred to nitrocellulose by the method of Southern.[58] A smear of radioactivity was observed over fragments varying in size from less than 1 to over 40 kb. There was no distinct band that hybridized with the 5200 bp sequence. Fragment C (900 bp) of this sequence did not show hybridization with any fragment of similar mobility in Hind III digests of DNAs from *Ae. speltoides, Ae. squarrosa,* and *T. monococcum.*[50] A smear resulting from hybridization with fragments in a wide range of molecular weights was observed. Many bands shared homology with the C fragments, indicating that the sequences related to this fragment are dispersed and have been amplified.

B. Ribosomal DNA Spacer Region

As shown earlier in Figure 4, the repeating units of the ribosomal DNA have noncoding sequences besides the sequences that code for 18S and 26S RNAs. The extra DNA in each of the repeating units has been termed as spacer.[65] There are some spacer sequences present in the primary transcripts and these are designated as transcribed spacer, while others that are not transcribed are termed as nontranscribed spacer. In most higher organisms sequences in the spacer region show considerable divergence.[65] The rDNA of wheat and related species has been investigated using restriction enzyme analysis, reassociation of the fragments, and Tms of molecular hybrids[5,61,66,67] Restriction enzyme digests of the ribosomal RNA showed that some of the spacer fragments present in 2x wheat species were absent in 6x wheat. The 4x species were very different from the 2x and 6x species.[5]

A wheat DNA clone pTA 250 has been analyzed in detail.[61,66,67] The results show extensive polymorphism in the spacer sequences between cultivars of 6x wheat and natural populations of 4x *T. dicoccoides.* High rates of divergence were found between closely related wheat species. The rate of divergence was different for different spacer regions; the 1.2 kb region preceding 18S rRNA gene was more conserved compared to other spacer regions. The transcribed spacer between 18S and 26S rRNA genes was poorly conserved. Tms of molecular hybrids between "130"bp repeated sequence and other "750"bp nonrepeated sequence of the rDNA spacer of wheat cultivar Chinese Spring with a number of diploid and 4x species of *Triticum, Aegilops,* and *Secale* were compared.[67] △Tm revealed a mean divergence of 3 and 2% nucleotides in the "130" and "750" bp sequences, respectively.

C. 5S rRNA Repeating Units

The unit coding for 5S rRNA gene (5S DNA) can be separated by actinomycin D/CsCl ultracentrifugation. About 10,000 copies of the coding sequences per nucleus were found in wheat.[60] There were two repeating units of 410 and 500 bp each organized in tandem arrays distal to the rDNA region.[5,60] Each fragment contains one 120 bp 5S RNA gene and spacer DNA. The tandem arrays of 420 bp units were located mainly on chromosome 1B.[5] The 5S rDNA from diploid, tetraploid, and hexaploid wheat species and *Aegilops* species were digested with Bam HI, separated by electrophoresis and hybridized with radioactive probe for 5S RNA. All the species examined except 2x wheats (*T. monococcum* and *T. boeoticum*) and *Aegilops speltoides* showed both 420 and 500 bp fragments. The 420 bp fragment was missing in 2x wheat and *Ae. speltoides.* This fragment from 2x *Aegilops* species (*longisimma, sharonensis, searsii,* and *squarrosa*) could not be differentiated from that of polyploid wheats.[5] Both repeating units have been sequenced.[68] The coding sequences of the 410 bp units were 120 bp long, while the 500 bp units carried a 15 bp nontranscribed tandem duplication. Otherwise, the two units consistently differed at three positions. The central spacer region in the two showed extensive divergence of the repeated sequences, while the 70 bp spacer region preceding the genes showed high homology. The transcription start point for wheat 5S rRNA genes, like most other prokaryotic and eukaryotic genes, was at purine preceded by pyrimidine. The terminator region of wheat 5S RNA gene was also A T rich with T residues predominant in the transcribed strand.

D. Repeated DNA Sequences in *Secale*

Secale is another genus of cereals in which repeated DNA sequences have been investigated in detail.[55,56,69-71] Part of the interest in repeated sequences is due to the presence of terminal as well as interstitial blocks of heterochromatin in rye and other species of *Secale*. These results are already summarized in Table 7. Four unrelated families having repeating units of 480, 610, 630, and 120 bp, respectively, have been investigated in *S. montanum, S. vavilovii, S. silvestre, S. africanum,* and *S. iranicum.*[70] Each species was unique in its complement, chromosomal distribution, and amount of the repeated sequences families. Species other than *cereale* have a lower amount of repeated sequences and heterochromatin as compared to rye. Restriction enzyme digests using Eco RI, Hind III, and Hae III were similar for different species, except for the 480 bp family, indicating that most families of repeated sequences are similar.

XII. ORIGIN AND EVOLUTION OF REPEATED DNA SEQUENCES IN CEREALS

A. Quantitative Changes in DNA and Repeated Sequences

During evolution and in the process of speciation, changes in the amount of DNA per cell may arise due to:

1. Polyploidy, which involves duplication of the entire basic chromosome complement of the species or of hybrids between two species as in amphiploidy.
2. Aneuploidy, i.e., addition or deletion of some chromosomes.
3. Changes in the number of accessory or so-called B chromosomes.
4. Gains or loss of DNA without any change in the number of chromosomes.[72]

The DNA content per cell in cereal species varies (Table 3); polyploidy has contributed to an increased amount of DNA in 4x and 6x wheats. However, on a per chromosome basis the DNA content in rye is higher than that in 2x wheat and other cereals.[54] This is also reflected in increased amount of repeated DNA in rye. Families of repeated sequences in *Secale* species show a direct relationship with the amount of heterochromatin in the chromosomes.[54,55,70,71,73]

1. Origin, Evolution, and Divergence of Repeated DNA Sequences

It is hypothesized that repeated DNA originates by the sudden, disproportionate replication of specific nucleotide sequences; this process is described as saltatory replication.[74,75] Britten and Kohne,[74] and others using their model, have proposed a cyclical model[4,6] to explain the organization pattern of the repeated sequences in relation to single copy sequences. The essential features of the model are

1. Families of many identical sequences are formed due to saltatory replication which is regarded as the major event in evolution.
2. These families diverge from each other due to mutations, deletions, translocations, and rearrangement of bases resulting in families of similar but not identical sequences. Some of these families further diverge to the extent that they qualify to be classified as nonrepeated or single copy sequences at the precision level of the techniques used.
3. Some such sequences are again amplified by saltatory replication to start a new cycle.

An essential tenet of this hypothesis is that the chromosomal DNA contents are maintained by a balance of sequence amplification and deletion.[4,6] The process has been referred to as "turning over" of the genome.[4] The relative rates of the two processes would determine

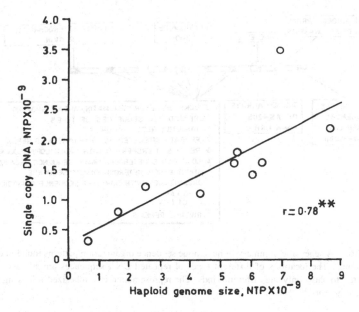

FIGURE 5. Single copy DNA content as a function of haploid genome size. Data are from Table 3. The proportion of single copy DNA is computed from 100 percent repeated DNA. Number of nucleotide pair (NTP) is calculated from the relationship of 1 pg DNA is approximately equivalent to 1×10^9 NTP. The line is a best fit following linear regression analysis. r = Correlation coefficient significant at (p = <0.01).

the genome size as well as the relative proportion of repeated and single copy sequences. Some crucial questions remain yet to be answered. What induces saltatory amplification of certain sequences? What is the time scale of the events visualized in the evolutionary history of the species?

A consistent relationship between single copy DNA and genome size has been observed in plant species.[4] The cereal species examined show a significant correlation (r = 0.78**) between genome size and the amount of single copy DNA (Figure 5). Cot required for 50% reassociation (Cot 1/2) of the slow (largely single copy sequences) reassociating DNA fraction of 2x wheat was less than that required for 4x and 6x wheats.[45] As Cot 1/2 is directly proportional to the amount of nonrepeated DNA,[76] increase implies a larger amount of nonrepeated DNA in the polyploid wheats. It was inferred that the "increase in the amount of nonrepeated DNA in the polyploid species (of wheat) probably indicates that the repeated sequences might have undergone considerable divergence during the course of evolution, and thus increasing the net amount of nonrepeated sequences, though the total DNA content remains unchanged".[45]

B. Sequence Organization Pattern in Cereal Chromosomes

In Figure 6 (a cereal chromosome) we have tried to take into consideration the different organizational patterns of the repeated sequences. The diagrammatic representations are based on several reports already discussed.[4,7,50,73]

During the course of evolution, unequal crossing over is believed to be responsible for the generation, maintenance, and variation of the tandemly repeated sequences.[77] The origin of the dispersed sequences is different. At least some of them have originated from transposable elements.[78,79] Members of a diverse array of repeated sequence families often show a high degree of homogeneity within a species, but show substantial differences between related species. Dover[80] has suggested that the "concerted" evolution of such sequences

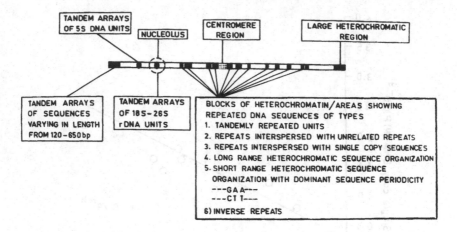

FIGURE 6.   A schematic summary of nucleotide sequence organization patterns found in cereal chromosomes. The locations of different types of repeated DNA sequences are arbitary. They are depicted to show only the different kinds. The representation is synthesized following work of different authors.[4-7,50,73]

can be brought about by some process of "molecular drive". It is visualized that certain members of a repeated sequence family preferentially convert other members of the family to their own sequence repeats. Sequences with the strongest drive become the predominant family in a relatively homogeneous array. The tandem array of telomeric heterochromatin in rye chromosomes is an example of homogenization of sequences and subsequent fixation.[71] The evolutionary advantage of these events remains unclear.

The sequence interspersion pattern in cereal genome indicates that most of the complex repeated sequences could have arisen from the amplification of compound sequences each containing repeated and nonrepeated sequences.[44,48-50,63,71] Amplification is further followed by sequence translocation and rearrangement. The origin of compound repeats in rye is explained by the insertion of elements into an array of simple repeats followed by amplification of the region containing the inserted sequence.[54,55]

Flavell et al.[50] have described the events leading to the evolution and divergence of cereal genome, especially the rye and wheat. The essential features of cereal evolution at molecular level are

1.   Only a small portion of the genome is responsible for coding and gene control. This is highly conserved.
2.   The repeated DNA sequences are not highly conserved and evolve by amplification, mutation, translocation, deletion, and rearrangement. It is mainly such molecular events that have contributed to chromosomal and species divergence. These events are also believed to prevent pairing of chromosomes at meiosis in interspecies hybrids. However, there is no experimental evidence relating repetitive sequences to pairing at meiosis. In general, it is now recognized that turnover of repeated DNA sequences has played an important role in the evolution and speciation of eukaryotes.[81] These molecular models, however, lack convincing experimental support at present.[81]

XIII. CONCLUSIONS

Repeated DNA will continue to be of immense interest in the future, and investigators will continue to try to establish its precise role in evolution, speciation, and gene regulation. For these investigations to succeed it would be necessary to ascertain the biological effects of the molecular events in the repeated sequences.

REFERENCES

1. **Stebbins, G. L.,** Cytogenetics and evolution of the grass family, *Am. J. Bot.,* 43, 890, 1956.
2. **Hutchinson, J. B.,** Crop plant evolution: a general discussion, in *Essays on Crop Plant Evolution,* Hutchinson, J., Ed., Cambridge University Press, London, 1965, 167.
3. **Britten, R. J. and Kohne, D. E.,** Repeated sequences in DNA, *Science,* 161, 529, 1968.
4. **Thompson, W. F., Murray, M. G., and Cuellar, R. E.,** Contrasting patterns of DNA sequence organization in plants, in *Genome Organization and Expression in Plants,* Leaver C. J., Ed., Plenum Press, New York, 1980, 1.
5. **Peacock, W. J., Gerlach, W. L., and Dennis, E. S.,** Molecular aspects of wheat evolution: repeated DNA sequences, in *Wheat Science — Today and Tommorrow,* Evans, L. T. and Peacock, W. J., Eds., Cambridge University Press, London, 1981, 41.
6. **Flavell, R.,** The molecular characterization and organization of plant chromosomal DNA sequences, *Ann. Rev. Plant Physiol.,* 31, 569, 1980.
7. **Flavell, R. B.,** Chromosomal DNA sequences and their organization, in *Encyclopedia of Plant Physiology New Series,* Vol. 14B, Parthier, B. and Boulter, D., Eds., Springer-Verlag, Basel, 1982, 46.
8. **Nagl, W., Jeanjour, M., Kling, H., Kühner, S., Michels, I., Müller, T., and Stein, B.,** Genome and chromatin organization in higher plants, *Biol. Zentralbl.,* 102, 129, 1983.
9. **Harlan, J. R.,** Barley, in *Evolution of Crop Plants,* Simmonds, N. W., Ed., Longman, London, 1976, 93.
10. **Goodman, M. M.,** Maize, in *Evolution of Crop Plants,* Simmonds, N. W., Ed., Longman, London, 1976, 128.
11. **Chang, T. T.,** Rice, in *Evolution of Crop Plants,* Simmonds, N. W., Ed., Longman, London, 1976, 98.
12. **Doggett, H.,** Sorghum, in *Evolution of Crop Plants,* Simmonds, N. W., Ed., Longman, London, 1976, 112.
13. **Feldman, M.,** Wheats, in *Evolution of Crop Plants,* Simmonds, N. W., Ed., Longman, London, 1976, 120.
14. **Harlan, J. R., DeWet, J. M. J., and Price, B. E.,** Comparative evolution of cereals, *Evolution,* 27, 311, 1973.
15. **Bennett, M. D. and Smith, J. B.,** Nuclear DNA amounts in angiosperms, *Philos. Trans. R. Soc. London Ser. B:,* 274, 227, 1976.
16. **Bennett, M. D.,** Nuclear DNA content and minimum generation time in herbaceous plant, *Proc. R. Soc. London Ser. B:,* 181, 109, 1972.
17. **Bennett, M. D. and Smith, J. B.,** The effects of polyploidy on the meiotic duration and pollen development in cereal anthers, *Proc. R. Soc. London Ser. B:,* 181, 1972.
18. **Goldberg, R. B., Hoscheck, G., and Kamalay, J. C.,** Sequence complexity of nuclear and polysomal RNA in leaves of the tobacco plant, *Cell,* 14, 123, 1978.
19. **Kiper, M., Bartels, D., Herzfeld, F., and Richter, G.,** The expression of a plant genome in hnRNA and mRNA, *Nucleic Acids Res.,* 6, 1961, 1979.
20. **Kohne, D. E.,** Evolution of higher organism DNA, *Q. Rev. Biophys.,* 3, 327, 1970.
21. **McCarthy, B. J. and Farquhar, M. N.,** The rate of change of DNA in evolution, in *Evolution of Genetic Systems,* Smith, H. H., Ed., Gordon & Breach Science Publ., New York, 1972, 1.
22. **Jelinek, W. R. and Schmid, C. W.,** Repetitive sequences in eukaryotic DNA and their expression, *Ann. Rev. Biochem.,* 51, 813, 1982.
23. **Burr, R., Burr, F. A., John, T. P. S., Thomas, M., and Davis, R. W.,** Zein storage protein gene family of maize — an assessment of heterogeneity with cloned messenger RNA sequences, *J. Mol. Biol.,* 154, 33, 1982.
24. **Tabata, T., Sasaki, K., and Iwabuchi, M.,** The structural organization and DNA sequence of wheat histone H4 gene, *Nucleic Acids Res.,* 11, 5865, 1983.
25. **Long, E. O. and Dawid, I. B.,** Repeated genes in eukaryotes, *Ann. Rev. Biochem.,* 49, 727, 1980.
26. **Bazetoux, S., Jouanin, L., and Hugust, T.,** Characterization of inverted repeated sequences in wheat nuclear DNA, *Nucleic Acids Res.,* 5, 751, 1978.
27. **Ingle, J., Pearson, G. G., and Sinclair, J.,** Species distribution and properties of nuclear satellite DNA in higher plants, *Nature (London) New Biol.,* 242, 193, 1973.
28. **Ingle, J., Timmis, J. N., and Sinclair, J.,** The relationship between satellite deoxyribonucleic acid, ribosomal ribonucleic acid gene redundancy, and genome size in plants, *Plant Physiol.,* 55, 496, 1975.
29. **Ranjekar, P. K., Pallotta, D., and Lafontaine, J. G.,** Analysis of plant genomes. III. Denaturation and reassociation properties of cryptic satellite DNAs in barley (*Hordeum vulgare*) and wheat (*Triticum aestivum,*) *Biochim. Biophys. Acta,* 520, 103, 1978.
30. **Dennis, E. S., Gerlach, W. L., and Peacock, W. J.,** Identical polypyrimidine-polypurine satellite DNAs in wheat and barley, *Heredity,* 44, 349, 1980.
31. **Appels, R., Driscoll, C., and Peacock, W. J.,** Heterochromatin and highly repeated DNA sequences in rye *Secale cereale, Chromosoma,* 70, 67, 1978.

32. **Huguet, T. and Jouanin, L.,** Wheat DNA: study on the heavy satellite in Ag^+-Cs_2SO_4 density gradient, *Biochem. Biophys. Res. Commun.*, 46, 1169, 1972.

33. **Wimpee, C. F. and Rawson, J. R. Y.,** Characterization of the nuclear genome of pearl millet, *Biochim. Biophys. Acta*, 562, 192, 1979.

34. **Iyengar, G. A. S., Gaddipati, J. P., and Sen, S. K.,** Characteristics of nuclear DNA in the genus *Oryza*, *Theor. Appl. Genet.*, 54, 219, 1979.

35. **Deshpande, V. G. and Ranjekar, P. K.,** Repetitive DNA in three *Graminae* species with low DNA content, *Hoppe-Seyler's Z. Physiol. Chem.*, 361, 1223, 1980.

36. **Gupta, V. S., Gadre, S. R., and Ranjekar, P. K.,** Novel DNA sequence organization in rice genome, *Biochim. Biophys. Acta*, 656, 147, 1981.

37. **Gupta, V. S. and Ranjekar, P. K.,** DNA sequence organization in finger millet (*Eleusine coracana*), *J. Biosci.*, 3, 417, 1981.

38. **Hake, S. and Walbot, V.,** The genome of *Zea mays*, its organization and homology to related grasses, *Chromosoma*, 79, 251, 1980.

39. **Bendich, A. J. and McCarthy, B. J.,** DNA comparisons among barley, oats, rye and wheat, *Genetics*, 65, 545, 1970.

40. **Ranjekar, P. K., Pallotta, D., and Lafontaine, J. G.,** Analysis of the genomes of plants. II. Characterization of repetitive DNA in barley (*Hordeum vulgare*) and wheat (*Triticum aestivum*), *Biochim. Biophys. Acta*, 425, 30, 1976.

41. **Bendich, A. F. and Anderson, R. S.,** Characterization of families of repeated DNA sequences from four vascular plants, *Biochemistry*, 16, 4655, 1977.

42. **Rimpau, J., Smith, D. B., and Flavell, R. B.,** Sequence organization in barley and oats chromosomes revealed by interspecies DNA/DNA hybridization, *Heredity*, 44, 131, 1980.

43. **Ranjekar, P. K., Lafontaine, J. G., and Pallotta, D.,** Characterization of repetitive DNA in rye (*Secale cereale*), *Chromosoma*, 48, 427, 1974.

44. **Smith, D. B. and Flavell, R. B.,** Nucleotide sequence organization in rye genome, *Biochim. Biophys. Acta*, 474, 82, 1977.

45. **Mitra, R. and Bhatia, C. R.,** Repeated and non-repeated nucleotide sequences in diploid and polyploid wheat species, *Heredity*, 31, 251, 1973.

46. **Sanchez De Jimenez, E. and Meyer Willerer, A. O.,** Analysis of the genetic complexity of hybrid plant, *Can. J. Bot.*, 56, 1291, 1978.

47. **Bendich, A. J. and McCarthy, B. J.,** DNA comparisons among some biotypes of wheat, *Genetics*, 65, 567, 1970.

48. **Flavell, R. B. and Smith, D. B.** Nucleotide organization in the wheat genome, *Heredity*, 37, 231, 1976.

49. **Smith, D. B. and Flavell, R. B.,** Characterization of the wheat genome by renaturation kinetics, *Chromosoma*, 50, 223, 1975.

50. **Flavell, R. B., O'Dell, M., and Hutchinson, J.,** Nucleotide sequence organization in plant chromosomes and evidence for sequence translocation during evolution, *Cold Spring Harbor Symp. Quant. Biol*, 45, 501, 1981.

51. **Renkawitz-Pohl, R. and Kunz, W.,** Under-replication of satellite DNA in polyploid ovarian tissue of *Drosophila virilis*, *Chromosoma*, 49, 375, 1975.

52. **Nathans, D. and Smith, H.O.,** Restriction endonucleases in the analysis and restructuring of DNA molecules, *Ann. Rev. Biochem.*, 44, 273, 1975.

53. **Bedbrook, J. and Gerlach, W. L.,** Cloning of repeated sequence DNA from cereal plants, in *Genetic Engineering, Principles and Methods*, Vol. 2, Setlow, J. and Hollaender, A., Eds., Plenum Press, New York, 1980, 1.

54. **Bedbrook, J. R., O'Dell, M., and Flavell, R. B.,** Amplification of rearranged sequences in cereal plants, *Nature (London)*, 288, 133, 1980.

55. **Bedbrook, J. R., Jones, J., O'Dell, M., Thompson, R., and Flavell, R. B.,** A molecular description of telomeric heterochromatin in *Secale* species, *Cell*, 19, 545, 1980.

56. **Appels, R., Dennis, E. S., Smyth, D. R., and Peacock, W. J.,** Two repeated DNA sequences from the heterochromatic regions of rye (*Secale cereale*) chromosomes, *Chromosoma*, 84, 265, 1981.

57. **Burr, B., Evola, S. V., and Burr, F. A.,** The application of restriction fragment length polymorphism to plant breeding, in *Genetic Engineering — Principles and Methods*, Setlow, J. K. and Hollaender, A., Eds., Vol 5, Plenum Press, New York, 1983, 45.

58. **Southern, E. M.,** Detection of specific sequences among DNA fragments separated by gel electrophoresis, *J. Mol. Biol*, 98, 503, 1975.

59. **Flamm, W. G.,** Highly repetitive sequences of DNA in chromosomes, *Int. Rev. Cytol.*, 32, 1, 1972.

60. **Appels, R., Gerlach, W. L., Dennis, E. S., Swift, H., and Peacock, W. J.,** Molecular and chromosomal organization of DNA sequences coding for the ribosomal RNAs of cereals, *Chromosoma*, 78, 293, 1980.

61. **Appels, R. and Dvořák, J.,** The wheat ribosomal DNA spacer region: its structure and variation in population and among species, *Theor. Appl. Genet.*, 63, 337, 1982.

62. **Flavell, R. B., Rimpau, J., and Smith, D. B.,** Repeated sequence DNA relationships in four cereal genomes, *Chromosoma,* 63, 205, 1977.
63. **Rimpau, J., Smith, D. B., and Flavell, R. B.,** Sequence organisation analysis of the wheat and rye genomes by interspecies DNA/DNA hybridisation, *J. Mol. Biol.,* 123, 327, 1978.
64. **Flavell, R., O'Dell, M., and Smith, D.,** Repeated sequence DNA comparisons between *Triticum* and *Aegilops* species, *Heredity,* 42, 309, 1979.
65. **Federoff, N. V.,** On spacers, *Cell,* 16, 697, 1979.
66. **Appels, R. and Dvořák, J.,** Relative rates of divergence of spacer and gene sequences within the rDNA region of species in the *Triticeae:* implications for the maintenance of homogeneity of a repeated gene family, *Theor. Appl. Genet.,* 63, 361, 1982.
67. **Dvořák, J. and Appels, R.,** Chromosome and nucleotide sequence differentiation in genomes of polyploid *Triticum* species, *Theor. Appl. Genet.,* 63, 349, 1982.
68. **Gerlach, W. L. and Dyer, T. A.,** Sequence organization of the repeating units in the nucleus of wheat which contain 5S rRNA genes, *Nucleic Acids Res.,* 8, 4851, 1980.
69. **Hutchinson, J. and Lonsdale, D. M.,** The chromosomal distribution of cloned highly reptetitive sequences from hexaploid wheat, *Heredity,* 48, 371, 1982.
70. **Jones, J. D. G. and Flavell, R. B.,** The structure, amount and chromosomal localisation of defined repeated DNA sequences in species of the genus *Secale, Chromosoma,* 86, 613, 1982.
71. **Jones, J. D. G. and Flavell, R. B.,** The mapping of highly-repeated DNA families and their relationship to C-bands in chromosomes of *Secale cereale, Chromosoma,* 86, 595, 1982. ·
72. **Rees, H. and Jones, R. N.,** The origin of the wide species variation in nuclear DNA content, *Int. Rev. Cytol.,* 32, 53, 1972.
73. **Appels, R.,** Chromosome structure in cereals: the analysis of regions containing repeated sequence DNA and its application to the detection of alien chromosomes introduced into wheat, in *Genetic Engineering of Plants — An Agricultural Perspective,* Kosuge, T., Meredith, C. P., and Hollaender, A., Eds., Plenum Press, New York, 1983, 229.
74. **Britten, R. J. and Kohne, D. E.,** Implications of repeated nucleotide sequences, in *Handbook of Molecular Cytology,* Lima-de-Faria, A., Ed., North-Holland, Amsterdam, 1969, 37.
75. **Britten, R. J. and Davidson, E. H.,** Repetitive and nonrepetitive DNA sequences and a speculation on the origins of evolutionary novelty, *Q. Rev. Biol.,* 46, 111, 1971.
76. **Laird, C. D.,** Chromatid structure: relationship between DNA content and nucleotide sequence diversity, *Chromosoma,* 32, 378, 1971.
77. **Smith, G. P.,** Evolution of repeated DNA sequences by unequal crossover, *Science,* 191, 528, 1976.
78. **Fritsch, E. F., Shen, C. K. J., Lawn, R. M., and Maniatis, T.,** The orgainzation of repetitive sequences in mammalian globin gene clusters, *Cold Spring Harbor Symp. Quant. Biol.,* 45, 761, 1980.
79. **Cameron, J. R., Loh, E. Y., and Davis, R. W.,** Evidence for transposition of dispersed repetitive DNA families in yeast, *Cell,* 16, 739, 1979.
80. **Dover, G.,** Molecular drive: cohesive mode of species evolution, *Nature (London),* 299, 111, 1982.
81. **Rose, M. R. and Doolittle, W. F.,** Molecular biological mechanisms of speciation, *Science,* 220, 157, 1983.
82. **Evans, G. M., Rees, H., Snell, C. L., and Sun, S.,** The relation between nuclear DNA amount and the duration of the mitotic cycle, in *Chromosomes Today,* Vol. 3, Plenum Press, New York, 1970.
83. **Paroda, R. S. and Rees, H.,** Nuclear DNA variation in Eusorghum, *Chromosoma,* 32, 353, 1971.
84. **Rees, H. and Walters, M. R.,** Nuclear DNA and the evolution of wheat, *Heredity,* 20, 73, 1965.
85. **Gerlach, W. L. and Bedbrook, J. R.,** Cloning and characterization of ribosomal RNA genes from wheat and barley, *Nucleic Acids Res.,* 7, 1869, 1979.
86. **Shepherd, N. S., Schwarz-Sommer, Z., Weinand, U., Sommer, H., Deumling, B., Peterson, P. A., and Saedler, H.,** Cloning of genomic fragment carrying the insertion element, Cin 1 of *Zea mays, Mol. Gen. Genet.,* 188, 266, 1982.
87. **Gupta, M., Bertram, I., Shepherd, N. S., and Saedler, H.,** Cin 1, a family of dispersed repetitive elements in *Zea mays, Mol. Gen. Genet.,* 192, 373, 1983.
88. **Liang, G. H., Wang, A. S., and Phillips, R. L.,** Control of ribosomal RNA gene multiplicity in wheat, *Can. J. Genet. Cytol.,* 19, 425, 1978.
89. **Gerlach, W. L. and Peacock, W. J.,** Chromosomal locations of highly repeated DNA sequences in wheat, *Heredity,* 44, 269, 1980.
90. **Miller, T. E., Gerlach, W. L., and Flavell, R. B.,** Nucleolus organizer variation in wheat and rye revealed by *in situ* hybridization, *Heredity,* 45, 377, 1980.
91. **Appels, R., Gustafson, J. P., and May, C. E.,** Structural variation in the heterochromatin of rye chromosomes in triticales, *Theor. Appl. Genet.* 63, 235, 1982.
92. **Appels, R., Driscoll, C., and Peacock, W. J.,** Heterochromatin and highly repeated DNA sequences in rye *(Secale cereale), Chromosoma,* 70, 67, 1978.

Chapter 3

HOMOLOGY OF NONREPEATED DNA SEQUENCES IN PHYLOGENY OF FUNGAL SPECIES

Mukti Ojha and S. K. Dutta

TABLE OF CONTENTS

I. INTRODUCTION

The interest in evolution and phylogeny has been constant and has evolved in parallel with our knowledge in other areas in biology. Numerous books and reviews have appeared from time to time, and these subjects have grown into a discipline. This paper focuses on primitive microorganisms (mainly fungi) and makes occasional reference to higher plants and animals. The fungi are an interesting group of organisms which appeared some 600 to 700 million years ago. They are highly adaptive forms and present a very flexible metabolic system. The study of evolution and phylogeny in these organisms is mainly based on the morphological and developmental features,[1,2] although other parameters such as ultrastructures,[3,4] cell walls,[5] enzyme aggregates,[6] DNA base compositions,[7] and nucleic acids[8] have also been used.

Homology, that is structural, physiological, or behavioral similarity, has been used as a criterion in establishing phylogenetic relationships between organisms. Phenotypic homology does not require genotypic homology because some characteristics arise through convergence. Convergence occurs when similar characteristics are acquired independently in two or more phylogenetic lines. The evolutionary relationships can be traced by measuring either the shared characters or divergence. To study the phylogenetic relationships, the ideal conditions would be (1) to compare the structure of the genes themselves, since they carry the evidence of change at the basic information level and (2) to examine their transcriptional and translational products.

In molecular terms, these comparisons would involve the nucleotide sequence organization of the genes and the stable RNAs or the amino acid sequences of the proteins. Comparative studies of sequence organization of amino acids in certain proteins (e.g., ferridoxin and cytochrome) have given information about phylogenic evolution.[9] Many other proteins have also been sequenced and compared. In addition to direct sequencing, investigators have used microcomplement fixation and electrophoresis to compare homology and divergence of a given protein from different sources. The former is based on the immunological cross reactivity (i.e., the sequence-immunology relationship), and the latter on the difference in charge and molecular weight of the protein due to sequence differences. However, simple estimates of amino acid differences between two proteins can sometimes underestimate the total number of mutations fixed because multiple substitution sometimes occurs at the same amino acid site. From the studies of proteins in phylogenetic evolution, it can be concluded that proteins have evolved at variable rates and that comparison is accurate only for the closely related organisms.[10]

Although the sequencing technique in the study of RNA is older than that for DNA, it has been successfully used in the study of evolution only recently. A very important contribution from the Woese group[11] is based on the study of nucleotide sequence analysis of 16S rRNA. In this method, the ^{32}P-labeled 16S rRNA were cleaved by T1 RNase, whose recognition sites are guanine bases at the 3' end, generating oligonucleotides of 1 to 20 bases. Oligonucleotides longer than 6 nucleotides were sequenced and arranged in groups of 6. A dictionary of 25-letter words was constructed, each word containing 6 letters represented by 6 nucleotides. For comparison between species, the dictionaries were compared and an association coefficient was established which expressed the proportion of nucleotide in the words being common in both dictionaries. The scheme defined further parameters for comparison between species, such as evolutionary depth, based on variation in S value. A value of 1 represented identity, and that of 0 indicated no relation. Shallow evolutionary depth represented a small variation of S in Enterobacteriaceae, but a deep S value (large variation of S) in Clostridiae. One very important contribution of this study is the finding of a group of bacteria, the methanogenic sulfur, the halophiles, and the thermoacedophiles that had deep S values and as a group were as closely related to eukaryotes as to other

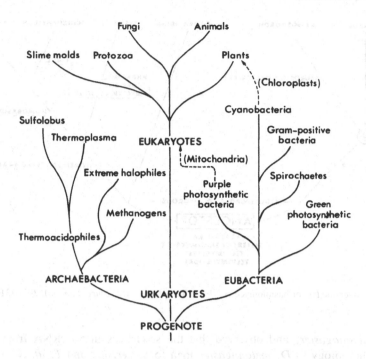

FIGURE 1. Phylogenetic tree of organisms shows position of fungi. (From Woese, C.R., *Sci. Am.*, 274, 98, 1980. With permission.)

bacteria. These bacteria were grouped as archebacteria as opposed to the other, the eubacteria. This discovery not only illustrates the progression of evolution in time scale as Woese points, but also indicates diverging lines early in evolution in primitive organisms. According to this scheme, three independent lines of evolution took place from a common ancestry "the progenotes", one leading to archebacterial type, another in the middle to the eukaryotic type, and the third to the eubacterial type (Figure 1).

Nucleotide sequence organization of another ribosomal RNA, the 5S rRNA, has also been used to study the phylogeny and evolution in eukaryotic microorganisms. In fungi, the 5S rRNAs have been sequenced and used to study the evolutionary relationships.[12,13] Walker and Ford-Doolittle[13] sequenced the 5S rRNAs from 15 basidiomycetes and used the sequence alignment procedure to group them into 5 clusters. The sequences differed by 9, 6 to 10, 0, and 2 to 14 within and 30 to 40, 24 to 30, 19 to 34, 20 to 40, and 18 to 41 nucleotides between clusters 1, 2, 3, 4, and 5, respectively. They observed that all species belonging to clusters 1 and 2 had simple septal pores, whereas those belonging to clusters 3 to 5 (except for *Exobasidium vaccini*) had dolipores. They concluded that the capped dolipores probably evolved from simple septum via capless dolipores. Templeton[14] constructed a phylogenetic scheme of basidiomycetes evolution, which essentially confirms Walker and Ford-Doolittle's[13] conclusion (Figure 2). In a more recent analysis of additional basidiomycetes, Gottschalk and Blanz[15] have shown that the 5S rRNA sequence analysis is of limited value for the differentiation within groups, particularly the cluster 5 of Walker and Ford-Doolittle.[13] Despite high differentiation in their host spectra, the 4 rust species of this group were found to have highly conserved 5S rRNA sequences.[15] In fact, *Coleosporium tussilaginis*, *Gymnosporangium claviforme*, and *Puccinia poarum* have identical 5S rRNA sequence. Similar conclusions were also drawn earlier by Huysmans et al.,[16] who stated that "5S rRNA is a low resolution phylogenetic marker yielding useful information only on a large time scale". Earlier, Mao et al.[17] compared the sequence organization of 5S rRNA from *Saccharomyces pombe* with two other species of yeasts, *S. cerevisiae* and *Torula utilis*, and with the fruitfly,

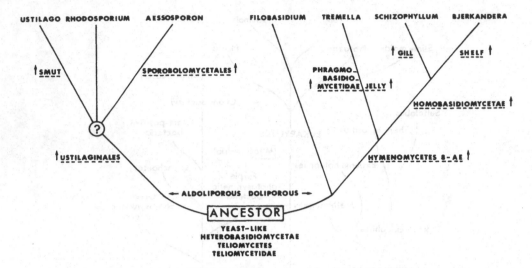

FIGURE 2.   Phylogenetic tree of basidiomycetes. (From Templeton, A., *Nature (London)*, 303, 731, 1983. With permission.)

Drosophila melanogaster, and observed that the sequences in 5S rRNA from *S. pombe* shared more homology to *D. melanogaster* than to *S. cerisiae* and *T. utilis*. All of these results indicate the limitation of the utilization of 5S rRNA sequences in the evaluation of phylogenetic relationships.

Considerable progress has been made in isolating defined genes and amplifying them by recombinant DNA technology in other organisms, either in bacteria or in yeast. Thus, it is now possible to obtain large quantities of any gene and analyze its sequence organization. This technique has been particularly useful in the analysis of individual genes and has given new information about our concept of genes. The information regarding the phylogenetic evaluation of species can be obtained by comparing expressed or unexpressed nucleotide sequences of these genes. But before discussing how changes in genes might have arisen during the course of time, we would like to examine certain information about the genomal DNA which might have some relevance to the phylogenetic relationships in fungi.

II. GENOME

A. Base Composition

The GC (guanine + cytosine) mol% of DNA has been used to identify the affinities between a wide range of bacteria, lower eukaryotes, higher plants, and animals. In fungi, Storck and Alexopoulos[7] and Storck[8] have reviewed the GC mol% and concluded on the basis of available information that zygomycetes on the average have the lowest GC content and the basidiomycetes the highest (the ascomycetes falling between these two groups). The GC content of hemiascomycetes varies from 29 to 50% and is closer to that of zygomycetes, whereas the euascomycetes have a range of 50 to 60% and are closer to the heterobasidiomycetes. The percent GC content of most deuteromycetes is close to that for ascomycetes.

The intrataxonomic heterogeneity in DNA was also analyzed in terms of standard deviation of frequency distribution of GC in taxons. A value equal to or less than 2% GC for species and 10% for the genera was found.[8] Higher values were characteristic for larger taxonomic groups, such as families, orders, and classes.

With respect to phylogeny, these studies revealed two main features, one with regard to the monophyletic origin of fungi and the other to the evolution of yeasts. According to the scheme of monophyletic origin, the fungi evolved from a primitive flagellate ancestor, a direct precursor of chytridiomycetes (Archemycetes according to the scheme of Gauman[2]). The zygomycetes evolved from chytrids and are direct precursors of the ascomycetes. The ascomycetes preceded basidiomycetes. The oomycetes are an exception to this scheme and probably arose from an algal ancestor. Taking the GC mol% data into consideration, Storck[8] argued "it would appear that fungal evolution was associated with progressive increase in GC content of the DNA". The average value of 53 mol% GC in oomycetes indicates that they are not on the main evolutionary line. With regards to origin and evolution in yeasts, these data reveal two points: (1) that one group of yeasts has a GC mol% closer to the zygomycetes than to the euascomycetes, indicating that they are more primitive than reduced forms of ascomycetes; (2) that one group has a higher GC mol% than ascomycetes and is considered to be related to heterobasidiomycetes. These two extreme variations can be taken as an indication of yeasts being degenerate forms of lower ascomycetes and primitive basidiomycetes. However, the higher GC content (51 to 63%) of chytridiomycetes[8,18] argues against the monophyletic origin of fungi, as concluded by Storck.[8] According to GC content, chytrids should be closer to the basidiomycetes in phylogeny.

B. Genome Size

The DNA content per cell, estimated by chemical means in a large number of organisms, agrees well with the accepted notion that the genetic complexity or genome size increased as the complex cellular organization of higher forms evolved.[19] Britten and Kohne[20] and Wetmur and Davidson[21] extensively studied the rate of reassociation of complementary DNA strands after dissociation and showed that the kinetics of renaturation was directly proportional to the sequence complexity of the reacting DNA molecules. Britten and Kohne[20] used the term "Cot $^1/_2$" to express the concentrations of reacting nucleotides expressed in mol/sec at which 50% reassociation occurred. The Cot $^1/_2$ value was found to be directly proportional to the sequence complexity of the genome. Thus, by known and unknown genomes, the Cot $^1/_2$ value of the unknown was used to determine its sequence complexity. Earlier, we reviewed the genome size of fungi representing different taxonomic groups.[22] Since then a few more fungi have been added to the list. In general, they all fall within a narrow range of approximately 1.4 to 3 × 10^7 nucleotide pairs. Although the genome sizes seem to follow the monophyletic origin of fungi, the narrow range of variation makes any definite conclusion difficult.

C. Genome Organization

Another aspect of the genome that has been extensively investigated in the eukaryotic genome is the organization of the repetitive sequences in the DNA. In prokaryotes, the entire sequences in the genome are transcribed and expressed as functional mRNA. There are only a few sequences that are repetitive, mostly genes coding for rRNA and tRNA. The eukaryotic genomes are much more complex as reassociation kinetics has indicated. It is composed of coding single copy sequences and families of repetitive sequences.[20] The latter could be very simple sequences such as the pure poly dAT present in large amounts in certain crabs.[23] Fast and middle or intermediate repetitive sequences are interspersed with single copy sequences at different places in the genome. These are mostly functionless genes as far as their coding capacity and final processing in the synthesis of protein are concerned. The exact pattern of interspersion is characteristic of different species and may be one of the following three types.

1. Short Period Interspersion

Single copy sequences (1000 to 2000 nucleotide pairs) interspersed with approximately 200 to 400 nucleotide pairs long repeat sequences. The short period interspersion pattern has been reported for representative species of all major animal phyla and flowering plants.[24,25]

Genomes showing this pattern also contain varying amounts of long repetitive sequences exceeding 1500 nucleotide pairs in length, some of which may be organized in a tandem array.[24] In eukaryotic microorganisms, this pattern has been reported for the slime mold, *Physarum polycephalum*,[26] and the cellular slime mold, *Dictyostelium discoideum*.[27] In *P. polycephalum*, repetitive sequences of approximately 600 bp are interspersed with single copy sequence 930 to 1300 bp long. In *D. discoideum*, half of the repetitive sequences are interspersed in the short period pattern, whereas the remaining half are organized as long blocks of over 2000 to 3000 nucleotide pairs in length. The long period repetitive sequences also contain the sequences coding for rRNA.

2. Long Period Interspersion
This pattern is found in certain insects with small genome sizes.[28,29] Single copy sequences, at least 10,000 nucleotide pairs long, are interspersed with repeat sequences of at least 6000 nucleotide pairs.

3. No Interspersion
This type appears to characterize fungi. These organisms show long period organization, but the highly and moderately repetitive sequences are organized as tandem arrays of precisely paired, regularly repeating units. This pattern has been found in *Achlya ambisexualis*,[30] *Phycomyces blakesleeanus*,[31] *Neurospora crassa*,[32] and *Schizophyllum commune*.[33] Compared with higher eukaryotes, the fungi as a group are characterized as having very few repetitive sequences. In some cases, the number is only sufficient to code for rRNA and tRNA genes.[34] Curiously, among the different classes of fungi, the ascomycetes, a group higher in the accepted evolutionary ladder, seems to have a smaller amount of repeated sequences (*Aspergillus nidulans* (2 to 4%),[34] *Saccharomyces cerevisiae* (5%),[35] *Neurospora crassa* (8%))[32,36] than phycomycetes (*Allomyces arbuscula* (20%),[37] *Phycomyces blakesleeanus* (30%),[31] *Achlya ambisexualis* (16%)[38]).

The phylogenetic significance of the sequence organization in fungi, similar to that in higher plants and animals, is not clear. The occurrence of the short period interspersion mode in the Myxomycete *P. polycephalum* and the acrasiale *D. discoideum* is interesting since they are not considered to be in the main line of fungal evolution. In this respect, they are a group apart from other fungal taxa (phycomycetes, ascomycetes, and basidiomycetes) showing a long period interspersion mode.

III. EVOLUTION OF NEW GENES

It is worthwhile here to discuss how polymorphism in the genes has evolved. There are at least five major sources of evolution of new genes from the existing ones.

A. Gene Duplication
This is probably one of the major sources of evolution of new genes. If a duplicate copy of a gene mutation can accumulate in one gene, the unaltered copy can maintain the original function of the gene. In time, the mutated gene provides the new activity of the modified gene. Among the genes that have been thought to arise in this way is one of the two actin genes in the sea urchin *Strongylocentrotus franciscanus*. These genes are physically linked and separated by about 5 kb. The two genes are extremely similar (they differ by only 1.7% of nucleotides in the coding region),[39] The number of actin genes in fungi are variable. The yeast *Saccharomyces cerevisiae* has a single actin gene,[40,41] while *Physarum polycephalum* contain 4,[42] and *Dictyostelium discoideum*[43,44] has 17. The 17 actin genes of *Dictyostelium* have been shown to contain transcribed and nontranscribed regions. The coding sequences show a large number of nucleotide differences but few amino acid changes. In the nontran-

scribed regions, the first 45 nucleotides in the 3' ends have substantial homology. This indicates that different families of actin genes arose by duplication of the progenitor gene. The conservation of the first 45 nucleotides of the 3' untranslated region could be due to selective pressure acting to maintain these sequences in evolution.[43]

The 5' untranscribed regions in another multigene family, the discoidin I gene, are also conserved since they share considerable homology.[44] It is believed that these genes also arose by duplication of the original gene. The occurrence of multiple copies of genes in higher organisms thus, would provide greater flexibility and selective advantage over prokaryotes in the sense that the organism would survive mutation in a functional gene.

B. Mutations Creating New Activities

One of the best known examples of this type is the lac Z gene of *Escherichia coli*. A deletion of this gene makes the organism unable to utilize lactose. However, a rare genetic event at a different locus termed ebg A (evolved B galactosidase) restores lactose metabolism and the organism becomes lactose-positive.[45,46] Another example of changes creating new activities by the fusion of old genes of related functions to form a new enzyme complex is the first two enzymes involved in the tryptophan pathway in enteric bacteria. In most nonenteric and some enteric bacteria, the enzyme is composed of a large and a small subunit.[47] The large subunit's gene has remained separate in all bacteria studied to date, but in some enteric bacteria, the gene for the small subunit has been fused with the gene immediately downstream from it, the one for the second enzyme in the pathway.[48,49] This result in the formation of a new complex of enzyme consisting of the large subunit of the first enzyme bound noncovalently to the fused polypeptide made from the small subunit of the first and second enzyme.

C. The Transposition and Insertion of New Sequences

The modification of genes through transposition is another event which occurs in both prokaryotes and eukaryotes. The primary sequences of transposable elements are highly conserved and they can be inserted into a large number of chromosomal (or plasmid) sites, thus promoting the evolution of plasmids and bacterial or eukaryotic chromosomes. Changes in attendant DNA sequences such as new promoters and terminators for transcription are necessary to make the insertion sequences functional. In fungi, transposable elements have been reported for yeasts and *Dictyostelium discoideum*. In yeast the transposable elements (Ty elements)[50] consist of a central region of 5.6 kb pairs flanked by direct repeats of 330 bp sequences called δ. There are 30 to 35 Ty elements per haploid yeast genome. Besides δ sequences associated with Ty elements, the yeast genome contains at least 100 solo sequences. The Ty elements are considered to move from one side to another through gene conversion, excision, and reintegration or by transposition. In *Dictyostelium*, Chung et al.[51] have described 40 copies of a similar 4.5 kb sequence. These sequences are scattered throughout the genome and are considered to have different flanking sequences in the same or different strains, indicating that the 4.5 kb sequence is a transposon. There is an indication that the sequence surrounding two discoidin I genes in this organism is also a transposon.[52] Another interesting case is the 5S rRNA genes in *Neurospora crassa*.[53] The 100 copies of this gene are not tandemly repeated and do not form part of a larger rRNA gene complex; instead, they are dispersed throughout the genome. These genes have both identical and divergent regions. There are three different types of these genes. A majority are α-type genes but there are also four minor types called B, B1, and genes. A majority of these genes have different flanking regions. It is believed that 5S rRNA genes in this organism may have evolved through repeated transposition.

D. Modification of Regulatory Devices

A common feature of microorganisms is their adaptability to the nutritional environment.

They are able to adjust the production of catabolic enzymes according to their need. An example of this is the substrate and end product induction and inhibition of the enzyme level and activities. Sometimes mutations occur in the regulatory gene which control the transcription of the gene and thereby derepress their synthesis; consequently, the enzyme is oversynthesized. In some cases, transposition of a gene is accompanied by a complete change in the regulatory apparatus. Thus, in *Pseudomonas putida* and *P. aeruginosa*, the A, B, and F genes of tryptophan are not at all responsive to the repressor produced by the tryp r gene.[54] Instead, the F gene has been left unregulated, while an entirely new regulator for the A and B genes has developed, making them inducible by their substrate rather than repressible by tryptophan.[55]

E. Genetic Recombination Through Sexual Exchanges

Sexuality and recombination provide another method for the evolution of genes. Fundamentally, they offer a means for selecting genes, since genes (or linked groups) are more feasible units for selection than the whole genome. Genes regulating the recombination frequency have been described and studied in detail in the yeasts *Neurospora*, *Ustilago*, and *Schizophyllum*.[56,57] In *Neurospora*, the controlling gene is not closely linked to the gene or region controlled and the allele giving lower recombination frequency is dominant over that giving higher. In *Schizophyllum commune*, Stamberg[58] showed that at least two regulatory genes are responsible for the control of recombination between the A and B incompatibility factor and that the genes are separate from the controlled regions and that they segregate and recombine with respect to one another.

IV. EVOLUTIONARY DIVERGENCE

Direct comparison of homologous DNA sequences enables us to evaluate the extent of sequence divergence in various functional and structural units of the genome. Mutations having no apparent effect on the organism are called "neutral mutations" or "silent substitutions". Jukes[59] estimates that half of the nucleotide substitutions occurring during evolutionary divergence of genes in animals, bacteria, and viruses are silent changes, and he believes that most of them are selectively neutral. Most "silent substitutions" occur in the third position of the codons.[59,60] A large number of silent nucleotide substitutions occur during the evolutionary divergence of lineage. Estimates have indicated that the rate of substitution at the third position of the codon is about four times greater than at the first and second positions. Mutations occurring in the DNA sequences directly involved in the synthesis of certain classes of RNAs such as ribosomal RNA could be lethal, and therefore would be eliminated from the population. The genes for rRNA belong to this class of highly conserved genes in which the divergence in the sequences is minimal even after an extended period of evolution.

Another class of DNA sequences which can be passed into the progeny are those which determine the templates for the proteins requiring definite amino acid sequences. Due to the redundancy of the code, some changes in these sequences can be tolerated and maintained in the evolution. Kohne[61] estimates that approximately 25% of the mutations can produce changes to be propagated, and the resulting difference after a long period of evolution will approach 17%.

A. Sequence Homology and Divergence

In the natural state, the genome (DNA and in some cases RNA) exists as a double-stranded molecule. The two strands are complementary and are held together by specific interaction between the individual nucleotides (A-T and G-C). The strands can be dissociated by certain treatments such as temperature and pH. Under proper conditions (pH, temperature, and salt concentration), the complementary strands reassociate to their original interacting base sequences and reform the double-stranded molecule. The rate of complementary sequence recognition (reassociation) depends upon the frequency with which a given sequence occurs. If the sequences are present in only one copy per genome (single copy sequences), an ideal second order reaction occurs.[20,21] When some sequences are present in more than one copy (repetitive sequences), they reassociate faster than the single copy sequences because of the greater probability of easily finding the complementary sequences. Theoretically, it is possible to compare the sequences between two genomes by making hybrid molecules of similar sequences in a heterologous reaction. This can be done by preventing homologous sequence recognition and formation of homoduplexes.

V. EXPERIMENTAL APPROACH

Two basic methods have been used to measure the nucleotide sequence homology: competitive reassociation of associated heterogenous DNA and cleavage of transcribed DNA sequences with restriction nucleases.

A. Competitive Reassociation of Dissociated Heterologous DNA

In this method, the DNA is denatured and challenged with radioactively labeled heterologous tracer DNA. Two methods of reassociation have been used. In the first, the immobilized DNA on solid support is challenged with radioactive heterologous DNA in solution. After a period of time, the solid support containing DNA is removed, treated with S1 nuclease to digest the tail end of the labeled reassociated DNA fragment, washed, and the percent hybridization determined by liquid scintillation counting. In the other method, the reaction is carried out in solution and the single stranded fragments are removed from the reassociated double-stranded fragments by differential binding to solid support; the single stranded fragments and the duplexes are then eluted with appropriate buffers. As outlined earlier, certain stringent requirements are necessary to avoid intrastrand and homologous pairing: (1) The fragment size should not be too long. The DNA should be sheared to fragments with an average length of 500 bp. (2) To achieve reproducible results and to obtain a true measure of base sequence evolution, particularly eukaryotic DNAs, the repeated sequences should be removed from the tracer DNA. For this, a knowledge of the property of reassociation kinetics of the DNA is essential. The repeated sequences are removed by homologous reassociation of the tracer DNA fragments to Cot values[20] — just enough to allow the duplex formation of the repeated sequences. This leaves the single copy sequences in the single strand form. The single-stranded molecules are then recovered by hydroxyapatite column chromatography and used as tracer fragments in heterologous reaction. (3) The ratio of tracer sequence to driver should be low enough to exclude their self-reassociation. In general, 1 part of the tracer to 1000 parts of the driver fragments should be used.

The hybrid duplexes formed after a given period of incubation (calculated to allow the duplex formation of all complementary sequences) are separated from the single-stranded molecules by hydroxyapatite chromatography. A step of S1 nuclease digestion should be used before the passage on hydroxyapatite to remove the tail ends as described above.

The sequence homology in heterologous hybridization and evolution assumes that all the sequences in the two genomes being compared have homology in the other species, all homologous sequences can form hybrids, and all degrees of genetic divergence can be detected.

B. Cleavage of Transcribed DNA Sequences Using Restriction Nucleases

The sequence homology within isolated genes or known DNA sequences can also be studied by restriction enzymes. These enzymes are nucleases with specific sequence recognition sites, and thus they generate fragments of a defined size. In practice, this is done as follows: the entire DNA of an organism is digested and then the different fragments are separated by electrophoresis. The fragment that is homologous to a particular gene is then identified by a DNA probe.[62] The DNA probe is the same piece of DNA as the gene under investigation, but is labeled with a radioactive isotope. In this case, any fragment that is partially or wholly homologous to the gene can be detected. It is clear that in this case only the sequences which are normally expressed and genetically functional can be used. Detailed discussions on the use of restriction enzymes for polymorphisms of specific genes (such as rDNAs) or specific DNA sequences are given in several other chapters of these volumes. Recently, this method has been extended to fungal species. Use of this approach for studies of polymorphism of rDNAs of heterothallic species of the genus *Neurospora* has enabled us to acquire the knowledge contained in the following paragraph.[63]

We have recently shown that about 300 bp sequences of the external spacer region present in *Neurospora crassa* are apparently deleted in the species of *N. intermedia* and *N. sitophila*, based on restriction patterns of 12 different enzymes and using two *N. crassa* rDNA clones in pBR322 plasmid. We have identified a Nru[1] site which was detected in the NTES (nontranscribed external spacer) regions of *N. sitophila* and of *N. intermedia*, but not present in that position in *N. crassa*. Russell et al.[64] have screened a *N. crassa* 74A wild-type strain and 30 other wild-type strains of *N. crassa*, *N. tetrasperma*, *N. sitophila*, *N. intermedia*, and *N. discreta*. Their data indicate that the rDNA repeat unit size was highly conserved and that all the strains have a conserved Hind III site near the 5' end of the 26S rRNA coding sequence; however, polymorphism in the number and/or position of Hind III sites in the nontranscribed spacer region was found between strains. Russell and co-workers concluded that restriction site polymorphism was strain-specific. Based on characterization with restriction endonucleases, Natvig et al.[65] have shown that plasmids from isolates of *N. tetrasperma* were more closely related to one another than to an evolutionarily homologous plasmid from *N. intermedia*. These same authors[66] have confirmed that four-spored isolates constituted a natural taxonomic group (*N. tetrasperma*). These results clearly establish that restriction analysis is a useful tool to study phylogenetic relationships of fungal species.

VI. DETERMINATION OF SEQUENCE DIVERGENCE

In hybrid duplex formation, the base sequence pairing all along the fragment may not be perfect because some sequences may not be complementary. This would result in certain mismatching. The extent of mismatched base pairs can be determined by the dissociation of the hybrid duplexes with the rise in incubation temperature. The temperature is raised progressively from what was used for hybridization, and the single-strand formation (due to the dissociation of hybrids) is determined by hydroxyapatite chromatography.[61] This gives the thermal denaturation profile of the hybrids. The midpoint transition (the temperature at which 50% of the hybrids remain as duplex) is determined by a plot of the percentage of hybrid molecules dissociated against temperature and is used for the estimation of base pair mismatching or sequence divergence in the heterologous duplexes.

A. Calibration of Sequence Divergence

Laird et al.[67] used synthetic nucleotides with specific deletions to study the duplex formation and their thermal stabilities. They calculated that a decrease in 1°C of Te50 (50% denaturation of DNA:DNA heteroduplexes) corresponds to a 1.5% difference in the base pairs. A further calibration of the Te50 value has been done against the absolute time scale to determine its evolutionary significance[61,68] using the paleontological data. For birds, the later authors[68] calculated that a δ Te50 value of 1 is equal to 4.5 to 5 million years; i.e., it takes 4.5 to 5 million years for the genome of two species to become different at 1% of

Table 1
SINGLE COPY NUCLEOTIDE SEQUENCE COMPLEMENTARITY BETWEEN SOME FUNGI

[32]P labeled DNA fragments	Unlabeled DNA fragments	Binding (%)	Normalized binding (%)	Tm (i)	Tm (i)	Ref.
Allomyces arbuscula	*A. arbuscula*	95	100	89.0	—	18
	A. macrogynus	70	73	86.8	—	
	Blastocladiella emersonii	55	58	86.8	—	
	Saprolegnia ferax	46	48	—	—	
Saprolegnia ferax	*S. ferax*	90	100	86	—	
	Achlya radiosa	51.3	57.0	83.5	2.5	
	Allomyces arbuscula	33.0	37.0	80	6.0	
	Blastocladiella emersonii	22.5	25.0	80	6.0	
	Neurospora crassa	39.6	44	—	—	
Neurospora crassa	*N. crassa*	93.7	100	90.5	0.3	76, 79—82
	N. intermedia	76.0	81.1	86.2	4.3	
	N. sitophila	78.5	83.8	86.5	4.0	
	Coprinus cinereus	14.3	15.0	82.6	7.9	
	Mucor azygospora	10.5	11.2	83.2	7.3	
	E. coli	0.4	0.43	—	—	
Coprinus cinereus	*C. cinereus*	95.05	100	100	—	80
	Neurospora crassa	9.05	9.47	—	—	
	N. intermedia	8.67	9.07	—	—	
	N. sitophila	10.10	10.57	—	—	
	N. tetrasperma	10.70	11.2	—	—	
	Mucor azygospora	8.57	8.97	—	—	
	E. coli	0.70	0.73	—	—	

their base pairs after they have diverged from a common ancestor. This calibration must be improved by additional evidence. More recently, Sibley and Ahlquist[69] have further discussed the usefulness of DNA:DNA hybridizations for phylogenetic studies. According to their calculations, the DNA "clocks" based on UAR (Uniform Average Rate), which is based on the statistical result of averaging over billions of nucleotides and millions of years, are real and keep excellent time. UARs of δ Te50 are measures of relative time. According to them, generation time has no effect on the average rate of DNA evolution. DNA clocks are certainly more dependable than protein clocks because each protein evolves at its own rate and rates vary with individual genes. DNA clocks, on the other hand, average across the entire genome.

B. Single Copy Sequence Homology and Divergence in Some Fungal Groups

Single copy sequence homology between distantly related filamentous fungi representing three major classes (Phycomycetes, Ascomycetes, and Basidiomycetes) and two subclasses of Phycomycetes (Chytridiomycetes and Oomycetes) is shown in Table 1. Although these results do not give any precise information about phylogeny, they do give some measure of affinity between distantly related groups. The Ascomycete *Neurospora* has approximately 11% of sequences in common with the Phycomycete (Zygomycete) *Mucor azygospora* and 15% with *Coprinus lagoupus*. The Oomycete *Saprolegnia ferax* shares 44% of sequences with *Neurospora crassa* and 37% with the Chytridiomycete, *Allomyces arbuscula*. The intergeneric sequence homology between members of the same family Saprolegniaceae (*S. ferax/A. radiosa*) and Blastocladiaceae (*A. arbuscula/Blastocladiella emersonii* is 57 and 58%, respectively.

Single copy sequence hybridization can be utilized with greater precision in the determination of homology and divergence in closely related species. We have used this to

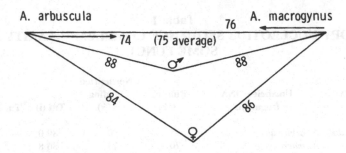

FIGURE 3. Relatedness between some zoospore fungi.[18]

examine two closely related species of the genus *Allomyces* and many species of *Neurospora*. In *Allomyces*, the single copy sequences common between *A. arbuscula*, *A. macrogynus*, two natural species, and two experimentally derived sexual hybrids, male and female obtained by interspecific crosses,[70] have been compared.[18]

As shown in the affinity diagram (Figure 3), the average sequence homology between the two parental types (75%) was lower than their hybrids (85 to 88%). The dissimilarities between the parental types could account for the polarity difference in sexual positioning, female gametangial morphology, and the intensity of carotenoid pigmentation in the male gametangia. The male and female strains hybridized to an equal extent with their parental types and had lower sequence dissimilarity (see Figure 3). These results provide molecular proof of the earlier conclusions drawn by Emerson and Wilson[70] that these strains are true hybrids. These results also indicate that the male strains share more sequences in common with the parental types than the female strains; however, the hybrid duplexes from male strains contain more divergent base pairs than the female strains.[37] A comparison of the ribosomal RNA cistron number in the hybrid strains has shown that the male strain has about 60% deletion of RNA cistrons as compared to the wild type and the female.[71] The fact that laboratory-derived stable strains with significant sequence divergence can be produced by sexual crossings poses some problem in the traditional estimation of absolute time based sequence divergence in evolution, since such interspecific mating may occur in nature and one can then find new species through genetic recombination and not through the accumulation of mutation which is a longer process.

A more extensive examination of the phylogenetic relationship has been done with the species of the genus *Neurospora*. This genus, designated by Shear and Dodge,[72] is classified into different groups mainly on the basis of mating reaction of its species. The heterothallic species typified by *N. crassa* have an asexual phase characterized by the production of conidia. The sexual developmental phase consists of perithecia, asci, and ascospores which develop only after mating interaction with a compatible strain. The pseudohomothallic strains, type species *N. tetrasperma*, have an asexual conidial phase and a sexual perithecial phase containing asci and ascospores. The perithecia develop without sexual interaction with another thallus. The true homothallic species lack an asexual conidial phase, and as the name suggests, the perithecia develop without sexual interaction with any other thallus. This group has members that differ in the number of pores in the ascospores. In *N. terricola* the ascospores have unipolar pores. *N. lineolata* represents the groups containing pores on both ends of the ascospores (bipolar pores). The matrix of percent heterologous competitive reassociation of *N. crassa* with the species of other groups is shown in Figure 4. These species can be distinguished on the basis of sequence homology and appear as clusters with respect to common single copy sequences. The heterothallic cluster shows that the species in this group share 84 to 86% of the sequences. The different isolates of *Neurospora* share between 97 and 98% of the sequences with the tracer *N. crassa*. The pseudohomothallic

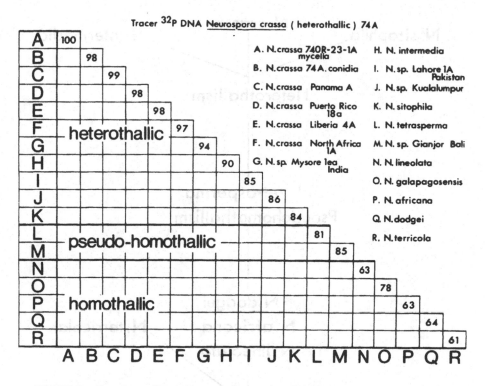

Tracer ^{32}P DNA <u>Neurospora crassa</u> (heterothallic) 74A

A. N.crassa 740R-23-1A mycelia
B. N.crassa 74A.conidia
C. N.crassa Panama A
D. N.crassa Puerto Rico 18a
E. N.crassa Liberia 4A
F. N.crassa North Africa 1A
G. N.sp. Mysore lea India

H. N. intermedia
I. N.sp. Lahore 1A Pakistan
J. N.sp. Kualalumpur
K. N. sitophila
L. N. tetrasperma
M. N. sp. Gianjor Bali
N. N. lineolata
O. N. galapagosensis
P. N. africana
Q. N. dodgei
R. N. terricola

FIGURE 4.   Homology of *Neurospora* species based on DNA:DNA reassociation studies.[79,80]

group, represented by *N. tetrasperma* and another isolate of *Neurospora* (*N. species*, Gianjor, Bali), has sequence homology ranging from 81 to 85%. However, the homothallic species have a relatively lower percentage of sequences in common with *N. crassa* (61 to 68%), except for *N. galapagosensis*, which shares 78% of the sequences. Reciprocal hybridization using representative tracer species gives essentially the same results. These molecular hybridizations confirmed what is known of the mating reactions; i.e., these species represent tight clusters and have a large number of single copy sequences in common. These conclusions find strong support when one compares the sequence homology data of the species of the same mating type. The hybridization reactions in homothallic species using *N. lineolata* and *N. galapagosensis* as tracers gave values of 91 to 97% and 94 to 100%, respectively. An exception to this in the homothallic cluster is *N. terricola*, which has diverged considerably from the other members of this group. This is illustrated by the single copy sequence homology and divergence (Te50) data (Figure 5). This is interesting, since *N. terricola* contains ascospores with only one pore, whereas other species have ascospores with pores on both ends. The interesting feature from the evolutionary point of view and phylogeny in *Neurospora* that has come from the reciprocal hybridization reactions is that the homothallic species have closer affinities to the pseudohomothallic species. Further, unlike homothallic species, the heterothallic species show greater diversity in DNA sequences (Figure 4). These results suggest the possible evolutionary sequence of mating type in *Neurospora*, homo-thallism-pseudohomothallism-heterothallism,[73] as is shown in Figure 5.

Another group of fungi in which sequence homology of single copy sequences has been extensively investigated to differentiate between various species and the strains of the same species is the yeasts.[74-76] The yeasts are a heterogenous group of unicellular fungi, reproducing vegetatively by budding and showing affinity to two major fungal taxa, the asco- and basidiomyces. The sexual phase in ascosporogenous yeasts (e.g., *Saccharomyces*) consists of the development of asci and ascospores. These types are considered to be primitive

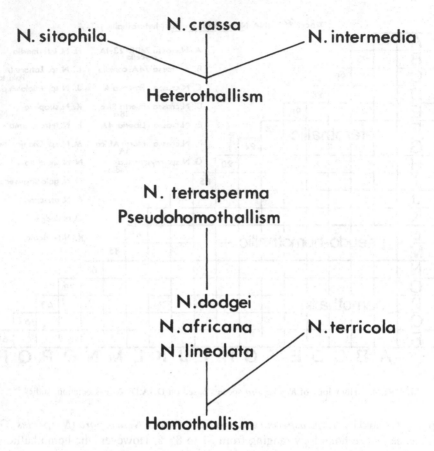

FIGURE 5. Evolutionary tree of the genus *Neurospora*.[73]

ascomycetes (see GC composition in this chapter). The yeasts showing basidiomycete affinity are normally asporogenous, although members of the family Sporobolomycetaceae produce oidia and arthrospores. The family Cryptococcaceae, which was previously classified as imperfect fungi, has now been placed in the basidiomycetes.[77] Besides these morphological criteria, the yeasts are also classified according to their biochemical, serological, and fertility reactions. Fertility reactions have been used particularly with the ascosporogenous yeasts. The sequence hybridization data from the literature indicates the following: (1) only close relationships can be deduced from the DNA reannealing experiments; (2) a homology of 80% or more should be considered as comprising species; (3) many phenotypically similar yeasts share a relatedness value of 10% or less,[74] therefore, an interspecific relationship can seldom be deduced from DNA complementary data. A curious finding was reported by Kurtzman et al.[75] in *Issatchenkia scultullata* var. *scultullata* and *I. scultullata* var. *exigua*, where sequence complementarity of only 24% permitted the production of 3.6% viable, fertile ascospores. This would mean that in some cases small sequence deletion would interdict, whereas large deletion would maintain the mating potential. (4) In yeasts, DNA complementarity levels between 20 to 80% are rarely encountered.[74-76]

The information about fossil fungi is not adequate to be used to construct an absolute time-based nucleotide change as has been successfully done using Te50 data as discussed previously.[61,68,69] There are about 645 fossil fungi recorded, appearing in the following order: Precambrian period (some 600 million years ago), Cambrian (500 million years), Chrytridiomycetes, and early Ordovician period (some 450 million years ago), the Zygomycetes. The Ascomycetes arose around the end of the Ordovician period and the beginning of the

Silurien (some 435 million years), and at about the same period one finds the ancestors of teliomycetes, principally Uridinales. The Acrasiales appeared late in the Permien Era.[78] Schopf[79] indicated the resemblance between an algo-oomycete ancestor and modern Ascomycetes dating back to the Precambrian Era.

VII. CONCLUSION

Attempts have been made to evaluate various parameters used for the study of phylogenetic relationships in fungi, but the discussion entered mainly on the properties of genomes in relation to evolution. From the data available on the dG and dC ratios obtained from diverse fungi as reviewed earlier, it can be concluded that these organisms do not follow the monophyletic pathway of evolution. Compared to higher organisms, fungi have smaller amounts of repetitive sequences and are mostly organized according to the long period interspersion mode, the two exceptions being the Myxomycetes and Acrasiales, where the repetitive sequences are organized according to the short period interspersion mode. The general mechanism of gene evolution such as by duplication, transposition and insertion, fusion, and recombination during sexual exchange is also applicable to fungi. Methods to study the phylogenetic relationship such as direct comparison of sequences by hybridization and restriction analysis or the sequencing of individual genes were also discussed.

ACKNOWLEDGMENTS

Some of the work published here was supported by the U.S. Department of Energy (SKD) and by the Swiss National Science Foundation (Prof. Gilbert Turian). We are thankful to Drs. Russell and Navtig for allowing us to see their unpublished work, and to Drs. Woese and Templeton for giving permission to reproduce their published figures.

REFERENCES

1. **Bessey, E. A.**, *Morphology and Taxonomy of Fungi*, 2nd ed., Constable & Co., London, 1952.
2. **Gauman, E.**, Les voies de l'evolution chez les champignons. Contribution a une discussion. *Ann. Biol.*, 23, 647, 1952.
3. **Moor, R. T.**, An alternative concept of fungi based on their ultrastructure. (8th Congr. Int. Microbiol.). *Rec. Adv. Microbiol.*, 49, 1971.
4. **Muller, E.**, *Taxonomy and Phylogeny of Fungi*, Springer-Verlag, Basel, 1980, 270.
5. **Bartnicki-Garcia, S.**, Cell wall chemistry, morphogenesis and taxonomy of fungi, *Ann. Rev. Microbiol.*, 22, 87, 1968.
6. **Hutter, R. and De Moss, J. A.**, Organisation of tryptophan pathway. A phylogenetic study of the fungi, *J. Bacteriol.*, 94, 1896, 1967.
7. **Storck, R. and Alexopoulos, C. J.**, DNA of fungi, *Bacteriol. Rev.*, 37, 126, 1970.
8. **Storck, R.**, DNA of fungi in evolution of genetics systems, *Brookhaven Symp. Biol.*, 23, 371, 1972.
9. **Schwartz, R. M. and Dayhoff, M. O.**, Origins of prokaryotes, eukaryotes, mitochondria and chloroplasts, *Science*, 199, 395, 1978.
10. **Wilson, A. C., Carlson, S. S., and White, T. J.**, Biochemical evolution, *Ann. Rev. Biochem.*, 46, 573, 1977.
11. **Woese, C. R.**, Archebacteria, *Sci. Am.*, 274, 98, 1980.
12. **Kumazaki, T., Hori, H., and Osawa, S.**, The nucleotide sequences of 5S rRNA from two Annelida species. *Perinercis brevicirris, Sabellastarte japonica* and Echiura species, *Urechis unicinclus, Nucleic Acids Res.*, 11, 3347, 1983.
13. **Walker, W. F. and Ford-Doolittle, W.**, 5S rRNA sequences from eight basidiomycetes and fungi imperfectii, *Nucleic Acids Res.*, 11, 7625, 1983.
14. **Templeton, A.**, Sytematics of Basidiomycetes based on 5S rRNA sequence and other data, *Nature (London)*, 303, 731, 1983.

15. **Gottschalk, M. and Blanz, P. A.,** Highly conserved 5S rRNA sequences in four rust fungi and atypical 5S rRNA secondary structure in *Microstroma juglandis, Nucleic Acids Res.,* 12, 3951, 1984.

16. **Huysmans, E., Dams, E., Vandenbergh, A., and DeWachter, R.,** The nucleotide sequences of the 5S rRNAs of four mushrooms and their use in studying the phylogenetic position of basidiomycetes among the eukaryotes, *Nucleic Acids Res.,* 11, 2871, 1983.

17. **Mao, J., Appel, B., Schaack, J., Sharp, S., Yamada, H., and Soll, D.,** The 5S RNA genes of *S. pombe, Nucleic Acids Res.,* 10, 487, 1982.

18. **Ojha, M., Dutta, S. K., and Turian, G.,** DNA nucleotide sequence homologies between some zoosporic fungi, *Mol. Gen. Genet.,* 136, 151, 1975.

19. **Holliday, R.,** The organisation of DNA in eukaryotic chromosome in *Symp. Soc. Gen. Microbiol., No. 20., Prokaryotic and Eukaryotic Cells,* Cambridge University Press, London 1970, 359.

20. **Britten, R. J. and Kohne, D. E.,** Repeated sequences in DNA, *Science,* 161, 529, 1968.

21. **Wetmur, J. G. and Davidson, N.,** Kinetics of renaturation of DNA, *J. Mol. Biol.,* 31, 349, 1968.

22. **Ojha, M. and Dutta, S. K.,** Nuclear control of differentiation in *Filamentous Fungi,* Vol. 3, Smith, J. E. and Berry, R. D., Eds., Arnold, London, 1977, 9.

23. **Smith, M.,** Deoxyribonucleic acid in crabs of the genus cancer, *Biochem. Biophys. Res. Commun.,* 10, 67, 1963.

24. **Davidson, E. H., Galau, G. A., Angerer, R. C., and Britten, R. J.,** Comparative aspects of DNA sequences organization in metazoa, *Chromosoma (Berlin),* 51, 253, 1975.

25. **Zimmerman, J. L. and Goldbert, R. B.,** DNA sequence organization in the genome of *Nicotiana tobacum, Chromosoma (Berlin),* 59, 227, 1977.

26. **Hardman, N., Jack, P. L., Fergie, R. C., and Gerrie, L. M.,** Sequence organization in nuclear DNA from *Physarum polycephalum.* Interspersion of repetitive and single copy sequences, *Eur. J. Biochem.,* 103, 247, 1980.

27. **Firtel, R. A. and Kindle, K.,** Structural organization of the genome of the cellular slime mold *Dictyostelium discoideum* interspersion of repetitive and single copy DNA, *Cell,* 5, 401, 1975.

28. **Crain, W. F., Eden, F. C., Pearson, W. R., Davidson, E. H., and Britten, R. J.,** Absence of short period intersperson of repetitive and non-repetitive sequence in the DNA of *Drosophila melanogaster, Chromosoma,* 56, 309, 1976.

29. **Wells, R., Royer, H. D., and Hollenberg, C. P.,** Non *Xenopus* like DNA sequence organization in the *Chironomus centans* genome, *Mol. Gen. Genet.,* 147, 45, 1976.

30. **Pellegrini, M., Timberlake, W. E., and Goldbert, R. B.,** Electron microscopy of *Achlya* deoxyribonucleic acid sequence organisation, *Mol. Cell Biol.,* 61, 136, 1980.

31. **Hershey, R. M., Jayaram, M., and Chamberlin, M. E.,** DNA sequence organisation in *Phycomyces blakesleanus, Chromosoma (Berlin),* 73, 143, 1979.

32. **Krumlauf, R. and Marzluf, G. A.,** Characterization of the sequence complexity and organization of the *Neurospora crassa, Biochemistry,* 18, 3705, 1979.

33. **Dons, J. J. M., DeVries, D. M. H., and Wessels, J. G. H.,** Characterization of the genome of the Basidiomycete *Schizophyllum commune, Biochem. Biophys. Acta,* 563, 100, 1979.

34. **Timberlake, W. E.,** Low repetitive DNA content in *Aspergillus nidulans, Science,* 202, 973, 1978.

35. **Lauer, G. D., Roberts, T. M., and Klotz, L. C.,** Determination of nuclear DNA content of *Saccharomyces cerevisiae* and implications for the organization of DNA in yeast chromosomes, *J. Mol. Biol.,* 114, 507, 1977.

36. **Dutta, S. K.,** Repeated sequences in fungi, *Nucleic Acids Res.,* 1, 1411, 1974.

37. **Ojha, M., Turler, H., and Turian, G.,** Characterization of *Allomyces* genome, *Biochim. Biophys. Acta,* 478, 377, 1977.

38. **Hudspeth, M. E. S., Timberlake, W. E., and Goldbert, R. B.,** DNA sequence organisation in the watermold *Achlya, Proc. Natl. Acad. Sci. U.S.A.,* 74, 4332, 1977.

39. **Johnson, P., Foran, D., and Moore, G.,** Organisation and evolution of sea urchin actin gene, *Mol. Cell Biol.,* 3, 1824, 1983.

40. **Gallwitz, D. and Saures, I.,** Structure of a split gene: complete nucleotide sequence of the actin gene in *Saccharomyces cerevisiae, Proc. Natl. Acad. Sci. U.S.A.,* 77, 2546, 1980.

41. **Ng, R. and Abelson, J.,** Isolation and sequence of the gene for actin in *Saccharomyces cerevisiae, Proc. Natl. Acad. Sci. U.S.A.,* 77, 3912, 1980.

42. **Schedl, T. and Dove, W. F.,** Mandelian analysis of the organization of actin sequences in *Physarum polycephalum, J. Mol. Biol.,* 160, 41, 1982.

43. **McKeown, M. and Firtel, R. A.,** Evidence for subfamilies of actin genes in *Dictyostelium discoideum* as determined by comparison of 3' end sequences, *J. Mol. Biol.,* 151, 593, 1981.

44. **Poole, S., Firtel, R. A., and Lamar, E.,** Sequence and expression of the discoidin I gene family in *Dictyostelium discoideum, J. Mol. Biol.,* 153, 273, 1981.

45. **Warren. R. A. J.,** Lactose-utilizing mutants of lac deletion strains of *E. coli, Can. J. Microbiol.,* 18, 1439, 1972.

46. **Hall, B. G. and Hartl, H.**, Regulation of newly evolved enzymes. I. Selection of a novel lactase regulated by lactose in *Escherichia coli, Genetics*, 76, 391, 1974.

47. **Zalkin, H.**, Anthranilate synthase, *Adv. Enzymol.* 38, 1, 1973.

48. **Henderson, E. J. and Zalkin, H.**, On the composition of anthranilate synthetase-anthranilate 5-phosphoribosyl-pyrophosphate phosphoribosyl transferase from *Salmonella typhimurium, J. Biol. Chem.*, 246, 6891, 1971.

49. **Yanofsky, C., Horn, V., Bonner, M., and Stasiowski, S.**, Polarity and enzyme functions in mutants of the first three genes of the tryptophan operon of *E. coli, Genetics*, 69, 409, 1971.

50. **Roeder, G. S. and Fink, G. R.**, Transposable elements in yeast, in *Mobile Genetic Elements*, Shapiro, J. A., Ed., Academic Press, London, 1983, 299.

51. **Chung, S., Zuker, C., and Lodish, H. F.**, A repetitive and apparently transposable DNA sequence in *Dictyostelium discoideum* associated with developmentally regulated RNAs, *Nucleic Acids Res.*, 11, 4835, 1983.

52. **Pool, S. J. and Firtel, R. A.**, Genomic instability and mobile genetic elements in regions surrounding two discoidin I genes of *Dictystelium discoideum, Mol. Cell Biol.*, 4, 671, 1984.

53. **Selker, E. U., Yanofsky, C., Driftmier, K., Matzenberg, R. L., Alzner-Deweerd, B., and Raj-Bhandari, U. L.**, Dispersed 5S rRNA genes in *N. crassa*: structure, expression and evolution, *Cell*, 24, 819, 1981.

54. **Manch, J. M. and Crawford, I. P.**, Ordering tryptophane synthase genes of *Pseudomonas aeruginosa* by cloning in *E. coli, J. Bacteriol.*, 146, 102, 1981.

55. **Calhoun, D. H., Pierson, D. L., and Jensen, R. A.**, The regulation of tryptophan biosynthesis in *Pseudomonas aeruginosa, Mol. Gen. Genet.*, 121, 117, 1973.

56. **Fincham, J. R. S., Day, P. R., and Radford, A.**, *Fungal genetics*, University of California Press, Berkeley, 1979.

57. **Ulrich, R. C. and Raper, J. R.**, Evolution of genetic mechanisms in fungi, *Taxon*, 26, 169, 1977.

58. **Stamberg, J.**, Genetic control of recombination in *Schizophyllum commune:* separation of the controlled and controlling loci, *Heredity*, 24, 306, 1968.

59. **Jukes, T. H.**, Silent nucleotide substitutions and the molecular clock, *Science*, 210, 973, 1980.

60. **Miyata, T., Yasunaga, T., and Nishida, T.**, Nucleotide sequence divergence and functional constraint in mRNA evolution, *Proc. Natl. Acad. Sci. U.S.A.*, 77, 7328, 1980.

61. **Kohne, D. E.**, Evolution of higher organism DNA, *Q. Rev. Biophys.* 33, 327, 1970.

62. **Botstein, D., White, R. L. Skolnick, M., and Davis, R. W.**, Construction of genetic linkage map in man using restriction fragment length polymorphism, *Am. J. Hum. Genet.*, 32, 314, 1980.

63. **Chambers, C., Crouch, R. J., and Dutta, S. K.**, Polymorphism in the ribosomal RNA genes in three heterothalic species of *Neurospora, Genetics*, 107, s18, 1984.

64. **Russell, P. J., Wagner, S., Rodland, K. D., Feinbaun, R. L., Russell, J. P., Breta-Harte, M. S., Free, S. J., and Metzenber, R. L.**, Organization of the ribosomal ribonucleic acid genes in various wild type strains and wild-collected strains of *Neurospora*, submitted to *Mol. Gen. Genet.*, 1984.

65. **Navtig, D. O., May, G., and Taylor, J. W.**, Distribution and evolutionary significance of mitochondrial plasmids in *Neurospora, J. Bacteriol.*, in press, 1984.

66. **Navtig, D. O. and Taylor, J. W.**, Phylogenetic analysis of *Neurospora* using cloned nuclear-DNA hybridization probes, *Neurospora Newslett.*, 31, 13, 1984.

67. **Laird, C. D., McConaughy, B. L., and McCarthy, B. J.**, Rate of fixation of nucleotide substitutions in evolution, *Nature (London)*, 224, 149, 1969.

68. **Sibley, C. G. and Ahlquist, J. E.**, The phylogeny and classification of the passerine birds, based on comparison of the genetic material, DNA, *Proc. XVIII Int. Ornith. Congress*, 1982.

69. **Sibley, C. G. and Ahlquist, J. E.**, The phylogeny of the hominoid primates, as indicated by DNA:DNA hybridization, *J. Mol. Evol.*, 20, 2, 1984.

70. **Emerson, R. and Wilson, C. M.**, Interspecific hybrids and the cytogenetics and cytotaxonomy of Eual-lomyces, *Mycologia*, 46, 393, 1954.

71. **Ojha, M. and Turian, G.**, Loss of rRNA genes during a phenotypic masculinizing mutation in *A. arbuscula, Mol. Gen. Genet.*, 166, 225, 1978.

72. **Shear, C. L. and Dodge, B. O.**, Life histories and heterothallism of the red bread-mold fungi of the *Monilia sitophila* group, *J. Agric. Res.*, 34, 1019, 1927.

73. **Williams, N. P., Mukhopadhyay, D., and Dutta, S. K.**, Homology of *Neurospora* homothallic species using nonrepeated DNA sequences, *Experientia*, 37, 1157, 1981.

74. **Price, C. W., Fuson, G. B., and Phaff, H. J.**, Genome comparison in yeast systematics: delimitation of species within genera *Schwanniomyces, Saccharomyces, Debanyamyces* and *Pichia, Microbiol. Rev.*, 42, 161, 1978.

75. **Kurtzman, C. P., Smiey, M. J., and Johnson, C. J.**, Emanation of the genus *Issatschenkia kudriavzev* and comparison of species by DNA reassociation, mating reaction and ascospore ultrastructure, *Int. J. Syst. Bacteriol.*, 30, 503, 1982.

76. **Baharaeen, S., Bentle, J. A., and Vishniac, H. S.,** The evolution of antartic yeasts, *Can. J. Microbiol.,* 28, 406, 1982.
77. **Lodder, J., Ed.,** *The Yeasts,* North Holland, Amsterdam, 1971.
78. **Locquin, M. V.,** *Les Champignons Fossils,* Vol. 1, Ph.D. thesis, Universite de Marie Curie, Paris, 1982.
79. **Schopf, J. W.,** Precambrian microorganisms and evolutionary events prior to the origin of vascular plants, *Biol. Rev.,* 45, 349, 1970.
80. **Dutta, S. K. and Ojha, M.,** Relatedness between major taxonomic groups of fungi based on the measurement of DNA nucleotide sequence homology, *Mol. Gen. Genet.,* 114, 23, 1972.
81. **Dutta, S. K., Sheikh, I., Choppala, J., Aulakh, G. S., and Nelson, W. H.,** DNA homologies among homothallic pseaudohomothallic and heterothallic species of *Neurospora, Mol. Gen. Genet.,* 147, 325, 1976.
82. **Dutta, S. K.,** DNA homologies among heterothallic species of Neurospora, *Mycologia,* 68, 388, 1976.

Chapter 4

CHLOROPLAST DNA AND PHYLOGENETIC RELATIONSHIPS

Jeffrey D. Palmer

TABLE OF CONTENTS

I. INTRODUCTION

During the last 25 years plant systematists have increasingly supplemented traditional biosystematic approaches with biochemical studies aimed at elucidating the phylogenetic significance of variation in the pattern and distribution of plant chemical constituents. The greatest number of these studies have involved the vast array of plant micromolecules (secondary plant products).[1-3] Other studies have analyzed protein variation through serological comparisons,[4] allozyme electrophoresis[2,5,6] and amino acid sequencing,[7] and DNA variation through DNA-DNA and DNA-RNA hybridization.[2,8]

The purpose of this chapter is to review the phylogenetic impact and promise of a relatively new set of molecular tools — DNA sequence and restriction endonuclease analysis — as applied to a specific DNA molecule, the chloroplast genome of flowering plants. The ability, through recombinant DNA technology, to obtain pure and virtually unlimited quantities of a given DNA sequence, together with the development of chemical and enzymatic methods for DNA sequencing, allows one to determine quickly and accurately DNA sequences of many thousands of base pairs. Although a number of chloroplast genes have been entirely sequenced, there have not yet been any chloroplast DNA sequence studies with the explicit purpose of exploring plant phylogeny. Nonetheless, limited phylogenetic conclusions can already be extracted from the published sequence studies, and this technique has immense potential for establishing higher order relationships among plants.

In contrast to DNA sequence analysis, restriction endonuclease analysis has already been used in a number of comparative chloroplast DNA studies that have provided a wealth of phylogenetic information. This review will focus on principles and approaches to analyzing chloroplast DNA variation, with primary emphasis given to restriction endonuclease studies. Examples of the kinds of phylogenetic insights these studies allow will be drawn from the literature, with molecular investigations in the genus *Brassica* presented as a case study.

II. OVERVIEW OF THE CHLOROPLAST GENOME

The reader should consult several recent reviews[9-13] for details beyond this brief summary and for references pertinent to the following facts and conclusions. Chloroplasts of land plant cells and of unicellular eukaryotic algae contain multiple (10 to 200) copies of a circular molecule ranging in size between 83 and 200 kb. Leaf cells, both light-grown and dark-grown, generally contain 10 to 20 times more plastid DNA than do nonleaf cells. However, the number of copies of the plastid genome per cell is remarkably constant over a wide range of leaf and leaf cell sizes. The increase in chloroplast number per cell observed during leaf expansion is therefore accompanied by a dilution of chloroplast genomes per chloroplast. Although the number of copies of the plastid genome, as well as its expression, vary with the developmental stage and differentiation of the plastid, the genome itself appears to be identical in organization and sequence in chloroplast, etioplast, proplastid, chromoplast, and leucoplast.

The structure of a typical chloroplast genome, from the cinnamon fern, *Osmunda cinnamomea*, is shown in Figure 1. The genome consists of one large and one small region of unique sequence DNA separated by the two segments of a large inverted repeat. Such an inverted repeat structure is found in the chloroplast genomes of all land plants and green algae examined, with the sole exception of one section of the family Leguminosae, where one entire segment of the inverted repeat has been deleted (see Section IV.B). Two distinct recombinational processes are associated with the presence of this large inverted repeat. Intramolecular recombination between segments of the repeat leads to frequent single copy sequence inversions, to the extent that an inverted repeat-containing chloroplast DNA is isolated as an equimolar population of two inversion isomers. Intermolecular recombination

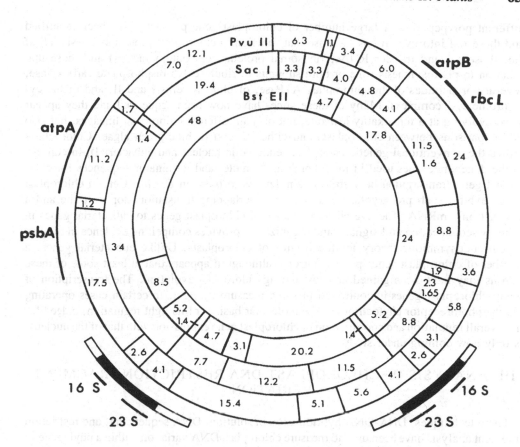

FIGURE 1. Physical map of the chloroplast genome of the cinnamon fern, *Osmunda cinnamomea*. Each concentric circle shows the position (given by the short radial lines) of cleavage sites for the indicated restriction endonuclease (Pvu II, Sac I, or BstEll) and the size (in kilobases) of the resulting restriction fragments. The two long, heavy black lines represent the minimum extent of the inverted repeat, while the open extensions of these lines represent its maximum extent. This map portrays the chloroplast genome in only one of the two orientations in which it exists (the single copy regions are inverted relative to one another in one half the native molecules[113,114]). The positions of the following genes are shown: ribosomal RNA genes (16S, 23S); gene for the large subunit of ribulose-1,5-bisphosphate carboxylase (rbcL); genes for the α and β subunits of the chloroplast ATPase (atpA and atpB); gene for a 32,000 dalton photosystem II polypeptide (psbA).[115]

within the repeat generates head-to-head circular dimers, a structure not found in genomes that lack the repeat. Results from a large number of studies indicate that major sequence rearrangements are extremely rare in chloroplast genomes that contain the inverted repeat, while more limited analysis suggests that rearrangement may be more frequent in the absence of the inverted repeat. The utility of these rearrangement mutations for phylogenetic studies will be discussed in Section IV.B.

In many land plants, the chloroplast and its genome are inherited maternally, and even in those plants with biparental plastid inheritance plastid fusion appears to be absent. The comparative study of maternally inherited genomes provides distinct phylogenetic insights, as discussed in Section IV.A. Fusion of chloroplasts and subsequent recombination of chloroplast genomes from both parents has been observed only in the green algal genus *Chlamydomonas*, which has emerged as the only system for performing chloroplast genetics.

The chloroplast genome is actively expressed: DNA-RNA hybridization experiments indicate that a large portion of the chloroplast genome from flowering plants and algae is transcribed into RNA. Moreover, isolated chloroplasts may synthesize as many as 100 different polypeptides. A large number of chloroplast gene products have been identified and these fall into two groups — those that function in chloroplast protein synthesis (all of the ribosomal and transfer RNAs, ribosomal proteins, elongation factors) and those that function in photosynthesis (one or both subunits of ribulose-1,5-bisphosphate carboxylase, several polypeptides of the chloroplast ATPase, of photosystems I and II, and of the cytochrome b_6-f complex). Many of these genes have now been sequenced and they appear to be evolving at a remarkably low rate, not only in different chloroplast lineages, but also in comparisons between chloroplasts and either *E. coli* or blue-green algae. Chloroplasts utilize the conventional genetic code (i.e., eukaryotic nuclear and eubacterial), in contrast to the degenerate ones used in mitochondria. Promoter and terminator sequences for chloroplast gene transcription bear striking similarities to those in *E. coli*. Certain chloroplast genes exhibit such prokaryotic features as an overlapping translation stop/start site and a polycistronic mRNA. The overall resemblance of chloroplast genes to eubacterial genes in primary sequence, control signals, and organization provides compelling evidence in support of the endosymbiotic theory for the origins of chloroplasts. Unlike eubacterial genes, a number of chloroplast genes possess introns, although it appears that at least some of these introns may have been gained and lost during chloroplast evolution. The transcription of many chloroplast genes is controlled in some measure by light, in certain cases operating via the photoreceptor phytochrome. The molecular basis for this light regulation, indeed for the overall regulation and coordination of chloroplast gene expression with that of the nucleus, is only now coming under study.

III. ANALYSIS OF CHLOROPLAST DNA RESTRICTION FRAGMENT VARIATION

Three techniques, DNA-DNA hybridization in solution, DNA sequencing, and restriction fragment analysis have been used to measure chloroplast DNA variation within a phylogenetic context. DNA-DNA hybridization has yielded only limited phylogenetic information when applied to chloroplast DNA (Section IV.B), and no further explication of its basic methods and principles[2,8] will be attempted here. DNA sequencing appears to possess immense potential for unraveling the pattern of evolution of major plant taxa. However, this potential is for the most part unrealized (Section IV.B), and therefore it appears premature to devote space here to phylogenetic aspects of DNA sequence analysis. Instead, the interested reader may consult several excellent comparative sequence studies of mitochondrial[14,15] and nuclear[16,17] genes. The third technique, analysis of restriction fragment variation, has already been widely applied to chloroplast DNA and has yielded important phylogenetic insights in a number of plant groups (Section IV). It therefore seems appropriate to review the basic techniques and principles for detecting variation in chloroplast DNA using restriction endonucleases and for analyzing this variation in a phylogenetically meaningful way.

Upholt[18] first described the restriction fragment phenotypes that are diagnostic for three types of mutations: base substitutions (point mutations), deletions/insertions (length mutations), and inversions. A point mutation has the potential to either create a new restriction site or lead to the loss of a preexisting one. Therefore, the restriction patterns of two DNAs that differ by a single restriction site change (normally the result of a single point mutation) will show three fragment differences: one DNA will possess a unique large fragment equal in size to the sum of two smaller fragments unique to the second DNA. The level of sequence variation encountered in chloroplast DNAs from related species has proven to be quite low, and as a result, in interspecific studies restriction site mutations are usually easily diagnosed by this simple kind of inferential analysis (see references in Section IV.A). This analysis becomes easier as more species are examined, for it is then often possible to find intermediate chloroplast genomes that bridge the gap between DNAs that have accumulated too many restriction site mutations to allow inspectional analysis alone.[19,20] Physical mapping of mutant restriction sites, or of the entire set of fragments produced by a given restriction enzyme, also greatly facilitates the mutational anlaysis of DNAs whose restriction patterns show complex differences.[19-23]

In theory, a restriction site mutation, which leads to three fragment differences, should be easily distinguishable from a length mutation, which produces only two restriction fragment differences in comparing two DNAs, i.e., the fragment carrying the length mutation will be larger in one DNA than in the other. However, in practice it turns out that the great majority of chloroplast DNA length mutations detected in restriction fragment comparisons are quite short (50 to 1200 bp) relative to the fragments normally studied (500 to 50,000 bp). One must then consider an alternative explanation, that a restriction site mutation occurred very near the end of a fragment and that this small new fragment escaped detection in the gel system used. In order to distinguish a small length mutation from a restriction site change near the end of a fragment some sort of mapping analysis must be performed. Where several restriction enzymes have been mapped, a deletion should show up as a size alteration of the same absolute magnitude and evolutionary direction within each fragment that maps to the altered locus.[21,23-25] If such complete mapping information is not available one can test a specific fragment alteration of uncertain origin by isolating the variable fragment and hybridizing it to a filter containing the two DNAs that differ, each digested with the same battery of enzymes. If the fragment alteration is due to length mutation, then the fragment should hybridize to fragments that for each enzyme differ by the same size and with the same evolutionary direction.

Depending on the precise nature of the analysis,[23-25] length mutations can assume a significant proportion of the total number of mutations detected in interspecific chloroplast DNA studies, and it is therefore critical that such mutations be correctly diagnosed relative to restriction site mutations. If not, and if the set of fragment alterations that are visualized with many restriction enzymes and which result from a single length mutation is instead counted as multiple independent mutations, then the total sequence divergence between two chloroplast DNAs will be grossly overestimated (see Reference 20 for discussion of one such case).

Inversions have an easily diagnosed restriction fragment phenotype. An inversion that includes a single restriction site will produce two new fragments equal in size to two fragments that are lost.[18] In practice, chloroplast DNA inversions, even small ones, are quite rare; in fact, the only inversion so far detected by comparative restriction analysis[23] is in a group of plants whose genomes appear unusually prone to rearrangement.[26,27] Thus, one normally expects to detect only point mutations and length mutations in analyzing restriction patterns of chloroplast DNA from related species and genera. It should be noted that even where chloroplast DNAs have diverged so extensively that their restriction patterns and maps no longer show any significant homologies, inversions can still be detected by comparing the overall arrangement of two genomes through heterologous filter hybridization.[27] Only fairly large inversions are detected in this type of analysis, and even though such events appear to be extremely rare over time (spans of tens and hundreds of millions of years), they nonetheless appear to be quite powerful phylogenetic markers (Section IV.B).

In spite of the large number of studies that have exploited chloroplast DNA restriction fragment variation for phylogenetic purposes, there has been relatively little effort in developing methods for constructing phylogenetic trees from this variation. Hence, the following discussion will focus on the methodology for phylogenetic reconstruction used by the author and his collaborators,[19,20,23,28] The approach taken in these studies is essentially cladistic in nature. Each restriction site mutation, and in one case also length mutation and inversion,[23] is treated as a separate character. The principle of parsimony[29,30] is used to construct phylogenetic trees in which the total number of independent mutations required

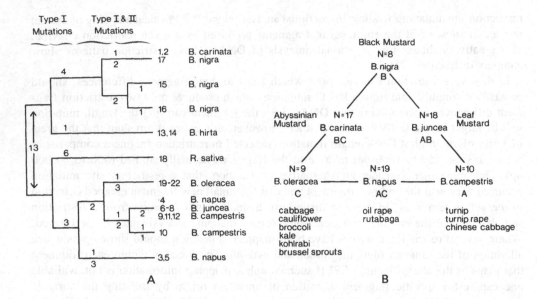

FIGURE 2.   (A) *Brassica* chloroplast DNA phylogeny. Numbers at termination of branches indicate accessions (see Table 1 of Reference 19). Numbers above branches indicate the number of Type I restriction site mutations specific to each branch, while numbers below branches indicate the number of Type II restriction site mutations. (B) Classical phylogeny for cultivated diploid and amphidiploid species of *Brassica* based on cytogenetic studies.[42] (From Palmer, J. D. et. al., *Theor. Appl. Genet.* 65, 181, 1983. With permission.)

to account for the observed distribution of different states of these characters is minimized.[31-34]

Figure 2A presents a phylogenetic tree, in this case based entirely on chloroplast DNA restriction site mutations,[19,20] which depicts the molecular relationships among 21 species and cultivars in the genus *Brassica*, plus radish, *Raphanus sativa*.[19] The level of restriction fragment variation encountered in this study necessitated a two-tiered approach for analyzing mutations. Certain enzymes, operationally designated Type I enzymes, cut the DNAs relatively infrequently and revealed sufficiently little variation to allow mutational analysis of all restriction fragment changes found in the 22 DNAs. Mutations found with these enzymes divided the DNAs into four major lineages, consisting of DNAs 1, 2, 15 to 17; 13, 14; 18; and 3 to 12, 19 to 22 (Figure 2A). The more complex patterns produced by enzymes operationally defined as belonging to the Type II class allowed further discrimination within each of these four lineages. The evolutionary direction (polarity) of Type II mutations was determined by a hybridization protocol using members of the other three lineages as outgroups.[19]

Figure 2A shows the most parsimonious tree which accounts for the 40 phylogenetically informative (shared by two or more DNAs) Type I and II mutations found.[19] Only a single case of parallel or convergent mutation is postulated by this tree. Such a low rate of convergence has been found in other interspecific studies,[23,28] and is expected given the low absolute rate of chloroplast DNA sequence change found in these studies and the absence of any strong imbalances in the transition-transversion ratio of chloroplast DNA point mutations (see data sets in Reference 35 to 37). The *Brassica* phylogenetic tree was rooted by assuming that the chloroplast genome evolves with a clocklike regularity[38,39] and hence that the numbers of mutations should be equal in all lineages (Figure 2A). In similar studies in *Lycopersicon*[28] and *Pisum*[23] such an assumption resulted in the same root as that determined by outgroup analysis. In the *Brassica* study,[19] the most appropriate outgroup, *Raphanus sativa*, fell well within the ingroup under the clock assumption. This result is not overly surprising given that *R. sativa* can still hybridize with certain *Brassica* species.[40]

IV. PHYLOGENETIC INFERENCES FROM CHLOROPLAST DNA SEQUENCE COMPARISONS

A. Interspecific Relationships

The majority of chloroplast DNA comparative studies have focused on closely related plants, usually species within a single genus. As an example of the kinds of phylogenetic insights such studies allow, I will first review in detail the conclusions reached by two groups of investigators working on the genus *Brassica*. Then, selected highlights from studies on a number of other genera will be briefly presented and discussed.

1. The Genus Brassica

Palmer et al.[19] and Erickson et al.[41] used a large number of restriction enzymes, 28 and 15, respectively, in order to analyze chloroplast DNA relationships among 6 cultivated diploid and amphidiploid *Brassica* species. Relationships for these species at the level of the nuclear genome, based on cytogenetic and crossing studies, are expressed by the triangle of U[42] (Figure 2B). Both groups of investigators divided the genus into two major sections based on chloroplast DNA homologies. One section contained the amphidiploid *B. carinata* and the diploid *B. nigra*, and the other section contained two amphidiploids, *B. juncea* and *B. napus*, and two diploids, *B. oleracea* and *B. campestris*. The mutational analysis performed by Palmer et al.[19] allowed them to construct a cladistically derived phylogenetic tree (Figure 2A), as described above, and also to quantitatively estimate genetic distances. The maximum sequence divergence between species within each of the two major sections was calculated as only 0.2 and 0.4%, respectively, whereas the divergence between the sections was 2.4%.[19] The chloroplast genome of *B. hirta* (white mustard) was placed in the same section with those of *B. nigra* and *B. carinata*, from which it differed by approximately 0.7% in nucleotide sequence (Figure 2A).[19]

One of the more unexpected results of the study by Palmer et al.[19] concerns the phylogenetic placement of radish, *Raphanus sativa*. The radish chloroplast genome was found to be significantly more closely related (1.1% divergence) to that of the section two species than the latter are to section one (Figure 2A). Although radish is normally placed in a separate genus from *Brassica*, it should be remembered that certain crosses can still be effected between the two groups.[40] This is evidence of not only a great deal of genetic similarity, but it also raises the possibility that cytoplasmic exchange has occurred through interspecific hybridization and introgression.

Highly concordant insights were obtained by both groups[19,41] into the origins of the amphidiploid species *B. carinata*, *B. juncea*, and *B. napus*. The *B. carinata* and *B. juncea* chloroplast genomes were essentially identical to those of the diploids *B. nigra* and *B. campestris*, respectively, with all restriction enzymes used in these studies. Since cytoplasmic DNAs, both chloroplast[41] and mitochondrial,[43] are maternally inherited in *Brassica*, it is readily concluded that the two amphidiploids arose through interspecific hybridization in which these diploids served as maternal parents. A variety of taxonomic studies have implicated *B. oleracea* and *B. nigra* as the other parents of *B. carinata* and *B. juncea*, respectively, and thus one can conclude by subtraction that these two diploids must have served as the paternal parents in these crosses (Figure 2).

A limited amount of intraspecific chloroplast DNA polymorphism was found in *B. nigra* and *B. campestris;* this enabled more precise inferences as to the specific sources of the *carinata* and *juncea* cytoplasms, respectively.[19] The complete identity of chloroplast DNA from both *B. carinata* accessions examined to that of a *B. nigra* line from India (DNA 17), all three of which differed by 6 restriction site mutations from *B. nigra* lines from Europe (DNA 16) and California (DNA 15), clearly implicates the Indian *nigra* or other very closely related *nigra* germplasm, as the donor of the *carinata* cytoplasm.[19] The differentiation found among *B. campestris* chloroplast genomes ruled out subspecies *trilocularis* (DNA 10) as a possible source of the *B. juncea* cytoplasm (Figure 2). Since the chloroplast DNAs of *B. carinata* and *B. juncea* were identical at all 3000 base pairs examined to those of specific accessions of *B. nigra* and *B. campestris*, respectively, it was possible to derive the quantitative conclusion that both of these hybridizations must have occurred very recently.[19]

Chloroplast DNA analysis indicates a complicated and unexpected origin for the cytoplasm of the amphidiploid *B. napus*, which at the nuclear level is derived by a cross between *B. oleracea* and *B. campestris* (Figure 2B). Two of the three *B. napus* lines examined by Palmer et al.[19] and 9 of the 12 examined by Erickson et al.[41] were shown to possess quite distinct chloroplast genomes from those of both diploids. The other *B. napus* lines have the *B. campestris* chloroplast genome and are all thought to result from recent backcrosses between *B. campestris* and *B. napus* performed in breeding programs.[41] Erickson et al.[41] tentatively concluded that the cytoplasmically distinct *napus* lines might have derived their cytoplasms from *B. oleracea*, based on the fact that these two shared slightly more enzyme patterns in common than did *B. napus* and *B. campestris*. Palmer et al.[19] used a greater number of restriction enzymes, and by determining the nature and polarity of individual mutations concluded that the *B. napus* cytoplasm actually diverged prior to the divergence of the *B. oleracea* and *B. campestris* cytoplasms. Most crucially, cladistic analysis showed that two derived mutations were shared by *B. oleracea* and *B. campestris* relative to all other *Brassica* species, including *B. napus*. To explain this result, Palmer et al.[19] postulated that either before or after the interspecific hybridization between *B. oleracea* and *B. campestris*, there occurred a series of introgressive hybridization events in which some unidentified *Brassica* species served as the maternal, cytoplasmic donor.

The results of these two studies on *Brassica* chloroplast DNAs are gratifying in several ways. First, it is comforting that two separate groups of investigators derived very similar results and conclusions by applying techniques of comparative restriction analysis. Second, many of their phylogenetic conclusions are highly concordant with those derived by various other taxonomic approaches (reviewed in Reference 44), including comparative morphology,[45] cytogenetics,[42] artificial resynthesis of hybrids[46,47] and molecular analysis of secondary chemical compounds,[48,49] proteins,[50-52] and nuclear DNA.[53] Nonetheless, it augers well for the continued use of chloroplast DNA analysis in systematic studies that a number of new and unexpected findings were obtained. Such findings include the placement of *R. sativa* within the genus *Brassica* and the suggestion of introgressive hybridization in the origin of *B. napus*. Moreover, these studies provide a degree of quantitative resolution that is hard to obtain by conventional approaches (Figure 2A; see Table 3 of Reference 19). Finally, that chloroplast DNA is maternally inherited in *Brassica*, as in most plants, allows insight into the direction of interspecific crosses that is virtually unparalled.

2. Other Genera

The closely related genera *Triticum* and *Aegilops* have received similar treatment to *Brassica* in terms of the variety of chloroplast DNA analyses that have been performed by several groups of investigators[25,54-57] and the kinds of questions, primarily relating to the origins of cultivated hexaploid (*T. aestivum*) and tetraploid (*T. dicoccoides*, *T. araraticum*, and *T. timopheevii*) wheat, that have been asked. Whereas a general consensus exists as to the donors of the A and D genomes of polyploid wheat, there is, despite the great variety of taxonomic approaches applied to the problem, little agreement as to the B and G genome donors. The chloroplast DNA studies of Ogihara and Tsunewaki[56,57] and Bowman et al.[25] are in general agreement that the diploid *Ae. longissima* is the donor of the B genome and cytoplasm to *T. aestivum* and *T. dicoccoides*, and that either the diploid *Ae. speltoides* or the conspecific *Ae. aucheri* donated the G genome and cytoplasm to the polyploid timopheevi wheats *(T. timopheevii*, *T. araraticum*, and *T. zuhkovsky*). Despite these interesting and potentially quite important conclusions, there are certain limitations to the data collection and analyses performed in these studies that have led to the suggestion[20] that more extensive chloroplast DNA examination is warranted before these conclusions are completely accepted.

Early molecular studies on the genus *Nicotiana* were quite limited in scope, but did at least point to the potential of chloroplast DNA comparisons for illuminating relationships.[58-60] More recently, Kung et al.[61] used the restriction enzyme Sma I to analyze the parentage of the amphidiploids *N. tabacum* and *N. rustica* and to define the Australian species of *Nicotiana* as a distinct, probably monophyletic lineage within the genus. Scowcroft[62] found a single EcoRI restriction site polymorphism that divided nine Australian populations of *N. debneyi* into two groups. This polymorphism proved crucial in following the assortment genomes following intraspecific somatic fusion.[63]

Examination of chloroplast DNA variation in eight species in *Lycopersicon* and two closely related species in *Solanum* provided a detailed phylogenetic outline[28] that generally agrees with results obtained from morphology and crossing studies,[64] but which provides a new level of quantitative resolution. This analysis[28] unambiguously supports the reassignment[64] of *S. pennellii* to *Lycopersicon* and neatly circumscribes the three red-orange fruited species in *Lycopersicon* — *L. esculentum* (the cultivated tomato), *L. pimpinellifolium*, and *L. cheesmanii* — as a single monophyletic lineage. The major surprise from molecular analysis[28] is that the chloroplast DNA polymorphism found within *L. peruvianum* encompassed both *L. chilense* and *L. chmielewskii*. The latter species is not normally thought to be closely related to *L. peruvianum*[64] and this result might reflect either cytoplasmic exchange between the two species through introgression, as postulated above in *Brassica*, or the fact that the reproductive isolation of the two species[64] is not a true measure of their overall genetic similarity.

Although little phylogenetic information was obtained in a study[24] of chloroplast DNA variation in the subsection Euoenothera of the genus *Oenothera*, this work is nonetheless of interest for two reasons. First, there are a set of unusual and well-characterized genetic compatibility relationships worked out between the nucleus and chloroplast, which are biparentally inherited in Euoenothera.[65,66] Second, the detailed and careful examination of chloroplast DNA deletion/insertion mutations performed by Gordon et al.[24] is an excellent model for this type of analysis.

An investigation of chloroplast DNA relationships in the genus *Pisum*[23] is noteworthy for the emphasis placed upon the intraspecific resolution afforded by chloroplast DNA analysis. Considerable intraspecific discrimination was obtained in a survey of 13 cultivars of *P. sativum* (the garden pea) and between and even within wild populations of *P. elatius* and *P. humile*. In particular, very strong evidence was found in support of the conjecture by Ben-Ze'ev and Zohary[67] that the garden pea was domesticated primarily from northern populations of *P. humile*.

Other less detailed and informative studies that have utilized chloroplast DNA restriction analysis to investigate interspecific relationships have been published for *Pelargonium*,[68] *Coffea*,[69] *Petunia*,[70] *Zea*,[71] and *Pennisetum*.[72] A preliminary report has appeared on an extensive study in progress on chloroplast DNA variation in *Atriplex*.[73]

B. Relationships Above the Species Level

Four studies have utilized restriction fragment and map comparisons in order to deduce evolutionary relationships among different genera within a family. Although the number of taxa compared in these studies and the amount of phylogenetic information obtained were quite limited, it is gratifying that the conclusions reached are in general agreement with those based on other approaches. In the case of the studies by Vedel et al.[74] and Fluhr and Edelman,[21] this is despite the fact that genetic distances were estimated solely from the proportion of shared restriction fragments, an approach fraught with danger when applied

Table 1
DISTRIBUTION OF THE CHLOROPLAST
DNA INVERTED REPEAT WITHIN THE
PLANT KINGDOM[9,11-13,80]

+ Inverted repeat	− Inverted Repeat
Angiosperms	
33 Families	1 Family — Leguminosae
70 Genera	8 Genera
200 Species	16 Species
Gymnosperms	
Ginkgo biloba	
Ferns	
2 Families	
2 Genera	
4 Species	
Bryophytes	
Marchantia polymorpha	
Algae	
Chlamydomonas reinhardtii	*Euglena gracilis*
Chlorella ellipsoidea	
Cyanophora paradoxa	

to chloroplast DNA (see Section III). Vedel et al.[74] concluded that among four cereal grains, wheat (*Triticum aestivum*) and rye (*Secale cereale*) were most closely related, the next most closely related was barley (*Hordeum vulgare*), and oats (*Avena sativa*) were most distantly related. In studies on the Solanaceae, Fluhr and Edelman[21] found somewhat greater chloroplast DNA homologies between *Nicotiana tabacum* and *Petunia parodii* than between either species and *Atropa belladonna*. More rigorous comparison of chloroplast DNA restriction maps and mutations enabled Poulsen[75] to show that wheat and barley are more closely related to each than to maize (*Zea mays*). Similarly, Palmer et al.[22] found that the molecular distance between *Phaseolus vulgaris* and *Vigna radiata*, members of the subtribe Phaseolinae, is approximately half that between either species and *Glycine max*, a member of the subtribe Glycininae.

Chloroplast genomes from different families, orders, and classes usually have accumulated so many point mutations that it is no longer possible to find sufficient restriction map homologies in order to deduce evolutionary relationships. Instead, three other approaches have been used to compare distantly related chloroplast DNAs. The first is to examine their comparative sequence organization in order to find major structural rearrangements, which, although rare, can be very powerful phylogenetic markers. One such rearrangement is the loss of the large inverted repeat found in most chloroplast genomes (Table 1) from members of one section of the subfamily Papilionoideae of the family Leguminosae. Species in the tribes Phaseoleae (*Vigna, Phaseolus, Glycine*) and Genisteae (*Lupinus*) have retained the repeat, while all those examined from the Vicieae (*Pisum, Vicia, Lathyrus*), Cicereae (*Cicer*), Trifolieae (*Medicago, Trifolium, Melilotus*), and Tephrosieae (*Wisteria*) have lost the repeat structure.[22,26,27,76-80] This event appears, therefore, to have occurred at a fairly early stage during the evolution of the Papilionoideae.

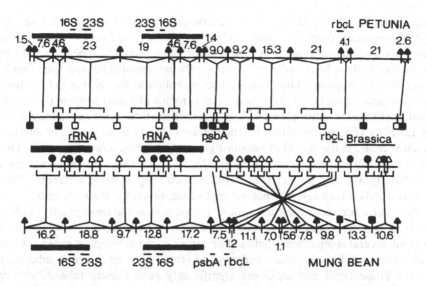

FIGURE 3.   Comparative sequence arrangement of the *Brassica*, petunia (*Petunia hybrida*), and mung bean (*Vigna radiata*) chloroplast genomes. (Top panel) Cloned Pst I restriction fragments from petunia chloroplast DNA were each labeled with ^{32}P by nick-translation and hybridized to replica nitrocellulose filters containing Sac II, Sal I, and Sac II-Sal I fragments from *Brassica hirta* chloroplast DNA, Sac II and Sac II-Sal I fragments from *Brassica campestris* chloroplast DNA, and Sac II fragments from *Raphanus sativa* chloroplast DNA. (Bottom panel) Cloned Pst I, Sal I and Pst I-Sal I fragments from mung bean chloroplast DNA were each labeled with ^{32}P and hybridized to replica nitrocellulose filters containing Bgl I fragments from *Brassica juncea* chloroplast DNA and Hpa I fragments from *Raphanus sativa* chloroplast DNA. The extent of the petunia (mung bean) fragments used as hybridization probes is indicated by the two lines that converge below (above) the fragments, while the size of each fragment is given above (below) in kilobases. The *Brassica* fragments to which the petunia (mung bean) probe fragments hybridize are indicated by the lines leading from the petunia (mung bean) fragments to the *Brassica* fragments. These maps portray the chloroplast genome in only one of the two orientations in which it exists (the single copy regions are inverted relative to one another in one half the native molecules [113]). Gene nomenclature is given in the legend to Figure 1. Restriction sites shown: (▲) Pst I, (■) Sal I, (□) Sac II, (●) Bgl I, and (△) Hpa I. (From Palmer, J.D. et al., *Theor. Appl. Genet.* 65, 181, 1983. With permission.)

Three other major sequence rearrangements among angiosperms have been revealed by performing heterologous filter hybridizations, in which cloned restriction fragments from one chloroplast genome are hybridized to filter-bound DNA of a second. A number of such hybridizations are summarized in Figure 3 and these show that chloroplast DNA from *Petunia hybrida* is essentially unrearranged relative to that of various *Brassica* species, whereas both taxa differ from *Vigna radiata* by a large inversion approximately 50 kb in size.[19] More extensive phylogenetic examination has shown that this 50 kb inversion is shared (and also derived) by all species examined from 12 genera and 6 tribes of the subfamily Papilionoideae of the family Leguminosae.[22,27,80] Species from the legume subfamilies Mimosoideae and Cesalpinoideae and from related families in the Rosidae should also be examined to see whether they contain the same inversion. A 20-kb chloroplast DNA inversion is shared by 3 genera of the Poaceae,[27,75,81,82] and a 30-kb inversion by 6 tribes of the Asteraceae.[80] Again, related families and orders should be examined to establish the phylogenetic boundaries of these macromutations.

The second approach used in comparing extremely divergent chloroplast genomes is DNA-DNA hybridization performed in solution, which measures the average amount and degree of nucleotide sequence homology between two DNAs.[2,8] This approach is rather complicated to perform, has yielded only limited phylogenetic insight and shows little future promise. One major observation from the three studies[27,83,84] that have applied this technique to chloroplast DNA is that in general, all dicot chloroplast genomes appear roughly equally diverged relative to those from different families, whereas members of the same family have significantly greater sequence homologies. The exception to this is that chloroplast DNA from *Vigna radiata* (mung bean) is no more similar to that of *Pisum sativum* (pea) and *Vicia fava* (broad bean) than to chloroplast DNA of species from three other subclasses of dicots.[27] This may reflect a very ancient origin for the legumes relative to all dicots, or alternatively, a significant increase in the rate of chloroplast genome evolution among legumes. The other major result from these studies is that the molecular divergence between monocots and dicots is slightly but significantly greater than between dicots representing different subclasses. This result suggests a very early, if not monophyletic, origin for the monocots.

So far, there have been no chloroplast gene sequence studies that are explicitly phylogenetic in nature. Nonetheless, certain conclusions can be drawn by considering the aggregate results obtained from several independent studies. For example, the chloroplast genes for the large subunit of ribulose-1,5-bisphosphate carboxylase (rbcL) and the β and ε subunits of the chloroplast ATPase (atpB and atpE) are significantly more closely related between two dicots, *Nicotiana tabacum*[85,86] (subclass Asteridae) and *Spinacia oleracea*[35,87] (Caryophyllidae) than between either dicot and a monocot, *Zea mays*.[88,89] This result also provides strong support for the notion that the monocots are a distinct lineage that arose before extensive divergence within the dicots. The rbcL genes from the above-mentioned angiosperms also show quite strong sequence homologies with the same genes from a green alga[90] and two blue-green algae.[91,92] Indeed, the remarkable sequence homologies found between several chloroplast genes and genes from *E. coli* and blue-gree algae[11-13] provide some of the strongest evidence in favor of an endosymbiotic origin for chloroplasts.[93-95]

V. GENERAL UTILITY OF CHLOROPLAST DNA FOR SYSTEMATIC STUDIES

In this section I summarize the major advantages and disadvantages of using chloroplast DNA as a molecular marker for systematic studies at a variety of taxonomic levels. Particular attention will be paid to the relative merits and systematic value of studying chloroplast DNA as opposed to mitochondrial and nuclear DNAs.

Several features make chloroplast DNA a fairly "easy" molecule to use in systematic studies. Typically, several hundred to several thousand molecules of chloroplast DNA are present in a leaf cell.[11,96,97] As a result it is relatively straightforward to isolate large amounts of sufficiently pure chloroplast DNA from many angiosperms.[98,99] Although plant nuclear DNA is at least as easy to isolate as chloroplast DNA, very little mitochondrial DNA is present in plant cells and its purification is a formidable task for most species. The small size of the chloroplast genome is advantageous in two ways: the entire array of fragments produced by many restriction enzymes is conveniently visualized on a single agarose gel and individual genes can be readily identified and isolated for sequencing studies. The much larger sizes of plant nuclear[100] and mitochondrial[101] genomes make it impossible to satisfactorily analyze the complex patterns of the total genome as revealed by agarose gel electrophoresis. Instead, cloned sequences must be used as hybridization probes in order to reveal variation in only a portion of the genome. Moreover, the fact that plant nuclear DNAs are several orders of magnitude more complex than chloroplast DNAs makes it relatively difficult to isolate and clone specific nuclear genes.

Several features of its evolution increase the systematic value of the chloroplast genome, particularly in comparison to the nuclear genome. Most nuclear genes in animals[16,17,102-104] and in plants,[105,106] even those once thought to be "single copy", are actually members of small repeated gene families. A number of evolutionary processes such as gene duplication and deletion, concerted evolution, and pseudogene formation have been associated with such repeat families. All of these processes tend to distort the evolutionary history of DNA sequences relative to that of organisms. Therefore, particular care must be taken to understand as completely as possible the evolutionary history of a given nuclear gene and its family members before using sequence changes in these genes to imply organismal phylogeny. In contrast, there is no evidence that any of these processes occur in chloroplast DNA in such a way as to confound phylogenetic interpretation. The two repeat elements present in the only significant repeat family in angiosperm chloroplast genomes, i.e., the large inverted repeat discussed previously, do undergo concerted evolution, but this appears to occur so rapidly as to be unresolvable within interspecific[19,21,24,28] and even laboratory[107] time scales. The net result is that the two repeats evolve essentially as one genetic unit with a single, undistorted evolutionary history. The chloroplast genome is evolving quite slowly at the nucleotide sequence level.[11-13,19,27,28,85,86] This fact, together with the absence of any mutational imbalances, such as the extreme transition-transversion bias found in animal mitochondrial DNA,[14,15,108] is reflected by the extremely low incidence of parallel and convergent restriction site mutations found in studies at the interspecific level.[19,23,28] Different portions of the chloroplast genome are evolving at different rates,[11-13,85,86] thus providing a range of molecular yardsticks with which to measure evolutionary distances and determine relationships.

The conservative evolution of chloroplast DNA is also its major disadvantage for phylogenetic studies, since this tends to limit the amount of useful sequence variation that can be found intraspecifically. In spite of this limitation, in several of the studies reviewed in Section IV.A, sufficient intraspecific variation was found as to allow further pinpointing of the wild sources from which several crop plants were domesticated.

The ability to trace the evolutionary history of a genome whose inheritance is usually maternal[109,110] provides unique advantages relative to biparentally inherited characters, i.e., the nuclear genome and the great majority of morphological and biochemical characters under its control. This feature is especially important given the widespread occurrence of interspecific hybrids and polyploid complexes among flowering plants.[111,112] Restriction site studies in *Brassica*,[19,41] *Triticum-Aegilops*,[25,56,57] and *Nicotiana*[61] have provided important insights into the origin and specific parentage of polyploid species and also the timing of hybridization events.

For several of these reasons, and as reviewed in Section IV.A, chloroplast DNA analysis has been and should continue to be most useful at the interspecific level, where most plant systematists work. Comparative restriction analysis is relatively inexpensive, simple, and so far has provided a wealth of phylogenetic information. Much of this information has confirmed preexisting phylogenetic hypotheses, thus helping to confirm the validity of chloroplast DNA analysis as a taxonomic tool. However, the molecular results have provided a level of quantitative resolution that is hard to obtain by conventional methods and, most importantly, have in a number of instances provided new and unexpected insights into plant evolutionary relationships.

Although restriction map comparisons can also be useful in evaluating relationships at the genus and family levels, the greatest progress in molecular systematics research above the genus level, particularly above the family level, will come through comparative DNA sequencing. With continuing improvements in the efficiency and ease of DNA sequencing, it is predicted that this technique will increasingly be used to answer questions of plant phylogeny. The ability to focus sequencing efforts on especially conserved[11-13,85,86] chloroplast genes should ultimately lead to unparalleled insight into the pattern of divergence and diversification of major plant taxa.

ACKNOWLEDGMENTS

I thank J. E. Boynton and N. W. Gillham for their hospitality and encouragement during the writing of this chapter, and M. E. Zolan for critical reading of the manuscript.

REFERENCES

1. **Crawford, D. J. and Giannasi, D. E.,** Plant chemosystematics, *Bioscience,* 32, 114, 1982.
2. **Giannasi, D. E. and Crawford, D. J.,** Plant chemosystematics, *Evol. Biol.,* in press.
3. **Harbone, J. B.,** Flavonoids and the evolution of the angiosperms, *Biochem. Syst. Ecol.,* 5, 7, 1977.
4. **Fairbrothers, D. E.,** Perspectives in plant serotaxonomy, *Ann. Mo. Bot. Gard.,* 64, 147, 1977.
5. **Gottlieb, L. D.,** Electrophoretic evidence and plant populations, *Prog. Phytochem.,* 7, 1, 1981.
6. **Gray, J. C.,** Fraction 1 protein and plant phylogeny, in *Systematics Association,*-Special volume 16, *Chemosystematics: Principles and Practice,* Bisby, F. A., Vaughan, J. G., and Wright, C. A., Eds., Academic Press, New York, 1980, 167.
7. **Boulter, D.,** The evaluation of present results and future possibilities of the use of amino acid sequence data in phylogenetic studies with special reference to plant proteins, in *Systematics Association,*-Special volume 16, *Chemosystematics: Principles and Practice,* Bisby, F. A., Vaughan, J. G., and Wright, C. A., Eds., Academic Press, New York, 1980, 235.
8. **Belford, H. S., Thompson, W. F., and Stein, D. B.,** DNA hybridization techniques for the study of plant evolution, in *Phytochemical Society Symposium: Phytochemistry and Angiosperm Phylogeny,* Young, D. A. and Siegler, D. S., Eds., Praeger Press, New York, 1981, 1.
9. **Bohnert, H. J., Crouse, E. J., and Schmitt, J. M.,** Chloroplast genome organization and RNA synthesis, *Encycl. Plant Physiol.,* 14B, 475, 1982.
10. **Bottomley, W. and Bohnert, H. J.,** The biosynthesis of chloroplast proteins, *Encycl. Plant Physiol.,* 14B, 531, 1982.
11. **Whitfeld, P. R. and Bottomley, W.,** Organization and structure of chloroplast genes, *Ann. Rev. Plant Physiol.,* 34, 279, 1983.
12. **Gillham, N. W., Boynton, J. E., and Harris, E. H.,** Evolution of plastid DNA, in *DNA and Evolution: Natural Selection and Genome Size,* Cavalier-Smith, T., Ed., John Wiley & Sons, New York, 1985, 299.
13. **Palmer, J. D.,** Evolution of chloroplast and mitochondrial DNA in plants and algae, in *Molecular Evolutionary Genetics,* MacIntyre, R. J., Ed., Plenum Press, New York, 1985, 131.
14. **Brown, W. M., Prager, E. M., Wang, A., and Wilson, A. C.,** Mitochondrial DNA sequences of primates: tempo and mode of evolution, *J. Mol. Evol.,* 18, 225, 1982.
15. **Aquadro, C. F. and Greenberg, B. D.,** Human mitochondrial DNA variation and evolution: analysis of nucleotide sequences from seven individuals, *Genetics,* 103, 287, 1983.
16. **Edgell, M. H., Hardies, S. G., Brown, B., Voliva, C., Hill, A., Phillips, S., Comer, M., Burton, F., Weaver, S., and Hutchinson, C. A. III.,** Evolution of the mouse beta globin complex locus, in *Evolution of Genes and Proteins,* Nei, M. and Koehn, R. K., Eds., Sinauer Assoc., Sunderland, Mass., 1983, 1.
17. **Kazazian, H. H., Jr., Chakravarti, A., Orkin, S. H., and Antonarakis, S. E.,** DNA polymorphisms in the human beta globin gene cluster, in *Evolution of Genes and Proteins,* Nei, M. and Koehn, R. K., Eds., Sinauer Assoc., Sunderland, Mass., 1983, 137.
18. **Upholt, W. B.,** Estimation of DNA sequence divergence from comparison of restriction endonuclease digests, *Nucleic Acids Res.,* 4, 1257, 1977.
19. **Palmer, J. D., Shields, C. R., Cohen, D. B., and Orton, T. J.,** Chloroplast DNA evolution and the origin of amphidiploid *Brassica* species, *Theor. Appl. Genet.,* 65, 181, 1983.
20. **Palmer, J. D.,** Phylogenetic analysis of chloroplast DNA variation, *Ann. Mo. Bot. Gard.,* in press.
21. **Fluhr, R. and Edelman, M.,** Conservation of sequence arrangement among higher plant chloroplast DNAs: molecular cross hybridization among the Solanaceae and between *Nicotiana* and *Spinacia, Nucleic Acids Res.,* 9, 6841, 1981.
22. **Palmer, J. D., Singh, G. P., and Pillay, D. T. N.,** Structure and sequence evolution of three legume chloroplast DNAs, *Mol. Gen. Genet.,* 190, 13, 1983.
23. **Palmer, J. D., Jorgensen, R. A., and Thompson, W. F.,** Chloroplast DNA variation and evolution in *Pisum:* patterns of change and phylogenetic analysis, *Genetics,* 109, 195, 1985.
24. **Gordon, K. H. J., Crouse, E. J., Bohnert, H. J., and Herrmann, R. G.,** Physical mapping of differences in chloroplast DNA of the five wild-type plastomes in *Oenothera* subsection *Euoenothera, Theor. Appl. Genet.,* 61, 373, 1982.

25. **Bowman, C. M., Bonnard, G., and Dyer, T. A.,** Chloroplast DNA variation between species of *Triticum* and *Aegilops*. Location of the variation on the chloroplast genome and its relevance to the inheritance and classification of the cytoplasm, *Theor. Appl. Genet.*, 65, 247, 1983.
26. **Palmer, J. D. and Thompson, W. F.,** Rearrangements in the chloroplast genomes of mung bean and pea, *Proc. Natl. Acad. Sci. U.S.A.*, 78, 5533, 1981.
27. **Palmer, J. D. and Thompson, W. F.,** Chloroplast DNA rearrangements are more frequent when a large inverted repeat is lost, *Cell*, 29, 537, 1982.
28. **Palmer, J. D. and Zamir, D.,** Chloroplast DNA evolution and phylogenetic relationships in *Lycopersicon*, *Proc. Natl. Acad. Sci. U.S.A.*, 79, 5006, 1982.
29. **Farris, J. S.,** Outgroups and parsimony, *Syst. Zool.*, 31, 328, 1982.
30. **Farris, J. S.,** The logical basis of phylogenetic analysis, in *Advances in Cladistics*, Platnick, N. and Funk, V. A., Eds., Columbia University Press, New York, 1983, 7.
31. **Avise, J. D., Lansman, R. A., and Shade, R. O.,** The use of restriction endonucleases to measure mitochondrial DNA sequence relatedness in natural populations. I. Population structure and evolution in the genus *Peromyscus*, *Genetics*, 92, 279, 1979.
32. **Ferris, S. D., Wilson, A. C., and Brown, W. M.,** Evolutionary trees for apes and humans based on cleavage maps of mitochondrial DNA, *Proc. Natl. Acad. Sci. U.S.A.*, 78, 2432, 1981.
33. **Templeton, A. R.,** Phylogenetic inference from restriction endonuclease cleavage site maps with particular reference to the evolution of humans and the apes, *Evolution*, 37, 221, 1983.
34. **Templeton, A. R.,** Convergent evolution and non-parametric inferences from restriction fragment and DNA sequence data, in *Analysis of DNA Sequence Data*, Weir, B., Ed., Marcel Dekker, New York, 1983, 151.
35. **Zurawski, G., Perrot, B., Bottomley, W., and Whitfeld, P. R.,** The structure of the gene for the large subunit of ribulose-1,5-bisphosphate carboxylase from spinach chloroplast DNA, *Nucleic Acids Res.*, 9, 3251, 1981.
36. **Zurawski, G., Bohnert, H. J., Whitfeld, P. R., and Bottomley, W.,** Nucleotide sequence of the gene for the M_r 32,000 thylakoid membrane protein from *Spinacia oleracea* and *Nicotiana debneyi* predicts a totally conserved primary translation product of M_r 38,950, *Proc. Natl. Acad. Sci. U.S.A.*, 79, 7699, 1982.
37. **Tohdoh, N. and Sugiura, M.,** The complete nucleotide sequence of a 16S ribosomal RNA gene from tobacco chloroplasts, *Gene*, 17, 213, 1982.
38. **Wilson, A. C., Carlson S. S., and White, T. J.,** Biochemical evolution, *Ann. Rev. Biochem.*, 46, 573, 1977.
39. **Thorpe, J. P.,** The molecular clock hypothesis: biochemical evolution, genetic differentiation and systematics, *Ann. Rev. Ecol. Syst.*, 13, 139, 1982.
40. **Karpechenko, G. D.,** Hybrids of *Raphanus sativa* x *Brassica oleracea* L., *J. Genet.*, 14, 375, 1924.
41. **Erickson, L. R., Straus, N. A., and Beversdorf, W. D.,** Restriction patterns reveal origins of chloroplast genomes in *Brassica* amphiploids, *Theor. Appl. Genet.*, 65, 201, 1983.
42. **U, N.,** Genomic analysis in *Brassica* with special reference to the experimental formation of *B. napus* and peculiar mode of fertilization, *Jpn. J. Bot.*, 7, 389, 1935.
43. **Palmer, J. D., Shields, C. R., Cohen, D. B., and Orton, T. J.,** An unusual mitochondrial DNA plasmid in the genus *Brassica*, *Nature (London)*, 301, 725, 1983.
44. **Prakash, S. and Hinata, K.,** Taxonomy, cytogenetics and origin of crop *Brassica*, a review, *Opera Bot.*, 55, 1, 1980.
45. **Berggren, G.,** Reviews on the taxonomy of some species of the genus *Brassica*, based on their seeds, *Sv. Bot. Tidskr.*, 56, 65, 1962.
46. **Olsson, G.,** Species crosses within the genus *Brassica*. I. Artificial *Brassica juncea* Coss., *Hereditas*, 46, 171, 1960.
47. **Olson, G.,** Species crosses within the genus *Brassica*. II. Artificial *Brassica napus* L., *Hereditas*, 46, 351, 1960.
48. **Dass, H. and Nybom, H.,** The relationships between *Brassica nigra*, *B. campestris*, *B. oleracea*, and their amphidiploid hybrids studied by means of numerical chemotaxonomy, *Can. J. Genet. Cytol.*, 9, 880, 1967.
49. **Vaughan, J. G.,** A multidisciplinary study of the taxonomy and origin of *Brassica* crops, *Bioscience*, 27, 35, 1977.
50. **Gatenby, A. A. and Cocking, E. C.,** The evolution of fraction 1 protein and the distribution of the small subunit polypeptide coding sequences in the genus *Brassica*, *Plant Sci. Lett.*, 12, 299, 1978.
51. **Uchimiya, H. and Wildman, S. G.,** Evolution of fraction 1 protein in relation to origin of amphidiploid *Brassica* species and other members of the Cruciferae, *J. Hered.*, 69, 299, 1978.
52. **Coulthart, M. and Denford, K. E.,** Isozyme studies in *Brassica*. I. Electrophoretic techniques for leaf enzymes and comparison of *B. napus*, *B. campestris* and *B. oleracea* using phosphoglucomutase, *Can. J. Plant Sci.*, 62, 621, 1982.

53. **Verma, S. C. and Rees, H.,** Nuclear DNA and the evolution of allotetraploid *Brassica, Heredity,* 33, 61, 1974.

54. **Vedel, F., Quetier, F., Dosba, F., and Doussinault, G.,** Studies of wheat phylogeny by EcoRI analysis of chloroplastic and mitochondrial DNAs, *Plant Sci. Lett.,* 13, 97, 1978.

55. **Vedel, F., Quetier, F., Cauderon, Y., Dosba, F., and Doussinault, G.,** Studies on maternal inheritance in polyploid wheats with cytoplasmic DNAs as genetic markers, *Theor. Appl. Genet.,* 59, 239, 1981.

56. **Ogihara, Y. and Tsunewaki, K.,** Molecular basis of the genetic diversity of the cytoplasm in *Triticum* and *Aegilops.* I. Diversity of the chloroplast genome and its lineage revealed by the restriction pattern of ct-DNAs, *Jpn. J. Genet.,* 57, 361, 1982.

57. **Tsunewaki, K. and Ogihara, Y.,** The molecular basis of genetic diversity among cytoplasms of *Triticum* and *Aegilops* species. II. On the origin of polyploid wheat cytoplasms as suggested by chloroplast DNA restriction fragment patterns, *Genetics,* 104, 155, 1983.

58. **Vedel, F., Quetier, F., and Bayen, M.,** Specific cleavage of chloroplast DNA from higher plants by EcoRI restriction nuclease, *Nature (London),* 263, 440, 1976.

59. **Atchison, B. A., Whitfeld, P. R., and Bottomley, W.,** Comparison of chloroplast DNAs by specific fragmentation with EcoRI endonuclease, *Mol. Gen. Genet.,* 148, 263, 1976.

60. **Rhodes, P. R., Zhu, Y. S., and Kung, S. D.,** *Nicotiana* chloroplast genome. I. Chloroplast DNA diversity, *Mol. Gen. Genet.,* 182, 106, 1981.

61. **Kung, S. D., Zhu, Y. S., and Shen, G. F.,** *Nicotiana* chloroplast genome. III. Chloroplast DNA evolution, *Theor. Appl. Genet.,* 61, 73, 1982.

62. **Scowcroft, W. R.,** Nucleotide polymorphism in chloroplast DNA of *Nicotiana debneyi, Theor. Appl. Genet.,* 55, 133, 1979.

63. **Scowcroft, W. R. and Larkin, P. J.,** Chloroplast DNA assorts randomly in somatic hybrids of *Nicotiana debneyi, Theor. Appl. Genet.,* 60, 179, 1981.

64. **Rick, C. M.,** Biosystematic studies in *Lycopersicon* and closely related species of *Solanum,* in *The Biology and Taxonomy of the Solanaceae,* Linnean Soc. Symp. Ser. No. 7, Hawkes, J. W., Lesh, R. N., and Skelding, A. D., Eds., Academic Press, New York, 667, 1979.

65. **Kutzelnigg, H. and Stubbe, W.,** Investigations on plastome mutants in *Oenothera.* I. General considerations, *Sub-Cell. Biochem.,* 3, 73, 1974.

66. **Herrmann, R. G. and Possingham, J. V.,** Plastid DNA — the plastome, in *Results and Problems in Cell Differentiation,* Vol. 10, Chloroplasts, Reinert, J., Ed., Springer-Verlag, Basel, 1980, 45.

67. **Ben-Ze'ev, N. and Zohary, D.,** Species relationships in the genus *Pisum* L., *Isr. J. Bot.,* 22, 73, 1973.

68. **Metzlaff, M., Borner, T., and Hagemann, R.,** Variations of chloroplast DNAs in the genus *Pelargonium* and their biparental inheritance, *Theor. Appl. Genet.,* 60, 37, 1981.

69. **Berthou, F., Matthieu, C., and Vedel, F.,** Chloroplast and mitochondrial DNA variation as indicator of phylogenetic relationships in the genus *Coffea* L., *Theor. Appl. Genet.,* 65, 77, 1983.

70. **Kumar, A., Cocking, E. C., Bovenberg, W. A., and Kool, A. J.,** Restriction endonuclease analysis of chloroplast DNA in interspecies somatic hybrids of *Petunia, Theor. Appl. Genet.,* 62, 377, 1982.

71. **Timothy, D. H., Levings, C. S., III, Pring, D. R., Conde, M. F., and Kermicle, J. L.,** Organelle DNA variation and systematic relationships in the genus *Zea:* teosinte, *Proc. Natl. Acad. Sci. U.S.A.,* 76, 4220, 1979.

72. **Clegg, M. T., Rawson, J. R. Y., and Thomas, K.,** Chloroplast DNA variation in pearl millet and related species, *Genetics,* 106, 449, 1984.

73. **Palmer, J. D., Osorio, B., Thompson, W. F., and Nobs, M. A.,** Chloroplast DNA evolution in *Atriplex, Carnegie Inst. Wash. Year Book,* 81, 96, 1982.

74. **Vedel, F., Lebacq, P., and Quetier, F.,** Cytoplasmic DNA variation and relationships in cereal genomes, *Theor. Appl. Genet.,* 58, 219, 1980.

75. **Poulsen, C. R.,** The barley chloroplast genome: physical structure and transcriptional activity *in vivo, Carlsberg Res. Commun.,* 48, 57, 1983.

76. **Kolodner, R. and Tewari, K. K.,** Inverted repeats in chloroplast DNA from higher plants, *Proc. Natl. Acad. Sci. U.S.A.,* 76, 41, 1979.

77. **Koller, B. and Delius, H.,** *Vicia faba* chloroplast DNA has only one set of ribosomal RNA genes as shown by partial denaturation mapping and R-loop analysis, *Mol. Gen. Genet.,* 178, 261, 1980.

78. **Chu, N. M., Oishi, K. K., and Tewari, K. K.,** Physical mapping of the pea chloroplast DNA and localization of the ribosomal RNA genes, *Plasmid,* 6, 279, 1981.

79. **Chu, N. M. and Tewari, K. K.,** Arrangement of the ribosomal RNA genes in chloroplast DNA of Leguminosae, *Mol. Gen. Genet.,* 186, 23, 1982.

80. **Palmer, J. D. and Thompson, W. F.,** Unpublished data, 1984.

81. **Howe, C. J., Bowman, C. M., Dyer, T. A., and Gray, J. C.,** The genes for the alpha and proton-translocating subunits of wheat chloroplast ATP synthase are close together on the same strand of chloroplast DNA, *Mol. Gen. Genet.,* 190, 51, 1983.

82. **De Heij, H. T., Lustig, H., Moeskops, D. J. M., Bovenberg, W. A., Bisanz, C., and Groot, G. S. P.,** Chloroplast DNAs of *Spinacia, Petunia* and *Spirodela* have a similar gene organization, *Curr. Genet.,* 7, 1, 1983.

83. **Lamppa, G. K. and Bendich, A. J.,** Chloroplast DNA sequence homologies among vascular plants, *Plant Physiol.,* 63, 660, 1979.

84. **Bisaro, D. and Siegel, A.,** Sequence homology between chloroplast DNAs from several higher plants, *Plant Physiol.,* 65, 234, 1980.

85. **Shinozaki, K. and Sugiura, M.,** The nucleotide sequence of the tobacco chloroplast gene for the large subunit of ribulose-1,5-bisphosphate carboxylase/oxygenase, *Gene,* 20, 91, 1982.

86. **Shinozaki, K., Deno, H., Kato, A., and Sugiura, M.,** Overlap and cotranscription of the genes for the beta and epsilon subunits of tobacco chloroplast ATPase, *Gene,* 24, 147, 1983.

87. **Zurawski, G., Bottomley, W., and Whitfeld, P. R.,** Structures of the genes for the beta and epsilon subunits of spinach chloroplast ATPase indicate a dicistronic mRNA and an overlapping translation stop/ start signal, *Proc. Natl. Acad. Sci. U.S.A.,* 79, 6260, 1982.

88. **McIntosh, L., Poulsen, C., and Bogorad, L.,** Chloroplast gene sequence for the large subunit of ribulose bisphosphate carboxylase of maize, *Nature (London),* 288, 556, 1980.

89. **Krebbers, E. T., Larrinua, I. M., McIntosh, L., and Bogorad, L.,** The maize chloroplast genes for the beta and epsilon subunits of the photosynthetic coupling factor CF_1 are fused, *Nucleic Acids Res.,* 10, 4985, 1982.

90. **Dron, M., Rahire, M., and Rochaix, J. D.,** Sequence of the chloroplast DNA region of *Chlamydomonas reinhardii* containing the gene of the large subunit of ribulose bisphosphate carboxylase and parts of its flanking genes, *J. Mol. Biol.,* 162, 775, 1982.

91. **Curtis, S. E. and Haselkorn, R.,** Isolation and sequence of the gene for the large subunit of ribulose-1,5-bisphosphate carboxylase from the cyanobacterium *Anabaena* 7120, *Proc. Natl. Acad. Sci. U.S.A.,* 80, 1835, 1983.

92. **Shinozaki, K., Yamada, C., Takahata, N., and Sugiura, M.,** Molecular cloning and sequence analysis of the cyanobacterial gene for the large subunit of ribulose-1,5-bisphosphate carboxylase/oxygenase, *Proc. Natl. Acad. Sci. U.S.A.,* 80, 4050, 1983.

93. **Gray, M. W. and Doolittle, W. F.,** Has the endosymbiont hypothesis been proven? *Microbiol. Rev.,* 46, 1, 1982.

94. **Cavalier-Smith, T.,** The origins of plastids, *Biol. J. Linnean Soc.,* 17, 289, 1982.

95. **Gray, M. W.,** The bacterial ancestry of plastids and mitochondria, *Bioscience,* 33, 693, 1983.

96. **Possingham, J. V.,** Plastid replication and development in the life cycle of higher plants, *Ann. Rev. Plant Physiol.,* 31, 113, 1980.

97. **Possingham, J. V. and Lawrence, M. E.,** Controls to plastid division, *Int. Rev. Cytol.,* 84, 1, 1983.

98. **Palmer, J. D.,** Physical and gene mapping of chloroplast DNA from *Atriplex triangularis* and *Cucumis sativa, Nucleic Acids Res.,* 10, 1593, 1982.

99. **Hermann, R. G.,** The preparation of circular DNA from plastids, in *Methods in Chloroplast Molecular Biology,* Edelman, M., Hallick, R., and Chua, N.-H., Eds., Elsevier/North Holland, Amsterdam, 1982, 259.

100. **Flavell, R.,** The molecular characterization and organization of plant chromosomes and DNA sequences, *Ann. Rev. Plant Physiol.,* 31, 569, 1980.

101. **Ward, B. L., Anderson, R. S., and Bendich, A. J.,** The size of the mitochondrial genome is large and variable in a family of plants (Cucurbitaceae), *Cell,* 25, 793, 1981.

102. **Hewett-Emmett, D., Venta, P. J., and Tashian, R. E.,** Features of gene structure, organization and expression that are providing unique insights into molecular evolution and systematics, in *Macromolecular Sequences in Systematic and Evolutionary Biology,* Goodman, M., Ed., Plenum Press, New York, 1982, 357.

103. **Li, W. H.,** Evolution of duplicate genes and pseudogenes, in *Evolution of Genes and Proteins,* Nei, M. and Koehn, R. K., Eds., Sinauer Assoc., Sunderland, Mass., 1983, 14.

104. **Arnheim, N.,** Concerted evolution of multigene families, in *Evolution of Genes and Proteins,* Nei, M. and Koehn, R. K., Eds., Sinauer Assoc., Sunderland, Mass., 1983, 38.

105. **Berry-Lowe, S., McKnight, T. D., Shah, D. M., and Meagher, R. B.,** The nucleotide sequence, expression and evolution of one member of a multigene family encoding the small subunit of ribulose-1,5-bisphosphate carboxylase in soybean, *J. Mol. Appl. Genet.,* 1, 483, 1982.

106. **Shah, D. M., Hightower, R. C., and Meagher, R. B.,** Genes encoding actin in higher plants: intron positions are highly conserved but the coding sequences are not, *J. Mol. Appl. Genet.,* 2, 111, 1983.

107. **Myers, A. M., Grant, D. M., Rabert, D. K., Harris, E. H., Boynton, J. E., and Gillham, N. W.,** Mutants of *Chlamydomonas reinhardtii* with physical alterations in their chloroplast DNA, *Plasmid,* 7, 133, 1982.

108. **Brown, G. G. and Simpson, M. V.,** Novel features of animal mtDNA evolution as shown by sequences of two rat cytochrome oxidase subunit II genes, *Proc. Natl. Acad. Sci. U.S.A.,* 79, 3246, 1982.

109. **Kirk, J. T. O. and Tilney-Bassett, R. A. E.,** *The Plastids: Their Chemistry, Structure, Growth and Inheritance,* Elsevier/North Holland, Amsterdam, 1978.

110. **Sears, B. B.,** The elimination of plastids during spermatogenesis and fertilization in the plant kingdom, *Plasmid,* 4, 223, 1980.

111. **Clausen, J., Keck, D. D., and Hiesey, W. M.,** Plant evolution through amphiploidy and autoploidy with examples from the Madiinae, *Carnegie Inst. Wash. Publ.,* No. 564, 1945.

112. **Grant, V.,** *Plant Speciation,* Columbia University Press, New York, 1981.

113. **Palmer, J. D.,** Chloroplast DNA exists in two orientations, *Nature (London),* 301, 92, 1983.

114. **Stein, D. B., Palmer, J. D., and Thompson, W. F.,** Structural evolution and flip-flop recombination of chloroplast DNA in the fern genus *Osmunda,* submitted, 1985.

115. **Palmer, J. D. and Stein, D. B.,** Chloroplast DNA from the fern *Osmunda cinnamomea:* physical organization, gene localization and comparison to angiosperm chloroplast DNA, *Curr. Genet.,* 5, 165, 1982.

Chapter 5

rDNA: EVOLUTION OVER A BILLION YEARS

R. Appels and R. L. Honeycutt

TABLE OF CONTENTS

I. INTRODUCTION

Genes coding for rRNA[1] were among the first genes isolated in pure form, initially using the properties of actinomycin-D/CsCl gradients to distinguish between different DNA sequences,[2] and later by cloning in plasmids such as pMB9, pSC101, and pACY184,[3] and bacteriophages such as Charon 4, λgts.[4] In most organisms the rRNA genes are present as multiple copies, ranging from 5 to 10 in bacteria to several thousand in eukaryotes.[5] In eukaryotes the rRNA genes are tandemly arranged at specific chromosomal locations.[5] The repeated nature of these genes in addition to their restricted distribution in the genome has allowed their analysis in a wide range of organisms. As a result this gene unit is unique in the molecular detail available. Data from such a diverse group of organisms provide a good opportunity for assessing the changes which occur in a gene system during the course of evolution. In this review we examine recent advances in the analysis of the rDNA locus, with a particular emphasis on the spacer region, and how these studies are modifying our views on the evolution of such repeated genes.

II. EVOLUTIONARY TRENDS AT THE rDNA LOCUS — AN OVERVIEW

The rDNA locus in eukaryotes is complex and the major trends in the evolution of the locus (Figure 1) appear to be correlated with the need for greater amounts of ribosomes, and thus more efficient protein synthesis. The result is that in most eukaryotes 1 to 5 chromosomal locations contain extensive tandem arrays of the rDNA units. The amount of rDNA at a given locus is polymorphic within a species and in certain situations can change within a few generations[6-9] (see Section III.B.). In addition, as discussed later, extrachromosomal copies (or changes in the number of nuclear copies) of the genes at certain times of development occur in eukaryotes to augment the requirement for rRNA[10,11] (Section III).

The rDNA unit has component sequences which evolve at different rates. The actual rRNA genes show considerable sequence homology between distantly related eukaryotes with certain regions within the genes showing virtually no divergence, as discussed in Section V. This extreme conservation in sequence is not always located in the regions of RNA secondary structure or protein binding sites and the reasons for the conservation of many of the sites relate to as yet undefined aspects of ribosome structure and/or function.[12-14] The difference in size of the rRNA molecules between pro- and eukaryotes [small rRNA: 1487 nucleotides in *A. nidulans*,[15] 1541 in *E. coli*,[16] 1789 in *S. cerevisiae*,[17] 1807 in soybean (Eckenrode and Meagher quoted in Reference 18), 1825 nucleotides in *X. laevis*,[19] 1858 in rabbit,[20] 1869 in rat,[18] and 1871 in *D. discoïdeum*;[21,22] large rRNA: 2876 nucleotides in *A. nidulans*,[23] 2904 in *E. coli*,[16] 3392 in *S. cerevisiae*,[25] 3788 in *Physarum polycephalum*,[24] 4110 in *X. laevis*,[26] 4712 in mouse,[27] and 4718 in rat[28]] does not disrupt extensive regions of sequence homology between a wide range of organisms.[24]

A striking feature of the evolution of the rDNA region is the changing relationship between the small-large rDNA gene unit and the 5S genes, suggesting that in lower eukaryotes an important branching occurs with respect to the linkage of these two sets of genes[29] (Figure 1). The most primitive state of the gene system would appear to be no apparent linkage of small rRNA, large rRNA, and 5S genes as observed in *Thermoplasma acidiphilum*.[30] In some lower eukaryotes such as yeast the 5S genes are independently transcribed even though they are closely linked. In many lower eukaryotes and all higher eukaryotes examined the 5S genes are in independent arrays; in *Neurospora crassa*[31,32] and *Schizosaccharomyces pombe*[33] the 5S genes are independent of the rDNA region but are not clustered in tandem arrays. The highly favored independence of the repeated arrays of 5S rRNA genes in eukaryotes may reflect a biological role for 5S rRNA which extends beyond a possibly structural role in cross-linking the small and large ribosomal units.[34,35] Alternate biological

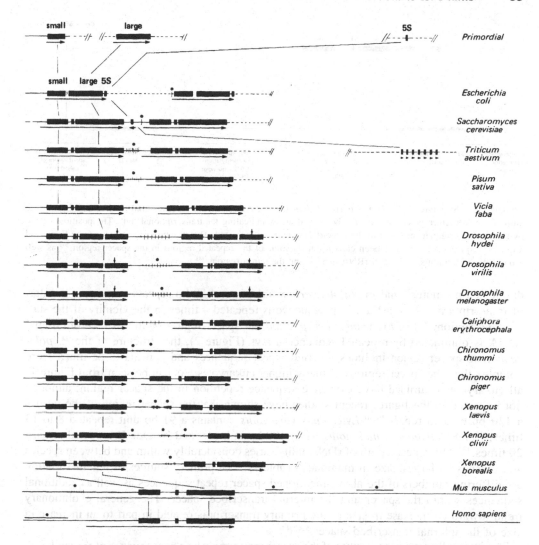

FIGURE 1. Evolutionary trends in the rDNA unit. The rDNA units of a number or organisms in which the spacer region has been analyzed are summarized diagrammatically. The units are drawn approximately to scale with horizontal arrows indicating the units of transcription. The vertical arrows in the *Drosophila* large (28S) rDNA gene indicate the position of intervening sequences (IVSs): the gaps shown in the insect large rRNA gene denotes the position of a post-transcriptional processing event which removes a portion of the RNA product. In the spacer region repetitive sequences are indicated (*). The sources of the data are as follows: primordial — a hypothetical representation, *Escherichia coli*,[16,398,399,401,405] *Saccharomyces cerevisiae*,[38,326] *Triticum aestivum* (Section III), *Pisum sativa*,[345] *Vicia faba*,[357] *Drosophila hydei*,[147] *Drosophila virilis*,[148] *Drosophila melanogaster* (Section III), *Caliphora erythrocephala*,[257] *Chironomus* sp.,[237] *Xenopus laevis* (Section III), *X. clivii, X. borealis*,[226] *Mus musculus* (Section III), *Homo sapiens*.[261,394,436]

roles for 5S rRNA molecules may have favored the separation of 5S and the other rRNA genes.

The strong evolutionary trend toward clustering of the rDNA gene units in tandem arrays has resulted in a spacer region between the rDNA units. In lower eukaryotes such as yeast and slime mold the 5S rRNA gene is located in this region (as discussed above), and in all organisms sequence repetition occurs in this spacer region. Even in *Escherichia coli* there are duplicate promoters for RNA polymerase, although these promoters share little DNA sequence homology.[16] The *Bacillus subtilis* rDNA operon, rrnB, also appears to have a

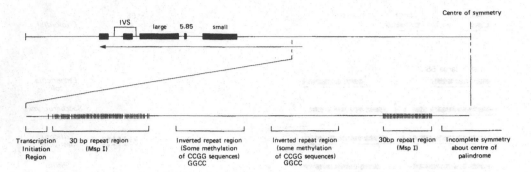

FIGURE 2.   Structure of *Physarum polycephalum* lower eukaryote extra chromosomal rDNA. One half of the palindromic structure is shown with the horizontal arrow indicating the transcriptional unit. The positions of the two intervening sequences (IVS) in the large rDNA gene are indicated. The structure was redrawn from Ferris and Vogt.[324] Sequence studies have been carried out on some of the repeated regions in the spacer region,[395] as well around the 3′ terminus of the 26S rRNA gene[423] and the intron regions.[428]

duplicated promoter[36] and in *Halobacterium halobium*, 4 80-bp repeats occur near the start of transcription.[37] In yeast a 15 bp sequence is repeated 4 times in the vicinity of the start of transcription.[38] In *Physarum polycephalum* the spacer region of the extrachromosomal rDNA is dominated by repeated sequence arrays (Figure 2); the structure of the *P. polycephalum* spacer region includes inverted repeat sequences and appears to be much more complex than the spacer regions of many higher eukaryotes. As can be seen from Figure 1, all eukaryotes examined have extensive sequence repetition in the spacer region; although not indicated in the figure, recent studies have shown that the spacer region of the rat has a 130 bp tandem repeat,[39,40] *Lytechinus variegatus* contains a 91 bp unit repeated 8 to 13 times,[41] and *Chironomus melanotus* has a 190 bp unit (defined by Dde I) repeated at least 20 times.[442] The repeat length of rDNA units varies considerably within and between species and reaches its largest size in mammals (Table 1). The primary sources of length variation are differing numbers of the above-mentioned spacer repeat sequences as well as additional sequences within the spacer and the internal transcribed spacer. The general evolutionary trend toward an increase in size of the primary transcript is related in part to an increase in size of the internal transcribed spacer.[5,42,43]

The internally repetitious nature of the spacer may simply be a consequence of the tandemly repeated arrangement of the rRNA units and may not have any functional significance.[44] However, sequencing of the repeated unit found in the spacer regions of *Drosophila* and *Xenopus* has indicated that these units share homology with the site for initiating transcription by RNA polymerase I (see Section III for details). Although this sequence homology is not found in the mouse (Section III), rat,[45] *Chironomus thummi thummi* (Section V), or man,[46,47] the *Drosophila* and *Xenopus* data have stimulated interest in the spacer region as a site for loading RNA polymerase I molecules for enhancing efficiency of transcription. This is analogous to the occurrence enhancer sequences and duplicate promoters for RNA polymerase in the rRNA gene units of *E. coli*.[16] The repeated sequence nature of the spacer region could well provide the basis for highly cooperative interactions involving proteins other than RNA polymerase I which are aimed at ensuring that once a given rDNA unit is made available for transcription, it is transcribed at maximum efficiency. In vitro transcription experiments have shown that eukaryote RNA polymerase I has a requirement for additional protein factors (some of which are species-specific) to initiate correct and efficient transcription[48-56,418,422] as is found for bacterial and the other eukaryote RNA polymerases.[57-59] It is hoped that site-directed mutagenesis on rDNA[60-62,417] coupled with in vitro studies of the type discussed will continue to elaborate on the biological characteristics of the rDNA system.

Table 1

STRUCTURE AND ORGANIZATION OF rDNA TRANSCRIPTIONAL UNITS[1]

Species	Unit length[a] (kb)	Intervening sequences[b]	Linked 5S genes[c]	No. of units[d]	Ref.
Prokaryotes[2]					
Acholeplasma laidlawii	6.0		Yes	2	291
Anacystis nidulans	6.7		Yes	2	292, 293
Bacillus subtilis	5.5		Yes	8—9	294, 296, 432
B. thuringiensis	5		Yes	2	297
Escherichia coli	5.6		Yes	7	16
Caulobacter crescentus	5.7		Yes	2	298
Methanococcus vanniellii	5		Yes + no	4	299, 300
Mycoplasma capricolum	6.0		Yes	1	291, 301
M. mycoides	6.0		Yes	2	291
Halobacterium halobium	5.7		Yes	1	302, 420
Rhodopseudomonas capsulata	Genes not linked		No	1	66
Thermoplasma acidphilum	Genes not linked			1	31
Thermus thermophilis	5		Close to 28S	2	303
Eukaryotes					
Algae					
Acetabularia mediterranea	6.6—12.8			1,900	304
A. major	8.6—10.2				305
A. cliftonii	11.4				185
A. calyculus	6.6				79
A. dentata	9.8				244, 409
A. exigua[f]	4.8 — 5.6				306
A. peniculus	9.8				244
A. ryukyuensis	7.7				244
Batophora oerstedii	5.9, 12.3				244
Cymopolia van bosseae	6.9				244
Chlamydomonas reinhardii	8		No	150	281
C. callosa	8				281
C. eguametos	11.3				281
C. globosa	8				281
C. intermedia	14.6				281
Dasycladus clavaeformis	6.2				244

Table 1 (continued)
STRUCTURE AND ORGANIZATION OF rDNA TRANSCRIPTIONAL UNITS[1]

Species	Unit length[a] (kb)	Intervening sequences[b]	Linked 5S genes[c]	No. of units[d]	Ref.
Protozoa					
Acanthamoeba castellani	12		No		307
Crypthecodinium cohnii	>7.5				308
Euglena gracilis	11.5		Yes	2,000	309
Euplotes aediculatus	7.5				283
Glaucoma chattoni	9.3				310 –
Leishmania donovani	14.3		No	170	311
Oxytricha fallax	7.5				283, 431, 433
O. nova	7.5				283
Paramecium tetraaurelia	7.8				312
Stylonychia pustulata	7.5				283
Stylonychia mytilus	6.8				313
Tetrahymena americanus	9.3				282
T. australis	9.6				282
T. borealis	9.0				282
T. canadensis	9.0				282
T. capricornis	9.3				282
T. cosmopolitanis	9.8	0.4			282
T. hyperangularis	10.1	0.4			282
T. pigmentosa	10.1	0.4			314
					282
T. pyriformis	9.3	0.4			315
T. thermophila	9.6	0.4			282
T. tropicalis	8.7				282
Trypanosoma brucei	>21	1.1			317
Fungi					
Achlya ambisexualis	>40		Yes	430	318
Aspergillus nidulans	7.8		No		319
Dictyostelium discoideum	42		Yes	200	30, 320, 413, 415
Mucor racemosus	9.6		Yes		321
Physarum polycephalum	30	0.7, 1.2	No	280	322, 324, 430
Saccharomyces cerevisiae	9		Yes	140	38, 325, 326, 425, 426
Schizosaccharomyces pombe	10.4		No		327
Neurospora crassa[g]	9		No	220	11, 32, 328

Species	Value			Page
N. discreta	9			328
N. intermedia	9			328
N. sitophila	9			328
N. tetrasperma	9			328
Torulopsis utilis	12	Yes		329
Flowering plants				
Brassica rapa (turnip)	10.2, 9.2			330
Citrus limon (lemon)	9.8			331
Claytonia caroliniana	9.5, 10.2, 10.5			332
C. virginica	10.2, 10.5			332
Clematis fremontii var. *richlii*	9.5, 10.2, 10.5			333
Cucumis melo (melon)	11.1			330
C. sativus (cucumber)	11.9, 10.4			330
Cucurbita pepo (marrow)	10.5, 9.8			330
C. pepo (pumpkin)	10.5, 9.8			330
Cymbidium spp. (orchid)	12.7, 11.2			330
Cytisus sp.	11.2			334
Daucus carota (carrot)	10.8, 11.3			335
Elytrigia elongata	9	No		336
Gaura demareei	9.4, 9.8			337
G. longiflora	9.4—10.6			337
Glycine max	7.8—9			338, 435
G. canescens	11.5, 12.5			339
G. clandestina	10.5			339
G. falcata	13.5, (12.3)			339
G. latifolia	10.5, (11.5, 13.0)			339
G. tabacina	11.0			339
G. tomentella	11.5, 12.5			339
Hordeum vulgare (barley)	9.5—10	No	2,900	81, 93
Haynaldia villosa	9	No		336
Lathyrus adoratus	12			334
Lilium henryi	11			340
L. speciosum				341
L. longiflorum				341
Linum usitatissimim (flax)	8.6	No	1,400—2,700	6, 342, 343
Lisianthius skinneri	11.5			344
L. jefensis	11.5			344

Table 1 (continued)
STRUCTURE AND ORGANIZATION OF rDNA TRANSCRIPTIONAL UNITS[1]

Species	Unit length[a] (kb)	Intervening sequences[b]	Linked 5S genes[c]	No. of units[d]	Ref.
L. peduncularis	11.9				344
L. sp. nova Sytsma	12.0				344
L. sp. nova Sytsma	12.4				344
Lupinus sp. (cv. Russell's lupine)	11—13				334, 345
L. luteus	8.8				346
Neonotonia wightii	8.3				339
Nicotiana glauca	11.3				347
Oryza sativa (rice)	7.5—7.8			850	348
Paris verticillata	15.6, 17.1				349
Petunia cv. Mitchell	8.5.9.7.10.4.9.3			No	350
Phaseolus vulgaris	11.4		No		345
Pisum sativum (30)[e]	8.4—11.9			3,900	345
Raphanus sativa (radish)	>11				351, 352
Secale cereale (rye)	9.0		No	2,900	81
Spinacea cleracea (spinach)	9.8				353
Teramnus uncinatus	10.5, 11.5				339
Trillium apetalon	13.7, 15.6, 17.1, 18.5				349
T. hagae	13.7, 15.6, 17.1, 18.5				349
T. kamtschaticum	15.6, 17.1, 18.5				349
T. tschonoskii	13.7, 14.7, 15.6, 17.1, 18.5				349
Triticum aestivum (wheat)	9.0, 9.1, 9.4		No	6,400	81
T. boeoticum	8.3—9.4		No		97
T. dicoccoides	8.6—9.4		No		97
T. durum	8.6, 9.4		No		97
T. longissimum	9.3, 9.4		No		97
T. monococcum	8.6, 9.4		No		97
T. searsii	9.4, 10		No		97
T. sharonensis	9.4		No		97
T. speltoides	9.4, 9.6		No		97
T. tauschii	8.6—9.4		No		97

Species					Ref.
Tripsacum laxum	9.4				354
Vicia benghalensis	9.5				334
V. dasycarpa	13				334
V. faba	8—13			4,800	355—357
V. grandifolia	8.8				334
V. sativa (4)[f]	8.5—10			1,900	345
V. tetrasperma	12.2				334
Trifolium repens	10.5				344
Wisteria sp.	11.4				344
Zea diploperennis	9.4		No		358
Z. luxurians	9.1		No		354
Z. mays (corn)	9.1		No		354
Z. perennis	9.4		No	3,000—9,000	354
Metazoa					
Invertebrates					
Nematoda					
Caenorhabditis riggsae	7				359
Caenorhabditis elegans	7			55	359
Arthropoda					
Acheta domesticus	35			170	360, 361
Artemia sp. (brine shrimp)	13.9			320	362
Attacus ricini	10.5				363
Bombyx mori	10.5	—[b]	No	240	364
Calliphora erythrocephala	11.5—13.5	6.1.2.9			257, 365, 366
Colymbetes fuscus	About 15				367
Chironomus melanotus	9—11				368
C. pallidivittatus	8.4				368
C. tentans	8.4		No	40—100	368
C. thummi piger	9.0		No		238
C. thummi thummi	9—16				238
Drosophila erecta	11		5	80	249
D. hydei	10.7—11.3	6	No	500—850	137, 155, 284
D. mercatorum	10.5,17.5	7	No		369
D. mauritiana	11				249
D. melanogaster	11	1—6.6	No	120—240	116
D. simulans	11			200—230	249
D. teissieri	11	5		150	249

Table 1 (continued)
STRUCTURE AND ORGANIZATION OF rDNA TRANSCRIPTIONAL UNITS[1]

Species	Unit length[a] (kb)	Intervening sequences[b]	Linked 5S genes[c]	No. of units[d]	Ref.
D. yakuba	11	5	No	130	249
D. virilis	11	5,10	No		148
Dystiscus marginalis	22			220	361
Locusta migratoria	18	7			370
Oncopeltus fasciatus	8.7—10.2				371
Phryne cincta	16				372
Rhynchosciara americana	9.5	3.5		100	373
Sarcophaga bullata	11	1—3, 5—7, 9—11		144	256
Sciara coprophila	8.4	0.9, 1.4		45	374, 382
Trichosia pubescens	6.9				375
Warramaba sp.	>14		No		236
Echinodermata					
Lytechinus variegatus	11.1, 11.7			260	376, 408, 437
	11—14				377
Paracentrotus lividus	10.5				378
Vertebrates					
Osteichtyes					
Misgurnus fossilis	20—25, 15—16		No	240	379
Xiphophorus helleri	>25			400	380
Brachydanio rerio	8.1				381
Amphibia					
Andrias davidianus	10.2				381
Notophthalmus viridescens	8.7—9.9				383
Pleurodeles waltlii	9.9				381, 384
Rana pipiens	9.6				385
Triturus alpestris	14.4				381
T. cristatus	12.8				381
T. helveticus	14.4				79
T. meridionalis	13		No		386, 387
Xenopus borealis	12.8		No	450	225
X. clivii	14.8		No		226

X. laevis	10.5—12	500—760	No	179
Aves				
Gallus domesticus	>25.5	200		388
Mammalia				
Bos taurus	32			389
Cricetulus griseus (Chinese hamster)	>24.3	250		390
Mesocricetus auratus (Syrian hamster)	>15			269
Mus musculus (mouse)	44	100	No	199
Rattus norvegicus (rat)	37.2	160	No	39, 391, 441, 434
Homo sapiens	30—37.5	50—200	No	235

1. This table should be viewed as an extension of Table 1 in Long and Dawid[5] with respect to the references for the numbers of rDNA units. If the reference given does not give the numbers of rDNA units, the reader is referred to Long and Dawid.[5]

2. Recently studies on a group of archaebacteria have been published.[392] In *Methanobacterium thermoautotrophicum, Halobacterium halobium,* and *Sulfolobus acidocaldarius,* close linkage of rRNA genes is found, as in eubacteria. Among the species *Thermoproteus tenax, Thermococcus celer, Thermofilum pendens, Desulfurococcus mobilis,* and *Desulfurococcus mucosus* the lengths between genes are more variable.

a. Many of the values shown were determined using probes for gene sequences and thus may represent minimum estimates of the unit lengths unless extensive restriction enzyme mapping of genomic DNA has been carried out. This problem arises because a segment of the spacer region may not be mapped if it is not joined to a gene sequence, where the unit has been cloned and spacer probes prepared, this problem is overcome. A partial digest with a restriction enzyme thought to define the repeat unit (assayed by gene sequences) can also establish the repeating unit from the resulting "ladder". For bacterial systems, the rDNA units are not in tandem and the figure is that required for encoding the genes in the operon. Where lengths in μM (from electron microscopic studies) were converted to lengths in kilobases, the conversion of $1 \mu M = 3$ kb was used.

b. All the intervening sequences indicated occur in the large rRNA gene. No intervening sequences to date have been located in the small rRNA gene.

c. Yes indicates that the 5S rRNA gene is part of the rDNA repeating unit as mapped in detail in, for example, yeast. No indicates that the 5S rRNA is located in tandem arrays independent of the rDNA gene. In most cases it has also been shown not to map to the same restriction fragments as the rRNA genes.

d. For protozoa the number estimated usually refers to extrachromosomal copies. Often only a single rDNA unit is integrated.

e. Number in brackets indicates the number of cultivars assayed.

f. *A. exigua* has unusual "head-to-head" arrays of rDNA units.[306] This alternating polarity suggests a series of palindromic arrangements of the rDNA units.

g. Extensive studies on different strains have been carried out and show little variation in length.[328]

h. 12% of the rDNA cistrons contain introns in the 28S rRNA gene,[393] one class in a position analogous to that found in, for example, *Drosophila melanogaster,* with a second unrelated class occurring closer to the 3' terminus.

In several of the examples outlined in Section III, the competition between rDNA units to provide the source of rRNA for the cell is striking. The dominance of some units (or arrays of units at a locus) over others may be a direct consequence of the nature of the spacer region and the interaction with the protein factors discussed above. This dominance can also extend to replication as shown by the pattern of inheritance of rDNA in *P. polycephalum*. In their analysis of the inheritance of the rDNA from strains 21 and 66 of *P. polycephalum*, Ferris et al.[63] found the rDNA characteristic of strain 66 appeared to have an advantage with respect to replication in the nucleoli of heterozygous plasmodia. As discussed in Section III, a similar situation occurs in *X. laevis* x *X. borealis* hybrids where the extrachromosomal rDNA in oocytes is dominated by the particular rDNA variant recovered from *X. laevis*.

In addition to the presence of transcribed and so-called nontranscribed spacer (NTS) regions in eukaryote rDNA repeats, some species (mainly dipterans and protozoa) have intervening sequences (IVS) in the large rRNA gene. The function of these IVSs is not clear. In some organisms such as *Drosophila* sp., the IVS is considered to lead to inactivation of the gene,[5] but in others this is clearly not the case and mechanisms for specifically splicing out the IVS from a precursor RNA have been elucidated.[64,65,410] Another interesting protozoan and dipteran characteristic (as well as some bacteria[66]) is that in the processing of precursor rRNA an additional gap is introduced into the large rRNA (Figure 1) in a region which undergoes secondary structure. This is a relatively late event in the processing of rRNA and the two halves of the large rRNA are subsequently held together by hydrogen bonding.[67,68] This does not appear to occur in all the eukaryotes. Although *Drosophila* carries out this type of processing it appears not to have the enzymes or co-factors required to remove certain IVSs.

Superimposed upon the above trends in evolution at the rDNA locus is the occurrence of extrachromosomal copies of rDNA in eukaryotes. The rDNA in mitochondria and chloroplasts generally resembles that in prokaryotes,[69,70] consistent with the generally accepted concepts of how these organelles originated; the occurrence of IVSs in both these systems appears to be a eukaryote characteristic. The rDNA IVSs in chloroplast DNA have been found in both the large rRNA gene and in the transcribed spacer between the small and large rRNA genes.[70] The extrachromosomal rDNA, not in organelles, which appears in certain developmental stages of eukaryotes is often derived from the chromosomal rDNA but has an arrangement which can differ from the chromosomal tandem arrays.[411] The origin of the rDNA on small circular DNAs (2.8 and 3.1 μm) in yeast[71] is not clear. The extrachromosomal rDNA of *Dictyostelium* and *Physarum*,[72] as well as several protozoans[73] is palindromic (see Figure 2). This structure has been postulated to reflect the mechanism used to generate these extrachromosomal rDNAs from the chromosomal rDNA unit.[74-76] In *Tetrahymena* and *Glaucoma* macronuclear rDNAs have characteristic termini featuring the sequence CCCCAA repeated 20 to 70 times as well as a specific array of single-stranded breaks. These characteristics are considered to be related to the mode of replication of the extrachromosomal rDNA.[73] The extrachromosomal rDNA in *X. laevis* is derived by a rolling circle mode of replication of an initial extrachromosomal replica of one or a few chromosomal rDNA units (see Section III). The result, in this case, is that the extrachromosomal rDNA occurs in tandemly arranged units.

The evolutionary trends at the rDNA locus suggest that this gene region is a valuable probe for phylogenetic relationships between particular groups of species. Recent studies along this line of investigation suggest, however, that some caution is required in interpreting the data because of the tandemly repeated nature of the locus. Rapid fixation (or "concerted evolution") of certain rDNA variants throughout the tandem array has the potential for yielding misleading results unless the structure of the rDNA units is understood in detail. While concerted evolution of a tandem array of repeated units of DNA is an important consideration in determining phylogenetic relationships, the "evolutionary divergence pro-

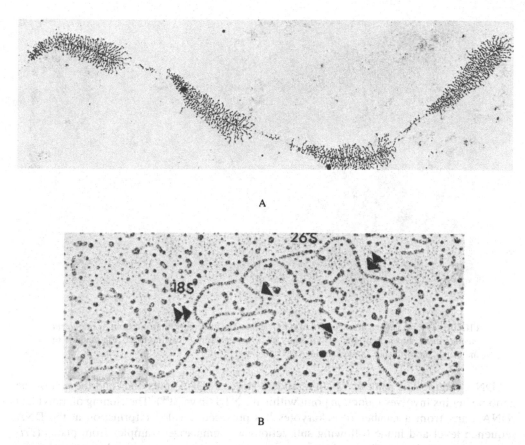

A

B

FIGURE 3. Electron microscopic visualization of rDNA genes. (A) Spreading of nucleolar chromatin to visualize the rRNA transcribed from the tandemly repeating units of rDNA.[396] (B) R-loop formation using purified rye rDNA and rRNA. The double-headed arrow indicates the DNA-RNA hybrid and the single-headed arrow the displaced DNA strand.[81]

file'' of the rDNA unit should be established prior to making phylogenetic statements. Such a profile shows that some parts of the spacer regions are relatively more conserved than others, with the gene regions most highly conserved. In Section V we evaluate the usefulness of such ''divergence profiles'' in evolutionary studies.

III. MOLECULAR ANALYSES OF THE rDNA UNITS FOUND IN PLANTS AND ANIMALS

The overall organization of rDNA units in higher eukaryotes is in the form of long tandem arrays in a ''head-to-tail'' configuration. This was first visualized directly by the electron microscopic analysis of nucleolar chromatin[77] (Figure 3A) and later using the R-loop technique[78] (Figure 3B). The ''head-to-tail'' arrangement results in a ''circular map'' when restriction enzyme sites are mapped in genomic rDNA; this has allowed the detailed mapping of rDNA units in eukaryotes by digesting genomic DNAs, transferring electrophoretically separated fragments to nitrocellulose filters, and hybridizing with appropriate ^{32}P labeled probes. Occasionally, rDNA units appear to be arranged in ''head-to-head'' configurations (Figure 4), and this could lead to heterogeneity as assayed by restriction enzyme mapping. The frequency of such unusual arrangements of rDNA units in eukaryotes is not clear at present and it has been pointed out[79] that configurations of the type shown in Figure 4 may not be

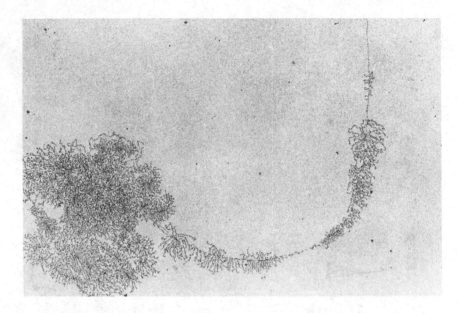

FIGURE 4.   An unusual arrangement of rDNA units. The nucleolar chromatin from *Acetabularia mediterranea* shows occasional rDNA units of inverse polarity ("head-to-head") in contrast to the usual "head-to-tail" tandem arrangement.[396]

of rDNA origin. The point at which a tandem array of rDNA units ends and the rest of the genome begins involves a junction point within the NTS (in yeast[80]). The cloning of individual rDNA units from a number of eukaryotes has provided detailed information at the DNA sequence level and in the following subsections we summarize examples from plants (*Triticum aestivum*), insects (*Drosophila melanogaster*), amphibians (*Xenopus laevis*), and mammals (*Mus musculus*).

A. The rDNA Loci of Wheat (*Triticum aestivum*)

The rRNA genes of wheat (*T. aestivum* cv. Chinese Spring) are located mainly on chromosomes 1B and 6B with a minor site located on chromosome 5D[81,82] (Figure 5). Although the rDNA is located in the distal one half to one third of the respective chromosomes, the genetic distance (determined by recombination frequency of the rDNA) from the centromere is very small (6B examined in detail[83]). Estimates for the numbers of rRNA genes on chromosome 1B range from 1300 to 1500, 6B from 500 to 3000, and 5D from 130 to 400 depending on the wheat variety considered.[84,438] In *T. aestivum* cv. Chinese Spring there are no detectable rRNA genes on chromosome 1A,[81] although in *T. aestivim* ssp. spelta this chromosome is a major location for rRNA genes.[85] Quantitative variation in rRNA gene numbers in wheat and related grasses is also evident from heterozygosity observed *in situ* hybridization experiments using radioactive probes, where grain counts consistently indicate differences between homologous sites.[85] Within the genus *Triticum*, most diploid and tetraploid species have two chromosomal locations for rDNA,[86,89] and in specific cases such as *T. araraticum*,[90] *T. dicoccoides*,[91] and *T. speltoides*[92] these sites have been designated 1B and 6B. The homologous group 5 chromosomes also carry ribosomal DNA in some diploid *Triticum* species.[89,92] Among hexaploid wheats as many as four chromosomal locations have been found.[87]

Mapping of the rDNA regions of *T. aestivum* was first carried out using a combination of R-loop analysis and hybridizing ^{125}I labeled-rRNA species to digests of genomic DNA.[81] These studies indicated a basic rDNA repeat unit of approximately 9.5 kb as defined by

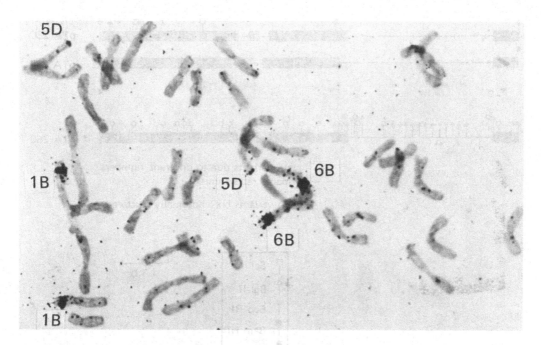

FIGURE 5. Chromosomal location of rDNA in wheat by *in situ* hybridization. The two pairs of major rDNA regions (1B, 6B) and one pair of minor chromosomal sites (5D) in hexaploid wheat *Triticum aestivum* are indicated. Probe used was ^{125}I-rRNA.[81]

EcoRI, and that a Bam HI site in the large (26S) rRNA gene was not accessible to digestion in all repeating units. The heterogeneity within the wheat rDNA was more clearly defined by Gerlach and Bedbrook,[93] who showed 3 length variants (9.0, 9.1, and 9.4 kb) existed; these authors also argued that methylation contributed to the lack of digestion of certain Bam HI sites in genomic DNA. Cloning of the 9.0 and 9.1 kb length variants was achieved by Gerlach and Bedbrook[93] using DNA enriched for rDNA genes on actinomycin-D/CsCl gradients; EcoRI segments of DNA were inserted into the EcoRI site of pACY184. The detailed structure for one of these clones, pTA250, as derived by Appels and Dvorak[94] is summarized in Figure 6. The spacer region was found to be dominated by the presence of 11 repeating units which are defined by the restriction enzymes Hae III and Hha I and are 131 to 133 bp in length. The repeating units are very similar as determined by sequencing 2 of the repeating units maximally different from each other by cross-hybridization criteria; they differed in 6 apparently randomly distributed positions. The 750 bp Hha I fragment near the start of the small (18S) rRNA gene very likely contains the site for transcription initiation by analogy with other systems, but this has not yet been demonstrated directly. We note that the sequence of 42 residues at the 3'-terminal of barley 18S rRNA has been determined,[95] and in view of the extremely high conserved nature of this region (see Section V), this can be assumed to be the same as the respective region of wheat 18S, rRNA. The first 18 residues ($^{3'}_{OH}$GUUACUAGGAAGGCGUCC) were determined directly from wheat 18S rRNA by Hagenbuchle et al.[96]

Among *Triticum* species,[97] as well as among individuals of a population of a single species, considerable spacer length variation occurs.[90,94] Variation is not random, however, and well-defined size classes segregate in the populations examined. Within the wheat varieties Chinese Spring, Hope, Timstein, and Cheyenne, specific size classes could be assigned to either chromosomes 1B, 6B, or 5D using the respective nulli-tetrasomic and chromosome substitution lines available.[94] In Chinese Spring, for example, the spacer lengths originating

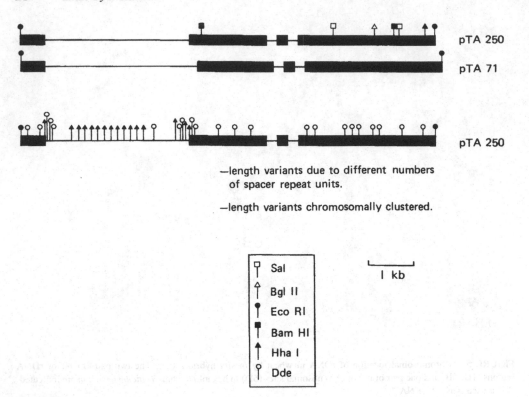

—length variants due to different numbers
of spacer repeat units.

—length variants chromosomally clustered.

Sal	
Bgl II	
Eco RI	
Bam HI	
Hha I	
Dde	

⊢———⊣
1 kb

FIGURE 6.   Summary map of the wheat rDNA unit[93,94] The black boxes are the rRNA genes, with the EcoRI site used to clone the unit occurring in the large rRNA gene. The sequence of 5.8S rRNA has been determined.[397] The references shown are 93 and 94.

from the 9.0 and 9.1 kb repeat units derive almost entirely from chromosome 6B, while the 9.4 kb variant derives from chromosome 1B. The cloned samples of the 9.0 and 9.1 kb variants (pTA250 and pTA71, respectively) differ in length due to a single 133 bp spacer repeat unit. A spacer length variant which gave rise to a characteristic Taq I fragment of 1.8 kb was assigned to chromosome 5D. As discussed in Section IV the length variation assayed above by restriction enzymes can also be assayed as the overall nucleotide sequence change in nucleic acid hybridization experiments.

The rDNA in wheat, as in other systems, is associated within nucleoli in interphase nuclei. The nucleoli are complex structures and have been studied at both the light microscopic[84,98] and electron microscopic[99] levels. In wheat, the size of the nucleolus associated with a given rDNA region is not simply correlated with the number of rDNA units. Chromosome 1B supports a nucleolus (and a metaphase secondary constriction) which is larger than that of chromosome 6B,[100] even though it has approximately half as many rDNA units. When a major rDNA site (either 1B or 6B) is removed, the remaining rDNA sites, including that on 5D, form larger nucleoli so that the mean number of nucleoli per nucleus decrease very little.[101,102] It is, furthermore, noteworthy that the introduction of an alien chromosome, chromosome IU from *Aegilops umbellulata,* has been shown to reduce the metaphase secondary constriction on chromosomes 1B and 6B.[103] The secondary constriction on chromosome IU in such material is prominent and correlated with the macronucleoli observed in interphase nuclei. Similar observations in triticales utilizing silver staining indicate the rDNA of IR is suppressed.[104] The modulation of rDNA activity of various chromosomal sites as measured cytologically is thus altered by genetic background. This competition between different rDNA regions to provide the source of rRNA for the cell is observed in

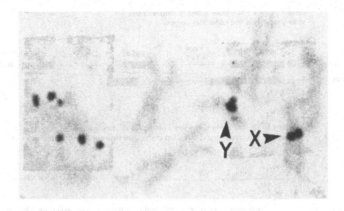

FIGURE 7.   Chromosomal localization of rDNA in *Drosophila melanogaster* by *in situ* hybridization. A neuroblast cell from a *D. melanogaster* male showing the rDNA regions on the X and Y chromosomes after hybridization with a ³H-labeled probe prepared from rDNA.[124]

many systems[84] (further examples are given in the following subsections). A corollary of the competition for activity between rDNA regions is that for much of the life cycle of wheat, significant numbers of the 2000 to 5000 rDNA units are inactive.[84] The inactive units are most likely located in the heterochromatin just proximal to the secondary constrictions.[105]

The methylation of wheat rDNA has been analyzed by Flavell et al.[106] using the restriction enzymes Hpa II (sensitive to methylation of C residues in the recognition sequence $\frac{CCGG}{GGCC}$) and Msp I (insensitive to methylation of the C residue which affects Hpa II[107]). These authors found varying levels of methylation among rDNA units with a major proportion having the $\frac{CCGG}{GGCC}$ sequence methylated. The number of rDNA units methylated increases as the number of rDNA units per cell increases in a way which suggests that excess rDNA is actually more efficiently methylated. This observation, taken together with the fact that wheat containing a 1U (from *A. umbellulata*, discussed above) substitution has the wheat rDNA preferentially methylated, suggests that methylation correlates with gene inactivity; as discussed by Flavell et al.[106] this agrees with observations in several other systems. It is interesting that the Hpa II site assayed by Flavell et al.[106] is in the vicinity of the start of transcription; the equivalent site in flax rDNA tends to be preferentially under-methylated and it has been speculated that methylation of this region may be particularly critical in determining gene activity.[108] While methylation is very likely one of the prerequisites for gene inactivity in vivo, it alone is probably not sufficient since in *Xenopus laevis* it has been demonstrated that highly methylated rDNA can be efficiently transcribed in oocytes.[109,110]

B. The rDNA Loci of *Drosophila melanogaster*

The rDNA loci of *D. melanogaster* are located on the X and Y chromosomes (Figure 7), and correspond to the genetically mapped *bobbed* loci.[111] The rDNA is located within heterochromatin and is in fact heterochromatic in its own right as judged from the properties of a segment of X chromosome rDNA manipulated genetically to be on its own within a euchromatic part of the genome.[112] At each of the chromosomal locations approximately 200 rDNA units are tandemly arranged in a "head-to-tail" fashion;[424] some changes in polarity of the blocks of rDNA units have been implied from genetic studies.[113,114] Not all rDNA units are coordinately transcribed, as visualized in electron microscopic studies of nucleolar chromatin in early embryogenesis,[79,115] and suggest an independent control for adjacent units.

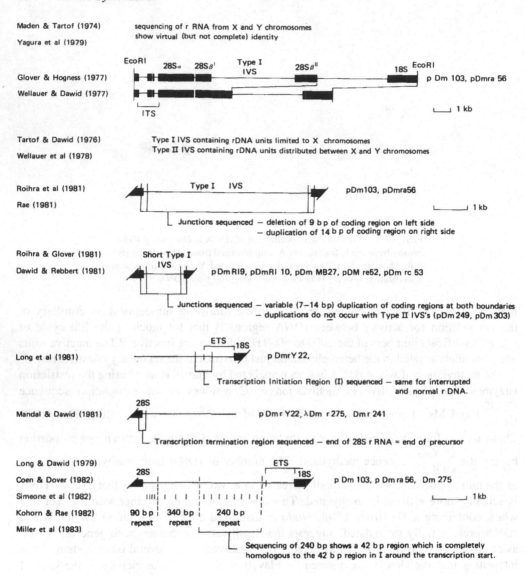

Maden & Tartof (1974)
Yagura et al (1979)
sequencing of r RNA from X and Y chromosomes show virtual (but not complete) identity

Glover & Hogness (1977)
Wellauer & Dawid (1977)
p Dm 103, pDmra 56

Tartof & Dawid (1976)
Wellauer et al (1978)
Type I IVS containing rDNA units limited to X chromosomes
Type II IVS containing rDNA units distributed between X and Y chromosomes

Roihra et al (1981)
Rae (1981)
pDm103, pDmra56
Junctions sequenced — deletion of 9 b p of coding region on left side
— duplication of 14 b p of coding region on right side

Roihra & Glover (1981)
Dawid & Rebbert (1981)
pDm RI9, pDmRI 10, pDm MB27, pDM re52, pDm rc 53
Junctions sequenced — variable (7—14 bp) duplication of coding regions at both boundaries
— duplications do not occur with Type II IVS's (pDm 249, pDm 303)

Long et al (1981)
p DmrY 22,
Transcription Initiation Region (I) sequenced — same for interrupted and normal r DNA.

Mandal & Dawid (1981)
p Dmr Y22, λDm r 275, Dmr 241
Transcription termination region sequenced — end of 28S r RNA = end of precursor

Long & Dawid (1979)
Coen & Dover (1982)
Simeone et al (1982)
Kohorn & Rae (1982)
Miller et al (1983)
p Dm 103, p Dmra 56, Dm 275
Sequencing of 240 bp shows a 42 b p region which is completely homologous to the 42 b p region in I around the transcription start.

FIGURE 8.   Summary diagram of the analyses carried out on *Drosophila melanogaster* rDNA. The references, in order down the figures, are 400, 47, 116, 117, 121, 252, 440, 402, 130, 403, 140, 141, 254, 255, 404, 119, and 406. The localization of the 5.8S and 2S ribosomal RNA sequences in the internal transcribed spacer region was carried out by Jordan and Glover.[421]

Cloning of the rDNA genes was achieved by Glover and Hogness[116] and Wellauer and Dawid[117] using plasmid vectors. The historical development of the structural analysis of *Drosophila* rDNA is given in Figure 8. The centerpoint of Figure 8, with respect to the subject of this review, is the discovery that the repeated sequence (defined by the restriction enzyme Alu I) found in the spacer region shares extensive sequence homology with the site of transcription initiation. Transcription can in fact occur within the spacer region,[118,119] a phenomenon first observed in *Xenopus* (as discussed later). Thus, it is possible that the spacer region has an important function in rDNA transcription even though it apparently changes rapidly in evolution. The evolutionary change in spacer and transcription initiation sequences correlates with a change in specificity of RNA polymerase I among *Drosophila* species; this contrasts with RNA polymerase II, which is very conservative in its recognition sites.[120] In in vitro transcription experiments, the RNA polymerase I of *D. melanogaster* does not appear to recognize the promoter of *D. virilis* rDNA.[48]

The clone pDm 103[116] contains an intervening sequence (IVS) in the large rRNA gene, 1.2 kb from the 3' end of the gene. This particular sequence, the first of many eukaryote IVSs characterized, was a representative of the major class of IVS in the large rRNA genes on the X chromosome. The 5 kb IVS in pDm 103 is present only in rDNA units on the X chromosome[121] and interrupts approximately one third of the large rRNA (28S) genes.[5] Other IVSs related in sequence to the above IVS, but smaller are found in the X chromosome rDNA units, and together the IVSs interrupt over half of the large rRNA genes. The major class of sequences has been referred to as type I IVSs, while the minor classes have been called type II IVSs. These sequences have some of the structural properties of transposable elements in that they are flanked by target site duplications[122] (Figure 8). The chromosomal distribution of the type I IVSs sequences is unusual in that early studies indicated these sequences were located outside the rDNA region.[123] *In situ* hybridization experiments demonstrated minor sites in the 102 C, D region of chromosome but within the X heterochromatin.[125] Hilliker and Appels[112] were unable to detect type I IVSs distal to the heterochromatic breakpoint of In(1)sc[4] using the cloned sequence present in pC2 (derived from the type I IVS in pDm103).[126] Using independently derived type I IVS clones Lifschytz and Hareven[127] were able to detect homology in the X heterochromatin distal to the In(1)sc[4] breakpoint. It is conceivable that the Lifschytz and Hareven clones contain a portion of a sequence not present in pC2; the arrays of type I IVSs appear to be complex as discussed in the following paragraph. Although neither Appels and Hilliker[125] nor Lifschytz and Hareven[127] detected type I IVSs proximal to the NO region by *in situ* hybridization, de Cicco and Glover[128] implied a low level of these sequences (not inserted into the 26S rRNA gene) in this region, or in the proximal portion of the NO, from their analysis of the Df(1) mal[12] chromosome.

Tandem arrays of the type I IVSs have been cloned[129] and these were found to have small segments of the large rRNA gene attached to them.[130] These arrays of type I IVSs also contain "insertions" which have short terminal sequence repetition and a dispersed genomic distribution characteristic of transposable (mobile) elements.[131,132] The arrangement of rDNA units with or without IVSs on the X chromosome has been investigated and suggests that although there is some interspersion of type I IVS⁺ and IVS⁻ rDNA units,[117,133,134] there is, at a chromosomal level, a tendency for type I IVS⁺ rDNA units to be clustered.[112,135] This type of clustering is much more clearly seen in *D. hydei*[134,136] and *D. neohydei*[137] and makes it simpler to envisage how IVS⁺ rDNA units are preferentially underreplicated (discussed below) and transcribed only at a very low level.[138,139] The virtual lack of transcription of type I IVS⁺ rDNA units cannot be accounted for by altered transcription initiation[140] or termination signals[141] and may thus reflect a property of an entire chromosomal region. Although rDNA units containing type I IVSs are not transcribed, RNA molecules do exist in vivo which are homologous to the type I IVS sequence.[138,139] Whether these originate from the tandem arrays of type I IVS sequences is not clear at present. Transcription of type II IVS containing rDNA units does appear to occur.[142-144]

The structural complexity of the rDNA locus in *D. melanogaster* is emphasized by the characterization of unusual rDNA containing segments of DNA (e.g., cDm207,[145] Dmrc52[132]). These molecules are characterized by rearrangements apparently involving the internal transcribed spacer region.[142] The rDNA unit recovered in Dmr Y24 has an intervening sequence in the 26S rRNA gene which is not located in the usual position 1.2 kb from the 3' end, but actually closer to this end.[146] The overall structure of the rDNA from *D. hydei*[147] and *D. virilis*[148] is similar to that of *D. melanogaster* and a comparison of the rDNA from different *Drosophila* species is discussed in Section V.

In considering evolutionary aspects of the rDNA locus, the various biological interactions involving the rRNA genes must be taken into account, and in *Drosophila* several studies have addressed this problem. A major reduction in rRNA production has severe effects as visualized by the bobbed phenotype;[111] in *D. hydei* the bobbed phenotype correlates directly with the number of rDNA units presumed to be inactivated due to the presence of an IVS in the large rRNA gene.[149] At a finer level the endoreduplication of chromosomal DNA which occurs in many tissues of *Drosophila* usually results in under-replication of rDNA,[111] apparently because only one of the two rDNA regions (the rDNA of one of the X chromosomes in females or of either the X or the Y chromosome in males) is endoreduplicated.[112,150,151] The controls operating on this differential endoreduplication of certain chromosomal rDNA loci have not been elucidated in detail but can be rationalized in terms of a competition between rDNA regions for a limiting nucleolus factor.[152] This competition model is supported by the results of deletion analyses by Hilliker and Appels,[112] which showed that X heterochromatin neighboring the rDNA region could modify the relationship between the X and Y rDNA regions; Endow[153] suggested that regions within the rDNA region rather than flanking heterochromatin modified dominance relationship. The studies on the differential endoreduplication of chromosomal rDNA loci under certain genetic conditions demonstrate that *Drosophila* maintains a finely balanced control over the number of rDNA units. It should be noted that in *D. hydei* the differential endoreduplication of certain chromosomal rDNA loci does *not* occur,[154] and further that the level of under-reduplication of IVS containing rDNA units in polytene tissues depends on the ratio of IVS$^-$ to IVS$^+$ rDNA units.[154] In diploid tissue increases in rDNA have been noted in response to sex heterochromatin deficiencies.[155,419]

The *bb* phenotype has been shown to be unstable in that males carrying the mutation can increase the amount of rDNA on the mutant chromosome if kept in a phenotypically bb combination.[5,111] After several generations the increased (magnified) rDNA is stably inherited; the product of the mei-41 gene (a meiotic mutant originally recovered as being defective in DNA repair and recombination) appears to be required for rDNA magnification.[156] Observations of this type, taken together with the phenotypic interactions of other physically distant loci such as *abnormal oocyte* (*abo*) with X rDNA and its surrounding heterochromatin,[112] indicate that DNA sequence changes in the rDNA region cannot be considered independent of the rest of the genome. It should be noted that although in special genetic situations the rDNA locus can be unstable it is generally stable as judged from experiments in which stocks with specific length variants were used as markers in crossing programs.[157]

C. The rDNA Loci of *Xenopus laevis*

The DNA in *X. laevis* can be divided into chromosomal and extra-chromosomal rDNA. The chromosomal rDNA consists of 450 to 800 tandemly repeated gene units which occur in the nucleolar organizer region.[158,159] Using *in situ* hybridization Pardue[160] confirmed the location of rDNA in the secondary constrictions of the largest subtelocentric pair of chromosomes. In addition to the normal occurrence of two nucleolar organizers, individuals heterozygous (1-nu) and null (o-nu) for the nucleolar organizers are known and have been used in developmental studies.[161-163,429] Although development is retarded in anucleolate individuals,[161] rRNA synthesis proceeds normally in individuals which have greatly reduced, but not totally depleted, copies of rRNA genes.[164] The lack of reduced rRNA synthesis during development is in part due to the presence of extrachromosomal copies of rDNA found in the oocyte. Extrachromosomal rDNA is amplified approximately 1000-fold in the oocyte and these copies are active only during oogenesis, thus enhancing the synthesis of rRNA during this stage of development.[165]

The chromosomal and extrachromosomal rDNA have the same basic molecular structure. Both have EcoRI restriction endonuclease sites which divide the rDNA repeat unit into two fragment classes, namely, a small fragment containing most of the 28S (large) rRNA gene and a larger fragment containing primarily the 18S (small) rRNA gene plus spacer.[166-168]

Repeat length heterogeneity resulting from length variation in the spacer region can be detected in both chromosomal and extrachromosomal rDNA, although certain quantitative differences are evident. All chromosomal repeat size classes can be seen in extrachromosomal rDNA, but the relative abundance of these size classes differs from chromosomal rDNA in individual females. The preference for amplifying a particular size class of extrachromosomal rDNA appears to be inherited since all siblings have the same frequency of a particular class.[169] This preference for amplifying a certain class of rDNA is particularly marked in interspecies hybrids formed between *X. laevis* and *X. borealis* where the hybrids primarily amplify *X. laevis* rDNA.[170]

A further difference between extrachromosomal and chromosomal rDNA is that the rDNA units of a given extrachromosomal rDNA molecule are homogeneous whereas length variants are more interspersed in chromosomal rDNA.[169,171] Data of this type prompted Wellauer et al.[169] to accept the rolling circle model for extrachromosomal rDNA amplification.[172] In this model a single rDNA repeat unit, in the form of a circle, is continuously replicated to generate a tandem array of identical rDNA repeating units.

A final difference between the two forms of rDNA is the occurrence of 5-methyl deoxycytosine residues in strands of chromosomal rDNA which are absent from the extrachromosomal rDNA strands.[173] In the following description of the molecular structure of *X. laevis* rDNA we make no further distinction between the two forms of rDNA.

The overall structure of the rDNA is described by a spacer region and a region giving rise to a primary precursor transcript. The precursor rRNA consists of an external transcribed spacer (ETS) preceding the 18S rRNA gene at the 5' end of the transcript, a 5.8S rRNA gene separated from both the 18S and 28S rRNA by internal transcribed spacers (ITS 1 and ITS 2), and the 28S rRNA gene at the 3' end of the transcript.[174] The structure of the rDNA has been determined at the nucleotide sequence level. The two major EcoRI fragments of the rDNA were first cloned in the bacterial plasmid pSC101[3] to produce CD18, containing mainly the 28S gene and CD30 containing the rest of the rDNA unit. The large EcoRI fragment in CD30 was transferred to the colicinegenic plasmid E1 (ColE1[176]) and renamed pXlr12.[175] Another spacer region EcoRI fragment (pX1r4) was cloned by Wellauer et al.,[167] transferred to the Col E1 plasmid, and renamed pXlr14.[177] These two clones, pXlr12 and pXlr14, provided the basis for most of the early work on the structural mapping of *X. laevis* rDNA (Figure 9).

The spacer of *X. laevis* rDNA varies in length from 2.7 (pXlr12) to 5.5 kb (pXlr14),[167,177] and this variation contributes directly to length heterogeneity seen in vivo within and between individuals.[167,178,179] Both heteroduplex mapping and restriction enzyme analyses of cloned rDNA indicate that the length variation is the result of the insertion or deletion of units of a repeating DNA sequence found in the spacer.[167,177] Botchan et al.[177] divided the spacer into four regions (A, B, C, and D; see Figure 9), differing with respect to their overall variability. Comparisons of four cloned fragments revealed the conservative nature of region A (in terms of length) relative to the length variation observed in regions B and D. Region B consists of multiple Sma I sites, thus denoting the repetitive nature of this spacer segment, and varying in length from 1 to 1.2 kb. Region D varies in length from 0.89 to 3.8 kb and is characterized by a regular distribution of Bam HI sites. This region accounts for most of the spacer length variation usually observed in vivo as typified by the comparison between pXlr12 and pXlr14 (Figure 9). Region C is defined as a region separating B and D. Botchan et al.[177] suggested that the spacer region originally consisted of a 15 bp repeat or multiples thereof which subsequently diverged to give the present structure.

Boseley et al.[174] provided more details on the restriction map of the spacer region using the clone pX1108. These authors recognized 3 repetitious regions (designated 1, 2, and 3; see Figure 9). Region 1 corresponds to region B of Botchan et al.[177] In addition to the regular order of Sma I sites this region consists of 100 bp repeating units as characterized by Hinf.

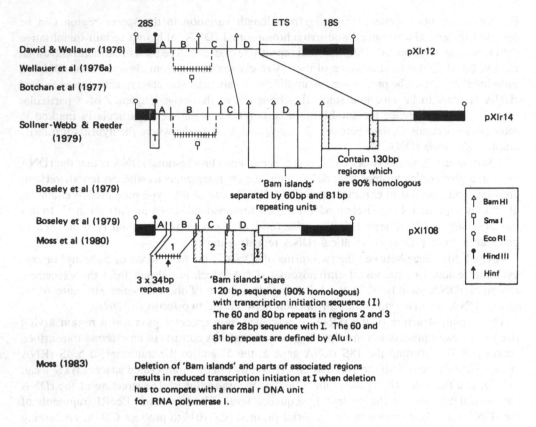

FIGURE 9. Summary diagram of the analyses carried out on the *Xenopus laevis* rDNA external region. The references, in order down the figure, are 175, 167, 177, 180, 174, 182, and 61.

Smaller repeating units are revealed by Ava I, Hpa II, and Hae III. The restriction enzyme, Alu I, defines repetitive regions 2 and 3 as consisting of alternating 60 and 81 bp repeats. Sequence data indicate that except for a 21 bp deletion/insertion, these two repeats are identical. In region 3 the 81 bp repeat has Sma I sites which are absent from the 81 bp repeats of region 2. The repetitive regions are separated by nonrepetitive sequences which center around Bam HI sites. Boseley et al.[174] refer to these sequences as "Bam HI islands". The sequences in the Bam HI islands are identical for at least 185 bp and are highly homologous to sequences present near the 5' end of the 40S precursor rRNA which is approximately 2.25 kb upstream from the EcoRI site in the 18S rRNA gene. This position for the initiation of transcription was also determined by Sollner-Webb and Reeder[180] for pXlr14. Boseley et al.[174] suggested that the Bam HI islands are duplicated sequences of the transcription initiation region which have been displaced into the spacer via saltations of the 60/81 bp repeating units. The sequence data did not support the suggestion by Botchan et al.[177] for the existence of a primitive 15 bp repeat precursor for the spacer region.

In addition to the sequence data provided by Boseley et al.,[174] most of the spacer plus external transcribed spacer of pXlr108 has been sequenced.[181,182] These sequence data have identified an additional repetitive region upstream from region 1 (also called B), which consists of 3 to 9 34-bp repeating units separated from the adjoining repetitive region by approximately 80 bp. Region 1 is characterized by 100 bp repeats;[174] variation between repeats results from base substitutions, deletions, and/or insertions. A 116 bp sequence separates the repetitive region 3 from the transcription site and contains an oligo-T tract.

Transcription termination has been mapped to the Hind III site at the 3' end of the 28S

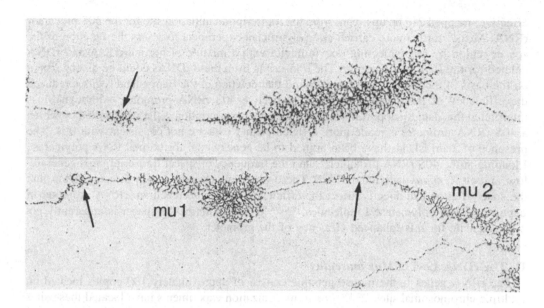

FIGURE 10. Transcription in the spacer regions of *Xenopus laevis* rDNA. The arrows indicate the transcription products originating from the spacer region.[185] Photograph provided by Dr. M. L. Trendelenburg.

rRNA gene (pXlr14,[180] pXlr108.[175,182] Bakken et al.[183] provided additional information on both transcription initiation and termination using a combination of electron microscopy, cloned sequences modified with respect to the initiation and termination sites, and microinjection of the cloned DNA into oocyte nuclei. For transcription termination a cluster of three T residues were found to be important. Two T residue clusters were located upstream from the transcription initiation site and a transcription termination (of transcription initiated in the spacer region) role was proposed for these sequences. The electron microscopic studies of Trendelenburg[184] suggest that transcription termination is a two-step process involving both the release of the precursor rRNA transcript followed by the release of RNA polymerase I molecules. Trendelenburg[184] defined the region of termination as consisting of three RNA polymerase I molecules with the first being associated with the precursor rRNA transcript.

Active transcription of the spacer region was observed at least 8 years ago using electron microscopic techniques[171,185-187] (Figure 10). The initiation of spacer transcripts maps occurs in the Bam islands.[171] The duplicated Bam islands are currently considered to represent multiple promoter regions and have become a focal point for recent research on the *Xenopus* spacer region. Transcription from the spacer promoters generally occurs at low frequency in most individuals and one site (α-type promoter) seems to be dominant. In some individuals a high frequency of spacer transcription is found.[171] Boseley et al.[174] suggested that the spacer repetitive regions may play a role in loading RNA polymerase I molecules for transcription, a concept first suggested by Mueller et al.[188] to account for the highly efficient transcription of *E. coli* rDNA.

Recently, Moss[61] proposed a model in which the actual transcriptional activity in the spacer provided a mechanism for shunting the RNA polymerase molecules toward the initiation site. S1 mapping indicated that spacer transcripts started at the transcription initiation sites in the Bam HI islands. The 3′ termination site for spacer transcription (90%

effective) mapped 213 bp upstream from the transcription initiation site for the 40S precursor rRNA. Moss[61] furthermore carried out a significant experiment to assess the function of the spacer region by microinjecting oocyte nuclei with a mixture of normal rDNA and rDNA deleted for the Bam island region. The transcripts from these rDNAs could be distinguished on the basis of their length and it was found that deletion of the Bam island regions reduced the efficiency of transcription from the respective 40S rRNA promoter. Although Moss interpreted this data to support his model that spacer transcription is the mechanism by which a 40S rRNA promoter is made more efficient, other data are not consistent with this. The presence of Bam islands have been argued to be nonessential for normal RNA polymerase I loading at the 40S rRNA promoter[183] and the frequency of spacer transcription is generally low among *Xenopus* individuals.[171,189] These observations have led to the suggestion that the spacer region can directly affect the efficiency of the 40S precursor rRNA promoter in capturing RNA polymerase I molecules.[190,191] Transcription of the spacer is apparently not a prerequisite for this enhanced efficency of the promoter.

D. The rDNA Loci of *Mus musculus*

The rRNA genes in the mouse genome consist of approximately 100 copies located on multiple chromosomal sites.[192-195] *In situ* hybridization experiments have located these sites on 5 different chromosomes (12, 15, 16, 18, and/or 19) with the number of chromosomes involved varying among different inbred strains of mice.[192,194]

In addition to variation in the location of rDNA sites and the relative ranking of these sites in terms of rDNA copy number, repeating units of rDNA also vary in length due to variation in a region called V rDNA. This restriction enzyme length polymorphism represents as many as 15 distinct fragment sizes with 4 to 6 major size classes per inbred strain.[196] Linkage mapping of 5 length classes has assigned them to 3 linkage groups, and in one instance 2 of the classes occur on chromosome 12. As pointed out by Arnheim et al.,[197] the localization of fragment classes to specific chromosomes indicates relatively little exchange of rDNA occurs among nonhomologous chromosomes.

The structural map of the rDNA repeating unit was determined originally by restriction enzyme analysis and ^{125}I labeled rRNA (5.8S, 18S, 28S) probes prepared from Balb/c mice. The size of the unit was estimated to be between 36[198] and 44 kb.[199] The restriction enzyme EcoRI produces three fragments which hybridize to 18S and/or 28S rRNA: (1) a fragment varying in size from 13 to 15 kb, containing most of the 18S rRNA gene, all the external transcribed spacer, and part of spacer; (2) a 6.6 kb fragment containing approximately 25% of the 18S rDNA, both internal transcribed spacers (ITS 1 and ITS 2), the 5.8S rDNA, and most of the 28S rDNA; (3) a 6.6 kb fragment containing the 3' end of the 28S rDNA and part of the spacer downstream from the 28S rDNA. As summarized in Figure 11 these three fragments in combination with detailed restriction enzyme maps have been the starting point for the structural analysis of the mouse rDNA repeating unit.

Fragment B was originally cloned in λgtWES following an enrichment of rDNA EcoRI fragments using RPC5 chromatography.[4] This fragment occurs in all strains of mice, and in recent years has provided the basis for the analysis of the internal transcribed spacer. A 3.7 kb fragment defined by EcoRI and Bam HI covers the ITS 1 and ITS 2 regions, the 5.8S rDNA, the 3' end of the 18S gene, and the 5' end of the 28S gene. This fragment has been cloned in pBR322 (pME B3[200]). The sequences surrounding the 4 rRNA processing sites in pre-RNA have been determined, and although the regions share little homology, sequences downstream from the 5.8S rDNA are conserved among vertebrates (85% for

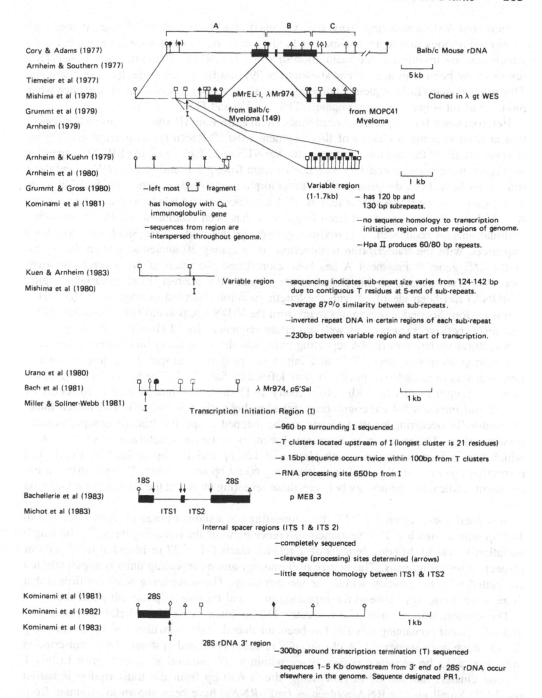

FIGURE 11. Summary of analyses carried out on the mouse rDNA region. The restriction analyses shown are drawn to scale, as indicated on the right side of the diagram. References on the left side are the source of the data summarized, with conclusions generally summarized on the right side. Where possible, specific names of λ and plasmid clones are given to aid in further examination of the literature. The restriction endonuclease sites shown are Bam HI (△), Bgl II (◆), Acc I (✗), Ava I (τ), Eco RI (○), Hind III (●), Hinf I (▲), Pst I (▲), Pvu II (■), Sal I (□), Sma I (△), Xho I (○). The references in order down the Figure are 199, 207, 4, 204, 206, 205, 196, 262, 208, 407, 209, 204, 213, 212, 211, 200, 201, 407, 203, and 202.

rodents and 73% comparing *Mus* and *Xenopus*). Bachellerie et al.[200] suggest that such conserved regions may represent specific binding or recognition sites for U3 nucleolar RNA which may be involved in the maturation of precursor rRNA. The entire ITS 1 and ITS 2 regions have been sequenced[201] and shown to be 999 and 1089 nucleotides long, respectively. The regions share little sequence homology but show some conservation of sequence when mouse and rat sequences are compared (ITS-1, 75% and ITS-2, 30%).

Heterogeneity for the presence or absence of an extra Bam HI site in fragment C suggests that at least two major classes of this fragment exist.[199] Recently, Kominami et al.[202] recovered clones of this fragment in the vector λgtWES and subcloned it in pBR322. Repetitive sequences have been located 1 to 5 kb downstream from the 3' end of 28S rDNA, and these sequences have been designated PR1 (polymorphic repetitive sequence 1). In addition to their location in the rDNA spacer region, PR1 sequences are found elsewhere in the genome. A 1.3 kb EcoRI-SmaI segment from fragment C has been subcloned and the transcription termination site sequenced. Approximately 300 bp surrounding the SmaI site have been sequenced with the transcription termination site mapping 30 nucleotides from the 3' end of the 28S gene.[203] Fragment A has been cloned and characterized by several investigators.[204-206] Two aspects of this fragment are of particular interest. First, a variable region (V-rDNA) has been identified with the length variation observed in fragment A localizing to this region. Second, a region upstream from the VrDNA region has been identified which contains repetitive sequences as well as certain sequences found elsewhere in the genome.

Structural variation of rDNA repeating units was shown to occur both within individuals and among strains of mice,[199,207] and initial mapping of fragment A suggested that this variation was localized to a specific region defined by Sal I.[205,206] The Sal I (VrDNA) region varies in length from 1 to 7 kb and as many as 15 discrete fragment classes (detected by Pvu II and includes Sal I recognition sites) have been identified in wild and inbred mice. The naturally occurring length variants can be mapped to specific linkage groups, as mentioned earlier. The variation in fragment A centers around a structural unit of "135 bp" which has in fact two major length classes of 120 bp and 130 bp defined by PvuII. The restriction enzyme HpaII reveals an alternating 60/80 bp arrangement;[208] Hybridization experiments indicate no homology between these repeating units and the transcription initiation site.[209]

Sequencing studies on the "135 bp" repeating units show a range of sizes from 124 to 142 bp with as much as 13% sequence difference between the repeating units.[209] The length variation is due to differing lengths of T residue tracts (11 to 27 residues) at the 5' end of respective repeating units. The degree of homology among repeating units is apparently not correlated with the position within the tandem array. The sequencing work confirmed that there is no homology between the repeating units and the transcription initiation site.

The transcription initiation site is located 230 bp downstream of the VrDNA region[209,210] and a fragment containing this site has been subcloned. Approximately 960 bp surrounding the site have been sequenced. A cluster of T residues is located upstream from transcription initiation, a 15 bp sequence occurs twice within a 100 nucleotide interval prior to this T residue cluster, and the RNA processing site is 650 bp from the transcription initiation site.[211-213] Small nuclear RNA molecules (snP1 RNAs) have been shown to originate from the spacer preceding the initiation site,[214] a situation somewhat analogous to that found in *Xenopus* (see Section II).

The expression of mouse rRNA genes has been examined in mouse-human hybrid cells and depending on the source of the cells used to form the hybrid, the mouse rRNA genes can be either active[215] or selectively inactive.[216] In these studies it is the electrophoretic mobility of mouse 28S rRNA which is distinguishable from human 28S rRNA and thus allows the activity of the different genes to be assayed. Infection by SV40 can reactivate transcriptionally inactive mouse rRNA genes,[217] suggesting that the apparent competition between the human and mouse rDNA units can be modulated by factors introduced during infection. As discussed in Section II, this appears to reflect the requirement for protein factors, in addition to RNA polymerase I, for efficient initiation of transcription of rDNA units.

IV. SUMMARY OF MOLECULAR APPROACHES IN THE DERIVATION OF PHYLOGENIES

At present three basic approaches are available for obtaining information at the DNA level which can be used to characterize the similarities and differences between species. We discuss these in increasing order of resolution, namely restriction enzyme analyses, hybridization and hybrid melting point (Tm) analyses, and finally sequencing studies. Each approach has its advantages and disadvantages in an evolutionary study of repeated sequence DNA such as that found at the rDNA locus. Ideally such a study should combine the three techniques.

A. Restriction Enzyme Analyses

Digestion of DNA samples with restriction endonucleases and separating the DNA fragments on a size basis using electrophoresis in an agarose or polyacrylamide gel is the first step in characterizing the rDNA of an organism. Transfer of the DNA fragments to nitrocellulose[218] and hybridization with radioactive rRNA (or a DNA sequence from a gene region from one of the organisms detailed in the preceding section) allows the preliminary mapping of the rDNA unit. A basic parameter which is essential to know in an uncharacterized system is the repeat size of the rDNA unit (see Table 1); with restriction enzyme digests this is best determined by a partial digest with an enzyme which cuts only once. Hexanucleotide recognition restriction endonucleases such as Bam HI, Hind III, EcoRI, and XbaI are often useful. The periodicity of the "ladder" which results from a partial digest of a tandem array of sequences gives the repeat length of the unit; the large size of some eukaryotic rDNA repeating units, it should be noted, precludes the use of such ladders.

In an evolutionary study the restriction enzyme analyses serve to map the rDNA unit and thus locate regions of variability within the unit. The restriction enzyme analyses per se do not provide useful information on the relationships between species. The reason for this is that in such analyses lengths of DNA segments are measured and a single mutation can lead to loss of a restriction site and a dramatic change in length of the DNA segment being assayed. It has been estimated that sequence divergences of 3 to 10% are usually correlated with much higher divergences of fragment patterns (40 to 80%).[148] A corollary of this is that for the rDNA system, length variation within a species can be just as extensive as the variation observed between species.[83,94,197,219] The internally repeated sequence nature of the rDNA spacer region means that length variation in a restriction enzyme fragment is not always due to inactivation of a restriction enzyme site, but could also result from variation in the number of repeating units in the spacer.

In a study of members of the Triticeae to identify species which are closely related to the genomes of hexaploid wheat, *Triticum aestivum*, Peacock et al.[97] utilized EcoRI and Bam HI digests to characterize the rDNA unit. Double digestion generates three major fragments 0.9, 3.6, and 4.4 kb in length (see Figure 6). In the range of *Triticum* species (diploid through to hexaploid) the 3.6 and 0.9 kb fragments were invariant, as expected from the fact that they originate from the gene region, while the 4.4 kb fragment showed considerable variation. The 4.4 kb fragment contains the spacer region and a question in such a study is whether or not it is valid to conclude, on the basis of fragment length only, that the species which contain a fragment of this length is most closely related to the genome carrying the rDNA of hexaploid wheat. The authors found that among the species studied only *Triticum tauschii* (*Aegilops squarossa*) contained the 4.4 kb fragment and speculated that this known donor of the D genome of wheat also contributed to the B genome. A significant aspect of the study was that accessions of the species considered, on the basis of several other parameters, to be most closely related to the B genome (i.e., *T. speltoides*, *T. searsii*, *T. longissimum*, and *T. sharonense*) did not contain the 4.4 kb fragment. In contrast, Dvorak and Appels[90] found extensive variation in the length of a spacer fragment defined by Taq I in populations of *T. speltoides* and that the spacer length classes found in hexaploid wheat were segregating in these populations. Other analyses suggested that the spacer region of *T. speltoides* (among the diploid species tested) was most closely related to the rDNA spacers in hexaploid wheat (discussed in detail later). In a larger sample size Peacock et al.[97] would probably have found a spacer segment of the required length in particular accessions of *T. speltoides*, *T. searsii*, *T. longissiumum*, and *T. sharonense* examined.

The application of a restriction enzyme analysis of the rDNA region in relation to phylogeny has also been carried out in *Drosophila* sp.[220] and we can ask, once again, whether any valid relationship can be drawn between spacer length variation and phylogeny. Examination of published data indicates that extensive variation for spacer length in rDNA units exists within lines of *D. melanogaster* derived from a natural population.[219] Phylogenies of the type described by Coen et al.[220] cannot therefore be considered reliable because adequate sampling of populations of the species was not presented. The problem here is analogous to the one discussed above for analyzing the *Triticeae*.

The plant and insect examples discussed in this section indicate that length of a given sequence as defined by restriction endonucleases is not a useful taxonomic character unless, as pointed out by Kossel et al.,[221] many restriction endonucleases are examined. A corollary of this conclusion is that models of rDNA evolution based on restriction endonuclease length measurements alone need to be carefully re-examined.

B. Hybridization and Hybrid Melting Point (Tm) Analyses

It is common to find, in recent discussions of the application of nucleic acid chemistry to evolutionary studies, that the analysis of genome relatedness by hybrid melting point analysis is considered of "very limited taxonomic value".[221] While this is true for the traditional type of experiment using a heterogeneous fraction of DNA as a probe, we wish to show in this section that this is no longer the case if a cloned segment of DNA (approximately 100 bp in length) is used as a probe. Utilization of rRNA as probes in melting point analyses has provided a valuable parameter to quantify relationships between groups of bacteria.[222-224] Melting point analyses using cloned probes from a well-defined region of the genome such as the rDNA region allow hundreds of species to be examined within the time of a few weeks for a quantitative assignment of the degree of relatedness with respect to the sequence assayed. As discussed below this type of analysis has shortcomings but we argue that the technique has an important place in evolutionary studies, in combination with restriction enzyme analyses and sequence work.

A classic example where the melting point analysis was utilized in a well-defined situation, before the availability of cloned DNA, may be found in the analysis of *X. laevis* and *X. borealis* (*X. mulleri*) rDNA.[225] The highly purified rDNA from each species was hybridized with cRNA synthesized from either *X. laevis* or *X. borealis* rDNA in the presence of a large excess of unlabeled rRNA to ensure gene sequences did not hybridize the radioactive cRNA. Brown et al.[225] found a small amount of heterologous hybridization which melted approximately 7°C lower than homologous hybrids; this ΔTm suggested 10% mismatch among cross-hybridizing sequences. It is interesting to examine these early studies in relation to the structure of rDNA as it is known today for these two *Xenopus* species. The overall structure of the spacer regions of *X. laevis* and *X. borealis* is quite different at the restriction enzyme level. Sequence studies on the 245 bp preceding the transcription initiation site have demonstrated an overall mismatch of approximately 47%[226] with certain stretches (15 and

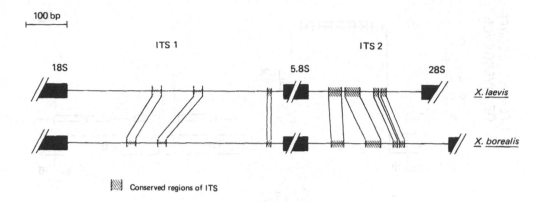

100 bp

ITS 1

ITS 2

18S

5.8S

28S

X. laevis

X. borealis

▨▨▨ Conserved regions of ITS

FIGURE 12. Comparison of the internal transcribed spacer regions of two *Xenopus* species. The data summarized[168,266,267] emphasize the distribution of conserved regions within the transcribed spacers.

18 bp long) showing complete homology. Furthermore, sequencing of the internal transcribed spacer regions (Figure 12) has shown the existence of well-defined, conserved, regions of homology. In relating this sequencing information to the early ΔTm data, the limitation of the ΔTm type analysis is clearly demonstrated: the analysis underestimates the degree of difference between two DNA sequences being compared. If the regions being compared are too dissimilar they will not cross-hybridize and thus will not be assayed with a given probe. We note that a lack of hybridization should be revealed as a marked quantitative difference in the amount of hybridization in the heterologous reaction relative to the homologous reaction, as was observed in the early *Xenopus* work.[225] The cross-hybridization between *X. laevis* and *X. borealis* spacer regions would tend to be dominated by the homologies specified above.

Recognition of the above shortcoming of the ΔTm type of analysis allows this problem to be minimized in an evolutionary study, as attempted by Dvorak and Appels in their analysis of the rDNA in species of the tribe *Triticeae*.[90,94,227] It is clear from the foregoing discussion of the *X. laevis* and *X. borealis* comparison that if probes approximately 100 bp long were subcloned from the spacer regions, then the ΔTm analysis would reveal a certain profile of sequence divergence along the length of the spacer region. Appels and Dvorak[227] determined such a sequence divergence profile for rDNA within the genus *Triticum* using, as probes, 11 different parts of the cloned rDNA region of wheat (pTA250; Figure 13a). The probes were 100 to 400 bp in length. Five *Triticum* species were compared to *T. aestivum*, the source of the probe, and ΔTm values for each probe allowed the species to be ranked with respect to their relatedness to *T. aestivum*. DNA samples were immobilized on nitro-cellulose filters for hybridization and Tm determinations. Furthermore the ΔTms could be plotted on a Y axis vs. an arbitrary "evolutionary distance" scale on the X axis to yield a series of lines readily described by linear regressions (Figure 13b). The data plotted in this way quantifies an evolutionary parameter of sequence divergence for each of the sequences and demonstrates that, as shown in the sequence comparisons of specific *Xenopus* cloned rDNAs, the various spacer regions have different levels of conservation. The data in Figure 13, it should be emphasized, measure the *average* situation for the 2000 to 4000 rDNA units in wheat species.

The ranking of the *Triticum* species for each of the probes shown in Figure 13 is remarkably constant with only the tightly grouped species of *T. searsii*, *T. tauschii*, and *T. dichasians* sometimes changing their relative ranking. One notable exception to this was *T. speltoides*, assayed with either an 18S or 26S rDNA probe, which showed a ΔTm of 1 to 2°C compared to no detectable ΔTm for all the other species examined. In view of the fact that all the spacer sequences suggest that *T. speltoides* rDNA is most closely related to *T. aestivum*

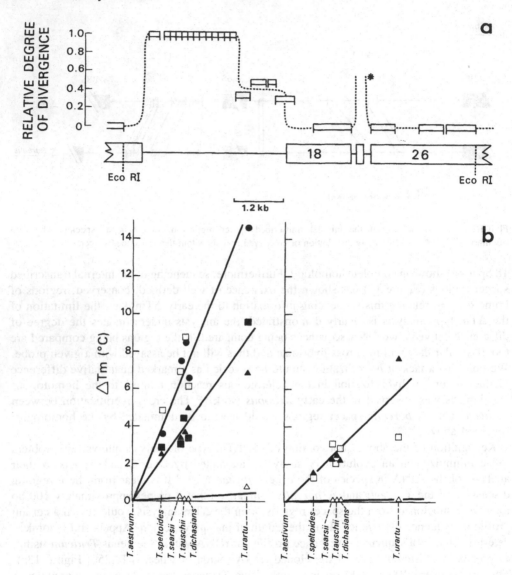

FIGURE 13. The evolutionary divergence profile of *Triticum* rDNA. The evolutionary diverge profile (a) was plotted using the restriction enzyme map of the rDNA clone pTA250 from wheat (see Figure 6 for details) and the degree of evolutionary change estimated from plots of the type shown in (b). The data in (b) are discussed by Appels and Dvorak[227]; a number of different probes were derived from pTA250 and used to hybridize the DNA from the 6 species indicated. The ΔTm of the nucleic acid hybrid was determined using *T. aestivum* as a standard. The ΔTm estimates are plotted on the Y axis, while the X axis is an arbitrary evolutionary distance between the species chosen so that the data could be analyzed as linear regressions. The maximum slope of the lines was subsequently normalized to a divergence of 1.0 in order that each probe could be assigned a relative degree of evolutionary divergence used to give the plot in the upper panel (a).

rDNA this result clearly indicates a situation requiring further analysis by cloning the rDNA from *T. speltoides*. This example also indicates the danger of relying on only a few sequences to develop an evolutionary relationship between species.

The use of the ΔTm parameter in an evolutionary study, in the case of the grasses examined by Dvorak and Appels, was valid in the sense that within-species variation of this parameter was less than between-species variation. It is thus, a more useful parameter than restriction enzyme length variation. In using the Tm parameter at a fine level of resolution (0.5°C) it has been noted[228] that the probe hybridized to the genomic DNA can yield a Tm significantly higher than the probe hybridized to itself. This is interpreted as indicating the assay of a hybrid in the genomic DNA which is only a portion of the probe; this problem is usually minimized by using a small probe (100 bp or smaller).

C. Sequence Analyses

In principle, the DNA sequence of a region of interest is the "ultimate" for an evolutionary study. This, however, is not feasible for the spacer region of rDNA units tandemly repeated hundreds or thousands of times even if an extremely large effort is mounted to obtain the data. In this regard it should be noted that direct estimates of the degree of homogeneity at the rDNA spacer regions within an individual have not been made and it is not clear how many rDNA units would need to be sequenced to describe the entire population of units. The cloning of many rDNA units from a number of organisms and the sequencing of them is difficult to justify on the grounds of an evolutionary study alone. If, however, a specific region of a cloned rDNA unit from a key organism is identified using a combination of the restriction enzyme and ΔTm approaches, as described in the preceding section, it may be possible to collect sequence information about this region from a number of species rather rapidly. A sequencing strategy which eliminates the need for cloning is likely to be most valuable for studying a repeated unit such as rDNA in many different species. The sequencing strategy developed by Qu et al.[229] is based on the observation that certain regions of the rRNA genes are highly conserved over extensive evolutionary distances. These regions are interspersed with divergent regions. The conserved regions from well-characterized rDNA units such as those described in detail in Section III can provide sequence "primers" by hybridizing to rRNA. The primer can, with the developing chemical DNA synthesis techniques, be made as a single strand segment corresponding to the sequence of the particular region of interest. The primer-rRNA complex provides a template for the enzyme reverse-transcriptase and this reaction, together with the use of dideoxy ribonucleotide triphosphates allows sequence information to be obtained in the region upstream from the primer using well-established techniques. This strategy can analzye the divergent regions of rRNA from a wide array of species at a nucleotide sequence level without cloning the rDNA each time. An analogous but more general approach has been described by Church and Gilbert.[230] In this case the standard chemical reactions for DNA sequencing[231] are carried out on restriction enzyme cut DNA (unlabeled). After separating DNA fragments on a sequencing gel they are transferred to nylon filters and hybridized with a suitable single-stranded, radioactive probe. The resulting ladders in the sequencing tracts give the sequence from the point of hybridization of the radioactive probe. Alternatively, rDNA can be highly purified on ac-tinomycin-D/CsCl gradients[93,232] and the strands of the rDNA (visualized by ethidium bromide staining) separated by gel electrophoresis. These strands of rDNA may then provide suitable material, using appropriate primers, for DNA sequencing of the spacer without first purifying individual rDNA units by cloning.

Kossel et al.[221] have argued that T_1-oligonucleotide mapping of rRNA sequences is a valuable taxonomic character to monitor. Although this method is limited to the RNA product of the gene it can contribute to a broad classification of organisms.

V. NATURE OF EVOLUTIONARY CHANGE AT THE rDNA LOCUS

A. Individual and Population Variation

Intra-individual, intrapopulational, and interpopulational (intraspecific) variation at the rDNA locus can be partitioned into several types of variation, including number of chromosomal sites (or chromosomal distribution of rDNA), gene copy number differences, repeat unit length variation, and sequence variation. The primary source of the location of repeat

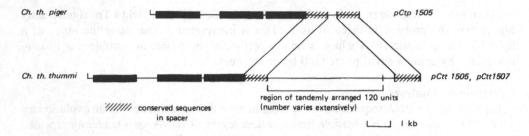

FIGURE 14.   Summary diagram of a comparison between the rDNA of two *Chironomus* species.[237]

length variation can be mapped to the spacer region as well as the external transcribed spacer (ETS), ITS-1 and ITS-2, and in certain cases the intervening sequences found in the large rRNA gene. In addition, some sequence variation has been mapped to gene regions (both small and large rRNA genes).

The location of rRNA genes and the number of rRNA genes at a chromosomal site show considerable intrachromosomal and interchromosomal variation. This type of variation is greater or more evident in organisms possessing multiple sites of ribosomal genes. There are 5 known sites of rDNA in humans (chromosomes 13, 14, 15, 20, and 21), and the copy number of rRNA genes at these 5 sites varies within and among individuals.[233,234,235] In addition, this variation in copy number is inherited.[234] As discussed in Section III, a similar variation in terms of chromosomal sites and copy numbers can be seen within and among varieties of wheat, *Triticum aestivum*, as well as within and among inbred strains of the mouse, *Mus musculus*. Similar variation has been seen in asexual species. In the hybrid parthenogenetic grasshopper species, *Warramaba virgo*, different combinations of chromosomal sites have been found for the two major groups of clones which are of separate origin.[236] Although certain chromosomal locations have been inherited directly from the sexual ancestors of the parthenogenetic groups, certain chromosomal sites of those original ancestors have been lost subsequent to the hybridization event and the formation of the parthenogenetic species. Within the asexual or parthenogenetic species, considerable inter-clonal (populational) variation in terms of rRNA gene copy number can also be observed.

By far the most common type of rDNA variation seen at the individual and populational level is repeat unit length variation as detected by restriction enzyme analysis, and this type of variation has been detected in plants, protozoans, insects, amphibians and mammals. This variation indicates that there is more than one class of rDNA repeating unit, and a large amount of such variation can be related directly to the spacer in several species has revealed the presence of repetitive sequences (Figure 1; see also Section III). These sequences consist of subunits defined by certain restriction enzymes, and the deletion or duplication of these subunits relates directly to length variation at the rDNA locus. Although intra- and interindividual length variation is not correlated with the number of chromosomal sites for the rDNA locus, interactions and patterns of variation between multiple sites in various species can be very different.

One illustration of how such spacer variation can be visualized is seen in the insect species *Chironomus thummi*. Analyses of *C. thummi* have shown that a tandem array of 120 bp repeating subunits defined by the restriction enzyme Cla I occur in a localized region of the spacer.[237,238] Considerable length heterogeneity (10 to 16 kb) has been seen in the subspecies *C. t. thummi* (both between strains and individuals), and this heterogeneity can be related to the number of 120 bp repeating units. Intraspecific variation between the subspecies *C. t. thummi* and *C. t. piger* has been shown to result from the presence or absence of 120 bp units (Figure 14). Some insight into the mechanism of the gain or loss of repeated units may be obtained by examining the *Chironomus* example. Repeating units defined by Cla I

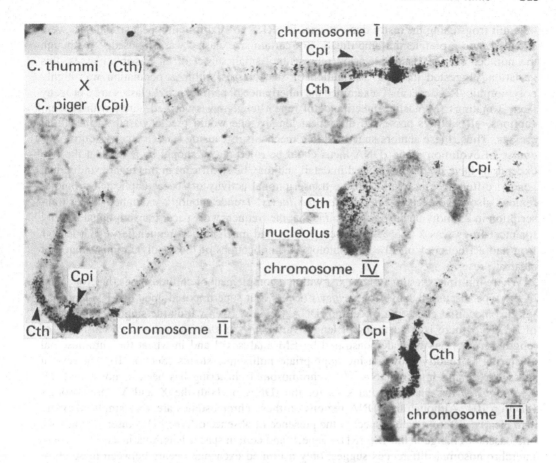

FIGURE 15.   Chromosomal distribution of the Cla-elements found in both the rDNA spacer and centromere region of *Chironomus thummi thummi*. *In situ* hybridization of cloned, highly repetitive, Cla-elements to the polytene chromosomes of an F_1 hybrid between *Ch. th. piger* and *Ch. th. thummi* is shown. The Cla-elements hybridize mainly to centromeric regions (C_{th} = *thummi*-homologue, C_{pi} = *piger*-homologue) of all chromosomes (I — IV), but in *Ch. th. thummi* also to the nucleolus and to many other chromosomal sites.

found in the spacer are homologous to a similar class of repeats in the centromere,[239] and these repeats have certain similarities to transposable elements. At the points of divergence of the spacer sequences of the *Chironomus* species, $\frac{AAAAAA}{TTTTTT}$ tracts were found at one end and $\frac{TTTTT}{AAAAAA}$ tracts were found at the other end, suggestive of a transposon-type mechanism having resulted in the presence of centromeric DNA in the rDNA spacer.[237] Consistent with this notion is the observation of numerous other chromosomal sites for this sequence (Figure 15). Whether this provides an appropriate model which can partially explain the deletion or addition of repeats in the spacer of organisms showing this type of variation remains to be seen. However, IVS seen in *Drosphila* appear to have transposition qualities,[240,403] and repeating elements in the spacer of *Mus musculus*[242] and human[241] have been found in other parts of the genome.

Although the rDNA locus occurs on only one pair of chromosomes in *X. laevis*, considerable repeat length variation within and between individuals has been detected (Section III), and the number of length variants is less discrete than the number seen in other organisms. As discussed in Section III, this length variation can be related directly to spacer variation, and results from the deletion or duplication of repetitive subunits. In a genetic analysis of

45 adult frogs using the restriction enzyme, EcoRI, 2 to 10 different repeat size classes were detected, and a preferential amplification of certain size classes was proposed.[179] Although the number of size classes detected represents a small subset of all possible classes, this variation suggested that the distribution of size classes within a population was highly polymorphic. Reeder et al.[178] examined the inheritance of particular size classes in 50 progeny from 3 matings. Mendelian inheritance of repeat lengths was verified, since with two exceptions, all siblings possessed the repeat lengths one would predict based on the initial crosses. Thus, these authors suggested that mechanisms causing sudden changes during the course of evolution at the rDNA locus could be ruled out; it should be noted that the two exceptions have not been analyzed in detail and may be significant in this regard. Individual genetic differences in relation to the transcriptional activity of spacer duplicated promoter regions also have been detected in *Xenopus laevis*. Trendelenburg[171] examined spacer transcription in 25 individual frogs and found that the frequency of spacer transcriptional activity for most frogs was 2 to 5%. However, 3 frogs had much higher frequencies and at least 1 frog had a frequency of 70%. The biological implications of these polymorphisms are not clear at present.

Where multiple sites for rDNA exist within a complement of chromosomes, heterogeneity of the type discussed above for *X. laevis* occurs, but superimposed upon this is a tendency for chromosomal clustering of certain rDNA variants. Even within the single rDNA region of *X. laevis* there is a clustering of length variants.[243] In *Batophora oerstedii* clustering of length variants has been demonstrated by EM analyses[244] and in wheat the chromosomal clustering is readily shown using appropriate nullisomic stocks (Section III). In several grasses[245,246] and human rDNA,[247,427] chromosomal clustering has been demonstrated. *D. melanogaster* has chromosomal sites for the rDNA on both the X and Y chromosomes (Section III). Although the rDNA regions on these chromosomes are very similar they are also clearly different with respect to the presence or absence of type I IVS inserts,[121] at least one basepair change in the 18S rRNA gene,[47] and certain spacer length variants.[220,248] These interchromosomal differences suggest only a limited exchange occurs between these chromosomes. The basis for the co-evolution of the rDNA units on more than one chromosme with respect to their overall similarity is most readily envisaged as a result of the combined effects of selective forces[249] and occasional exchange between the chromosomes. Recombination between the rDNA of the *Drosophila* X and Y chromosomes has been well studied at the level of generating X-Y translocations.[114,250,251] During the course of evolution, however, *double* exchange events or gene conversions must have occurred because the X and Y chromosomes have remained as separate entities. Repeat length variation in *Drosophila* species is discrete with at least 10 size classes known,[117,252] and the normal range of this spacer associated variation is between 3 to 6 kb.[148,219] Intervening sequences are major contributors to this length variation. Rae[253] has proposed a model involving unequal crossing over, with the 14 bp duplications flanking the IVSs (see Figure 8) serving as regions of homology for generating IVSs twice the length of the original as well as a 28S rRNA gene lacking the IVS. Variation or heterogeneity in length can also be related to the number of 250 bp repeats (defined by Alu I) in the spacer,[254] and like *Xenopus* these repeats share homologies with the transcription initiation site.[119,255] In general, length variation of these types if characteristic for *Drosophila*[148] and other dipterans including *Chironomus*,[237] *Sarcophaga*,[256] and *Calliphora*.[257]

Two mammals, man and mouse, demonstrate certain features of spacer repeat length variation at the population level which are worth discussing in light of the *Drosophila* data. In man, repeat length heterogeneity resulting from variation in spacer length is discrete with five known size classes varying in amount (copy number) from individual to individual,[207,258-261] and this type of heterogeneity is known for other primates as well.[262,439] A major variable region has been mapped 1.5 kb downstream from the 3' end of the 28S rRNA gene,[259] and the restriction enzymes (Bgl I or Bam HI) demonstrate length polymorphism.[258,259] Krystal and Arnheim[258] indicate that different nucleolar organizers (on different chromosomes) have the same length variants, thus suggesting interchromosomal exchange between different NORs. In mouse, 15 different size classes resulting from the deletion or duplication of 135 bp repeats (defined as Sal I) are known,[197,199,207] and variation has been mapped to a major VrDNA region (see Figure 11) of the spacer. The number and amount of these size classes have been shown to vary from individual to individual as well as between strains.[197,207] Unlike man, however, interchromosomal exchange in mouse appears to be limited and interchromosomal divergence in terms of fragment length polymorphisms is greater since certain fragment classes can be assigned to specific chromosomes.[196] Arnheim[263] has suggested that the difference between mouse and man relates to the chromosomal location of the rDNA region. The centromeric location of rDNA in mouse is argued to result in some conversion to avoid the translocation problem. The clear differentiation of rDNA loci in the situations of the type found in mice and in wheat may therefore reflect the presence of more efficient intralocus homogenization mechanisms (e.g., unequal crossing-over, demonstrated experimentally in yeast[264,265])or a more recent separation of the rDNA loci on an evolutionary time scale.

Several types of sequence differences in addition to fragment length variation such as that seen in the spacer also occur in the rDNA locus at the population level. The first such difference is restriction enzyme site polymorphisms. In man, two restriction enzymes (Hind III and EcoRI) vary in terms of the presence or absence of additional sites from one repeat to another. The Hind III polymorphism occurs as a result of the presence or absence of an additional enzyme site in the 28S gene,[259,262] and this polymorphism is old since it is widespread in other primate species.[262] Krystal et al.[235] determined the frequency of this polymorphism to be 30% for one Hind III site and 70% for two Hind III sites. The EcoRI site polymorphism has been mapped to the 5' end of the spacer[259] with an extra EcoRI site being present 80% of the time.[235,258] This polymorphism also occurs in chimpanzee, pygmy chimpanzee, and gorilla.[262] The second type of sequence variation is within individual variation resulting from sequence changes between subrepeats in the spacer. Unlike *Xenopus*, which has no sequence divergence between spacer subrepeat units, the mouse has 13% sequence divergence among the 13 copies of the 135 bp repeating unit.[209] Unfortunately, data of this kind for man and *Drosophila* are not available.

Microheterogeneity also occurs in the transcribed spacer regions. In *Xenopus laevis*, the external transcribed spacer (TS) and the internal transcribed spacers (ITS-1 and ITS-2) are not repetitious.[168,266] Thus, this type of heterogeneity is unlike that seen in the main spacer region with most of the differences between repeats resulting from basepair substitutions and small insertions and deletions.[168] No two transcription units have identical transcribed spacers out of all the cloned amplified, uncloned amplified, and cloned chromosomal rDNA repeats sequenced. From the 1100 nucleotides examined, 20 sites of variation were detected. Furlong and Maden[267] have found similar ITS microheterogeneity in *Xenopus borealis*.

B. Differentiation at the Species Level and Above

Interspecific comparisons of sequence divergence at the rDNA locus have confirmed early observations that different components of this locus evolve at different rates, and that these components have different limits of resolution relative to the level of phylogenetic inference being made. The most evolutionary conservative regions of the rDNA locus are the 18S (small), 5.8S, and 28S (large) rRNA genes, and these regions seem better as phylogenetic probes for higher taxonomic comparisons such as interordinal and above. The 3' ends of the 18S and 28S rRNA genes are highly conserved and sequence homology has been found between pro- and eukaryotes in these regions.[19,95,96,268,269] Out of the 670 nucleotides sequenced in the 18S gene, 1 bp difference was found between the 3′ ends of *Xenopus borealis* and *X. laevis*.[267] This same region is also conserved in more distantly related vertebrates since only 8 differences out of 230 bp sequenced were detected between *Rattus* and *Xenopus*; however, 42 bp differences were detected between the insects *Drosophila* and *Bombyx*.[182] In *D. melanogaster* the terminal 111 nucleotides upstream of the 28S rRNA gene (3′ termination site) were found to be 60% homologous with *Xenopus* and *Saccharomyces*, whereas no homology was detected downstream in the NTS.[141] Kominami et al.[203] examined 300 bp around the 3′-terminus of the 28S rRNA genes and found a 7 bp sequence which was closely related among mouse (GGTTTGT), *Drosophila* (GATTCGA), yeast (GATTTGT), and possibly *Xenopus*. Upstream of the 3′ termination site, mouse and *Xenopus* were 80% homologous with a drop in homology to 40% in the first 128 bp in the spacer.

Overall, the 18S gene seems to be more conserved than the 29S gene.[269,270] Sequence comparisons of the entire 18S genes of *Xenopus* and *Saccharomyces* (yeast) indicate extensive but interrupted areas of homology.[19] Using heteroduplex comparisons of two mammals, Triezenberg et al.[269] found high homology between the 18S genes of man and the Syrian hamster (*Mesocricetus auratus*), whereas the 28S genes, especially at the 5′ end, were more divergent with homologous tracts interrupted by tracts of low homology. These authors showed a greater decline in sequence homology at the 28S 5′ end as taxonomic distance increased. Similar trends were demonstrated by Gourse and Gerbi[268] in DNA-DNA hybridization comparisons among *Xenopus*, *Dictylostelium* (slime mold), *Saccharomyces* (yeast), and *E. coli*. Somewhat higher estimates of 28S 5′ end sequence homologies were found by sequencing the first 100 nucleotides of the 28S gene in *Mus*, *Xenopus*, and *Saccharomyces*.[271] *Mus* and *Xenopus* were 91% homologous with both showing 80% of their sequences in common with *Saccharomyces*. At the species level, only 1 bp substitution at the 5′ end of the 28S gene has been found between *Xenopus borealis* and *X. laevis*,[267] and the region of the 26S rRNA gene where the intervening sequence occurs in *Tetrahymena* was found to be 100% homologous between two species.[76]

Although somewhat less conserved than the 18S rRNA genes, sequence homology in the 5.8S gene can be seen between distantly related taxa. Homology of 70% has been found between yeast and *Xenopus*,[272,273] and this gene region is even more conserved among vertebrates.[200]

Direct sequencing around the 5′ transcription initiation site indicated that little homology exists between distantly related eukaryotes; however, more closely related species share certain homologous sequences. In comparisons of 3 lower eukaryotes (*D. discoideum*, *S. cerevisiae*, and *T. pyriformis*), 9 nucleotides downstream of the initiation site were found to be similar.[244] Long et al.[140] in their comparisons of *D. melanogaster*, *X. laevis*, and *S. cerevisiae* found a similar 9 nucleotides downstream. However, in both these studies the 9 nucleotides were not identical among the species examined and their position relative to the mapped initiation site varied. Again, little homology was found when mouse was compared to *Xenopus*, *Saccharomyces*, and *Drosophila*.[213,226] In mammals an increase in sequence homologies around the initiation site has been detected. Financsek et al.[275] found 77% homology upstream (167 bp examined) and 51% downstream (127 bp examined) of the initiation site in comparisons between the murid rodents *Mus* (mouse) and *Rattus* (rat). Likewise, human and mouse share a perfect 15 bp homology downstream of the initiation site.[46] Comparisons of 3 *Xenopus* species (*X. clivii*, *X. borealis*, and *X. laevis*) indicated that a 13 bp sequence around the initiation site was conserved. The overall sequence homology out of 245 bp around the initiation site was 82% for *X. laevis* to *X. clivii* and 63% for *X. laevis* to *X. borealis*.[226] Treco et al.[276] used this value of 63% for *X. laevis*-*X. borealis* comparisons to indicate that the rate of change in this region is about 1% nucleotide change every 0.4 million years. Although homologous regions have been found between different orders of mammals, this particular region probably has more phylogenetic resolving power at the familial level and below, and will probably be best at the generic level as shown by the *Xenopus* comparisons.

As indicated by early comparative studies of *X. laevis* and *X. borealis,* the rRNA gene regions are highly conserved relative to both transcribed and NTS sequences.[225] These spacer sequences and in certain cases the IVS are most effective as phylogenetic probes when one is comparing species within the same genus or populations within a species.

The most conserved part of the ITS has been found in ITS-2 immediately downstream of the 5.8S rRNA gene.[200] This particular region is conserved in vertebrates with a 13 nucleotide stretch being identical in mouse and rat and only two differences between these mammals and *Xenopus.* Similar comparisons of the ITS to more distantly related eukaryotes such as yeast show little sequence homology.[200,271] ITS-1 and ITS-2 have been totally sequenced for *Xenopus laevis* and *X. borealis*[267] and the mammal species mouse and rat.[201] Besides certain minor differences, ITS sequence divergence between the two *Xenopus* species as well as the two mammal species show similar patterns, and these patterns were mentioned earlier for *Xenopus* (Figure 12, Section IV). The ITSs are nonrepetitive and the two spacers (ITS-1 and ITS-2) are not related in sequence. In both cases, highly conserved sequences are shared between species, and these conserved sequences are interspersed with and laterally displaced by highly divergent sequences. Furlong and Maden[267] suggest that the displacement is the result of deletions, insertions, and possibly point mutations. The lengths of ITS-1 between species are similar, whereas ITS-2 lengths are different. In mouse the ITS-2 is 1089 bp and in rat 765 bp, and *Xenopus borealis* has a much larger ITS-2 than *X. laevis.* ITS-1 is more homologous (75%) than ITS-2 (30%) between rat and mouse. In contrast, ITS-1 (11%) is less homologous than ITS-2 (36%) in comparisons of the two *Xenopus* species. As have been found in comparisons of vertebrates in general, the most conserved region is the one located 3' to the 5.8S rRNA gene.

Comparisons of IVSs which insert in the 28S rRNA gene have been made for certain *Tetrahymena* species and these introns seem to be good phylogenetic probes for at least species level comparisons and possibly familial comparisons in *Drosophila. Tetrahymena thermophila* and *T. pigmentosa* are 93% homologous out of the 413 nucleotides sequenced for the IVS.[76] The types of changes between the two intervening sequences are found to be basepair substitutions (8 transitions, 14 transversions), and the 5' end was more conserved than the 3' end. Barnett and Rae,[277] using melting point analysis, indicated that the IVS of *D. virilis* and *D. melanogaster* differ in size, but share considerable sequence homologies even with more distantly related dipterans such as *Sarcophaga* and *Musca* (both of which are in the same suborder as the *Drosophila* species).

By far the most extensive data base for interspecific relationships at the rDNA locus comes from systematic comparisons of variation in the spacer. These comparisons have been based primarily on restriction enzyme analyses. Site variation as detected by these restriction enzymes has been used in conjunction with data on gene copy number and the chromosomal location of repeat classes to develop ideas concerning the overall mode of evolution at the rDNA locus. In some cases these restriction enzyme studies provide rather congruent phylogenies with respect to phylogenies produced by other data. However, the partitioning of variation in a phylogeny and the resulting phylogeny can sometimes be either vague or contrary to existing ideas concerning relationships.

Most evolutionary studies have confirmed the idea that the spacer region is the fastest evolving component of the rDNA locus. As discussed in Section IV, sequencing studies of certain spacer components in *Xenopus laevis, X. clivii,* and *X. borealis* have confirmed the divergent nature of the spacer relative to the gene regions.[226] Although the spacer-ETS boundaries around the transcription initiation site demonstrated homology between *Xenopus* species, little sequence conservation was found in the spacers of *X. laevis* and *X. clivii*. Only 8 nucleotides were held in common between two repetitive regions and 14 nucleotides between two additional regions.

In plants, assessments of relationships using spacer-specific probes and temperature melting experiments have provided a detailed description of the different rates of evolutionary divergence of the various components of the rDNA unit (see Section IV). Dvorak and Appels[90] ranked 19 *Triticum* and related species using 2 spacer probes, namely a 133 bp Hha I sequence which is repeated within the spacer and a 750 by Hha I sequence located in a unique position near the start of transcription (this sequence is probably equivalent to the ETS region; see Section III). Three species deserve detailed comments since they indicate that measurements of spacer sequence divergence can be correlated with the expected divergence between the respective species based on other taxonomic parameters. *T. dicoccoides* is a tetraploid in the *T. aestivum* lineage and shows a $\triangle$Tm of 1°C, using the 133 bp sequence, for the rDNA loci located on chromosomes 1 and 6B. *T. araraticum* is a tetraploid not in the same *T. aestivum* lineage as *T. dicoccoides* but still having its rDNA loci located on chromosomes 1 and 6B (as defined by meiotic pairing homology[90]), and showed a $\triangle$Tm of 2.7°C. *T. speltoides* is a diploid species belonging to a group of species in the section *Sitopsis* which are closely related to the species which originally donated the B genome of *T. aestivum*. The rDNA chromosomes of *T. speltoides* have been shown to be 1 and 6B (as defined by meiotic pairing[92]) and show a $\triangle$Tm of 3.5°C using the 133 bp probe. Qualitatively similar results were obtained using the 750 bp probe, although differences in $\triangle$Tm are not as great; it should also be noted that the $\triangle$Tm for the 133 bp probe are means based on DNA preparations from 46 *T. dicoccoides* individuals, 6 *T. araraticum*, and 51 *T. speltoides* individuals isolated from various natural populations. It is clear from these data that the $\triangle$Tm parameter of the rDNA spacer sequence correlates well with the evolutionary relatedness of the species as determined using independent criteria. The absolute time which has elapsed since the formation of the hexaploid *T. aestivum* from a *T. dicoccoides* × *T. tauschii* cross is at least 10,000 years, [278] and as the rDNA of *Triticum* species is characterized further, this should provide a time scale for the accumulation of nucleotide sequence change.

Restriction enzyme analyses at the rDNA locus have been used with varying degrees of success in other evolutionary studies. Wilson et al.[279] compared a 16 kb region surrounding the transcription initiation site among certain primates (man, pygmy chimpanzee, common chimpanzee, gorilla, gibbon, and rhesus monkey). The phylogeny produced from a numerical analysis was similar to the usual primate order, wherease that produced by a cladistic approach was somewhat different. The differences related to the placement of gibbon closer than orangutan to the other great apes and the placement of chimpanzee closer to man than gorilla. In this instance the conflict may be due to the small number of restriction sites available for anlysis. An earlier study by Nelkin et al.[280] on primates using restriction enzyme analyses on rDNA confirmed certain relationships depicted by Wilson et al.,[279] and demonstrated fairly good congruence with the known taxonomic relationships of certain additional taxa.

Similar restriction enzyme anlyses have been conducted on *Chlamydomonas* species,[281] *Tetrahymena* species,[282] and ciliated protozoans.[283] In the case of *Tetrahymena* the phylogenetic relationships determined by rDNA restriction enzyme analyses were different from existing phylogenies, and the apportionment of restriction fragments reveals considerable homoplasy (convergence and parallelism).

Information on divergence of spacer sequences in *Drosophila* is more complicated. Even though comparisons of two *Drosophila* subgenera (represented by *D. melanogaster* and *D. hydei*) revealed similar 250 bp repeating units in the spacer, the actual sequence homology in this region was very low when the degree of divergence was assayed using Southern blots and restriction enzyme analysis.[284] Species relationships as determined with Southern blots are higher within the subgenus *Drosophila*, and 20 to 30% homology of spacer sequences has been detected between *D. hydei* and *D. virilis* for species within the *D. virilis* group sharing high homology.[148] Again, no homology was detected between the subgenera *Sophophora* (*D. melanogaster*) and *Drosophila* (*D. virilis*). We might add that sequence relatedness was determined by hybridization intensities on Southern blots in the case of the above study, and no direct estimate of sequence homology among the virilis species group were provided. Nevertheless, a large number of restriction fragments were held in common between species. Tartof[249] has suggested that within the *Drosophila melanogaster* species group spacer sequences are as conserved as coding regions. Heteroduplex maps between *D. melanogaster* and *D. yakuba* show greater homology in the spacer than homologies between *X. borealis* and *X. laevis*. In addition, the melting point analysis of *D. simulans*, *D. melanogaster*, and *D. mauritiana* (all closely related) are the same with *D. yakuba*, *D. teissieri*, and *D. erecta* (more divergent taxa) being lower by 2.4 to 3.1°C. Again, the two closer related species (*D. teisseri* and *D. yakuba*)are identical. When spacer variation is examined for all species, the maximum divergence of any species from *D. melanogaster* is a 3.0%, thus suggesting sequence conservation.

Spacer variation within the *Drosophila melanogaster* species group has also been evaluated by Coen et al.,[220] and the patterns of variation as interpreted by these authors suggest that each species has primarily fixed characteristic variants resulting from length variation in the spacer. Within-species variation was considered less than between-species variation. These conclusions are misleading for several reasons. First, they are in conflict with Tartof's[249] data for the same species group which showed high similarity among even divergent species as far as the spacer is concerned. Second, as discussed in Section IV, Coen et al.[219] have published an analysis of spacer variation among 10 strains of *D. melanogaster* derived from the same wild population, and the range of fragment length variation seen among these 10 strains covers the entire range seen for the 7 sibling species of the *D. melanogaster* species group. Third, the fragment length variation at the rDNA locus was not partitioned in a phylogenetic manner by the authors.

As discussed by numerous authors,[227,263,276,285] the tandemly arranged units of the rDNA system appear to evolve in concert. It seems clear that mechanisms such as unequal crossing-over, gene conversion, and sequence transposition between sister and nonsister chromosomes[286-290,416] in combination with random genetic drift and selection, contribute to concerted evolution at the rDNA loci. However, as demonstrated throughout this review, the degree of homogeneity varies from one organism to another. The problem of explaining the evolutionary divergence of rDNA sequences between species may therefore be different from or at least as complicated as explaining homogeneity within an individual, population, or species. Despite the extensive studies on rDNA, relatively little is known (at a quantitative level) about how similar rDNA units are within individuals.[279] Few systematic studies of rDNA divergence among closely related species have been performed and our knowledge of how much sequence variation actually occurs in a population is limited. Although general patterns of rDNA variation have been established, it is evident that considerable work remains to be carried out before evolution at the rDNA locus is fully understood. In this review we have attempted to provide a framework for future evolutionary studies on the rDNA system so that patterns of evolution in this gene system can be related eventually to organismal evolution.

VI. CONCLUSION

Ribosomal RNA genes have been studied at the DNA level in 190 organisms ranging from bacteria to man. The details of these studies are summarized in Table 1 and those organisms in which the rDNA has been cloned and the spacer region analyzed are discussed in greater depth. The driving force for the evolving structure of the rDNA locus appears to be continually higher demands on the amount of rRNA required by organisms for their protein synthesizing machinery. Thus, in lower eukaryotes the rDNA is seen to be amplified in tandem arrays or as extrachromosomal copies while the 5S rDNA begins to be seen independently of the main rDNA unit. In higher eukaryotes the tandem arrays become longer, extrachromosomal copies of rDNA are confined to certain developmental stages, and the spacer regions (generated as a result of the tandem arrangement of the rDNA units) attain defined characteristics. The spacer regions house the transcription initiation signals and in both *Drosophila* sp. and *Xenopus* sp. the repeated sequences preceding transcription initiation contain extensive homology with the transcription initiation signal region. These regions appear to act as sites for sequestering RNA polymerase molecules to increase the efficiency of initiation and produce more rRNA per unit time. Other repeated sequences are also found in the spacer regions of mammals in particular.

The site of initiation of RNA polymerase I varies in sequence from organism to organism and this correlates with the high level of evolutionary change observed in the spacer region. The gene regions, in contrast are highly conserved. The rDNA gene system is therefore suitable for studying phylogenetic relationships among either closely or distantly related species. The appropriate probe can be chosen for the analysis from within either the spacer or gene region. The apparently rapid homogenization of the tandemly arranged rDNA units which occurs in both plants and animals is discussed in relation to using the rDNA gene system in an evolutionary study. The data available suggest that although the homogenization phenomenon necessitates caution in interpreting phylogenetic relationships, the latter can be inferred from the analysis of the rDNA system.

ACKNOWLEDGMENTS

The authors are grateful to Drs. W. Gerlach, J. Dvorak, A. J. Hilliker, D. R. Foran, and P. J. Russell for commenting on sections of this manuscript. Many researchers communicated their data to us prior to publication and we wish to thank all those who are acknowledged in the text as having provided a "personal communication". The photographs showing electron microscopic spreads of nucleolar chromatin (Figure 3a, 4, 10) were kindly provided by Dr. M. Trendelenburg, while Figure 15 was provided by Dr. E. R. Schmidt. The authors appreciate the opportunity to be able to feature these photographs.

REFERENCES

1. We have adopted the terms small and large rRNA genes rather than specifying whether they are a particular S value. Estimates of the size of the rRNA products vary for different organisms. The terms small and large rRNA are generally used in describing yeast mitochondrial rRNA genes and are convenient terms for this review since a wide range of organisms is discussed. Implicit in the use of these more general terms is the assumption that in all organisms the small and large rRNAs are the nucleic acids involved in the assembly of the small and large subunits of the ribosome, respectively.
2. **Kersten, W., Kersten, H., and Szybalski, W.,** Physicochemical properties of complexes between DNA and antibiotics which affect RNA synthesis (Actinomycin, Daunomycin, Cinerubin, Nogalamycin, Chromomycin, Mithramycin, Olivomycin), *Biochemistry,* 5, 236, 1966.
3. **Morrow, J. F., Cohen, S. N., Chang, A. C. Y., Boyer, H. W., Goodman, H. M., and Helling, R. B.,** Replication and transcription of eukaryotic DNA in *Escherichia coli, Proc. Natl. Acad. Sci. U.S.A.,* 71, 1743, 1974.
4. **Tiemier, D. C., Tilghman, S. M., and Leder, P.,** Purification and cloning of a mouse ribosomal gene fragment in coliphage lambda, *Gene,* 2, 173, 1977.
5. **Long, E. O. and Dawid, I. B.,** Repeated genes in eukaryotes, *Ann. Rev. Biochem.,* 43, 727, 1980.
6. **Cullis, C. A.,** Molecular aspects of the environmental induction of heritable changes in flax, *Heredity,* 38, 129, 1977.

7. **Kunz, W., Grimm, C., and Franz, G.,** Amplification and synthesis of rDNA: *Drosophila. Cell Nucleus.* 12, 156, 1982.

8. **Rodland, K. D. and Russell, P. J.,** Regulation of ribosomal RNA cistron number in a strain of *Neurospora crassa* with a duplication of the nucleolus organizer region, *Biochem. Biophys. Acta,* 697, 162, 1982.

9. **Rodland, K. D. and Russell, P. J.,** Segregation of heterogeneous rDNA segments during demagnification of a *Neurospora crassa* strain possessing a double nucleolar organizer, *Curr. Genet.,* 7, 379, 1983.

10. **Jacqmard, A., Kettmann, R., Pryke, J. A., Thiry, M., and Sachs, R. M.,** Ribosomal RNA genes and floral evocation in *Sinapis, Am. Bot.,* 47, 415, 1981.

11. **Dutta, S. K., Williams, N. P., and Mukhopadhyay, D. K.,** Ribosomal RNA genes of *Neurospora crassa:* multiple copies and specificities, *Mol. Gen. Genet.,* 189, 207, 1983.

12. **Gerbi, S. A.,** Fine structure of ribosomal RNA. I. Conservation of homologous regions within ribosomal RNA in eukaryotes, *J. Mol. Biol.,* 106, 791, 1976.

13. **Woese, C. R., Magrum, L. J., Gupta, R., Siegel, R. B., Stahl, D. E., Kop, J., Crawford, N., Brosius, J., Gutell, R., Hogan, J. J., and Noller, H. F.,** Secondary structure model for bacterial 16S ribosomal RNA: phylogenetic, enzymatic and chemical evidence, *Nucleic Acids Res.,* 8, 2275, 1980.

14. **Gerbi, S. A., Gourse, R. L., and Clark, C. G.,** Conserved regions within ribosomal DNA: locations and some possible function, *Cell Nucleus,* 10A, 351, 1982.

15. **Tomioka, N. and Sugiura, M.,** The complete nucleotide sequence of a 16S ribosomal RNA gene from a blue-green alga, *Anacystis nidulans, Mol. Gen. Genet.,* 191, 46, 1983.

16. **Morgan, E. A.,** Ribosomal genes in *Escherichia coli, Cell Nucleus.* 10A, 1, 1982.

17. **Rubtsov, P. M., Muskhanov, M. M., Zakharyev, V. M., Krayev, A. S., Skryabin, K. G., and Bayev, A. A.,** The structure of the yeast ribosomal RNA genes. I. The complete nucleotide sequence of the 18S ribosomal RNA gene from *Saccharomyces cerevisiae, Nucleic Acids Res.,* 8, 5779, 1980.

18. **Torczynski, R., Bollon, A. P., and Fuke, M.,** The complete nucleotide sequence of the rat 18S ribosomal RNA gene and comparison with the respective yeast and frog genes, *Nucleic Acids Res.,* 11, 4879, 1983.

19. **Salim, M. and Maden, B. E. H.,** Nucleotide sequence of *Xenopus laevis* 18S rRNA inferred from gene sequence, *Nature (London),* 291, 205, 1981.

20. **Connaughton, J. F., Rairkar, A., Lockard, R. E., and Kumar, A.,** Primary structure of rabbit 18S ribosomal RNA determined by direct RNA sequence analysis, *Nucleic Acids Res.,* 12, 4731, 1984.

21. **Olsen, G. J., McCarroll, R., and Sogin, M. L.,** Secondary structure of the *Dictyostelium discoideum* small subunit ribosomal RNA, *Nucleic Acids Res.,* 11, 8037, 1983.

22. **Ozaki, T., Hoshikawa, Y., Iida, Y., and Iwabuchi, M.,** Sequence analysis of the transcribed and 5′ non-transcribed regions of the ribosomal RNA genes in *Dictyostelium discoideum, Nucleic Acids Res.,* 12, 4171, 1984.

23. **Douglas, S. E. and Doolittle, W. F.,** Complete nucleotide sequence of the 23 rRNA gene of cyanobacterium, *Anacystis nidulans, Nucleic Acids Res.,* 12, 3373, 1984.

24. **Otsuka, T., Nomiyama, H., Yoshida, H., Kukita, T., Kuhara, S., and Sakaki, Y.,** Complete nucleotide sequence of the 26S rRNA gene of *Physarum polycephalum:* its significance in gene evolution, *Proc. Natl. Acad. Sci. U.S.A.,* 80, 3163, 1983.

25. **Georgiev, O. I., Nikolaev, N., Hadjiolov, A. A., Skryakin, K. G., Zakharyev, J. M., and Bayev, A. A.,** The structure of the yeast ribosomal RNA genes. IV. Complete sequence of the 25S rRNA gene from *Saccharomyces cerevisiae, Nucleic Acids Res.,* 9, 6953, 1981.

26. **Ware, V. C., Tague, B. W., Clark, C. G., Gourse, R. L., Brand, R. C., and Gerbi, S.,** Sequence analysis of 28S ribosomal DNA from the amphibian. *Xenopus laevis, Nucleic Acids Res.,* 11, 7795, 1983.

27. **Hassouna, N., Michot, B., and Bachellerie, J. P.** quoted in **Michot, B., Hassouna, N., and Bachellerie, J. P.,** *Nucleic Acids Res.,* 12, 4259, 1984.

28. **Chan, Y. L., Olvera, J., and Wool, I. G.,** The structure of rat 28S ribosomal ribonucleic acid inferred from the sequence of nucleotides in a gene, *Nucleic Acids Res.,* 11, 7819, 1983.

29. **Maizels, N.,** *Dictyostelium* 17S, 25S, 5S rDNA's lie within a 38,000 base pair repeated unit, *Cell,* 9, 431, 1976.

30. **Tu, J. and Zillig, W.,** Organization of rRNA structural genes in the archaebacterium *Thermoplasma acidophilum, Nucleic Acids Res.,* 10, 7231, 1982.

31. **Free, S. J., Rice, P. W., and Metzenberg, R. L.,** Arrangement of the genes coding for rRNA in *Neurospora crassa, J. Bacteriol.,* 137, 1219, 1979.

32. **Selker, E. U., Yanofsky, C., Driftmier, K., Metzenberg, R. L., Alzner-DeWeerd, B., and Rajbhandary, U. L.,** Dispersed 5S RNA genes in *N. crassa:* structure, expression and evolution, *Cell,* 24, 819, 1981.

33. **Mao, J., Appel, B., Schaack, J., Sharp, S., Yamada, H., and Soll, D.,** The 5S RNA genes of *Schizosaccharomyces pombe. Nucleic Acids Res.,* 10, 487, 1982.

34. **Azad, A. A.,** Intermolecular base-pair interaction between complementary sequences present near the 3′ ends of 5S rRNA and 18S (16S) rRNA might be involved in the reversible association of ribosomal subunits, *Nucleic Acids Res.,* 7, 1913, 1979.

35. **Kennedy, T. D., Hanely-Bowdoin, L. K., and Lane, B. G.,** Structural integrity of RNA and translational integrity of ribosomes in nuclease-treated cell-free protein synthesing systems prepared from wheat germ and rabbit reticulocytes, *J. Biol. Chem.*, 256, 5802, 1981.

36. **Stewart, G. C. and Bott, K. F.,** DNA sequence of the tandem ribosomal RNA promoter for *B. subtilis* operon rrnB, *Nucleic Acids Res.*, 11, 6289, 1983.

37. **Mankin, A. S., Teterina, N. L., Rubtsov, P. M., Baratova, L. A., and Kagramanova, V. K.,** Putative promoter region of rRNA operon from archaebacterium *Halobacterium halobium, Nucleic Acids Res.*, 12, 6537, 1984.

38. **Valenzuela, P., Bell, G. I., Venegas, A., Sewell, E. T., Masiarz, F. R., DeGennaro, L. J., Weinberg, F., and Rutter, W. J.,** Ribosomal RNA genes of *Saccharomyces cerevisiae, J. Biol. Chem.*, 252, 8126, 1977.

39. **Chikaraishi, D. M., Buchanan, L., Danna, K. J., and Harrington, C. A.,** Genomic organization of rat rDNA, *Nucleic Acids Res.*, 11, 6437, 1983.

40. **Mroczka, D. L., Cassidy, B., Busch, H., and Rothblum, L. I.,** Characterization of rat ribosomal DNA, *J. Mol. Biol.*, 174, 141, 1984.

41. **Wilson, F. E. and Stafford, D. W.,** Sea urchin DNA, *Cell Nucleus*, 10A, 271, 1982.

42. **Schibler, U., Wyler, T., and Hagenbuchle, O.,** Changes in size and secondary structure of the ribosomal transcription unit during vertebrate evolution, *J. Mol. Biol.*, 94, 503, 1975.

43. **Rungger, D. and Crippa, M.,** The primary ribosomal DNA transcripts in eukaryotes, *Prog. Biophys. Mol. Biol.*, 31, 247, 1977.

44. **Federoff, N. V.,** On spacers, *Cell*, 16, 697, 1979.

45. **Rothblum, L. I., Reddy, R., and Cassidy, B.,** Transcription initiation site of rat ribosomal DNA, *Nucleic Acids Res.*, 10, 7345, 1984.

46. **Miesfeld, R. and Arnheim, N.,** Identification of the *in vivo* and *in vitro* origins of transcription in human rDNA, *Nucleic Acids Res.*, 10, 3933, 1982.

47. **Yagura, T., Yagura, M., and Muramatsu, M.,** *Drosophila melanogaster* has different ribosomal RNA sequences on X and Y chromosomes, *J. Mol. Biol.*, 133, 533, 1979.

48. **Kohorn, B. D. and Rae, P. M. M.,** Accurate transcription of truncated ribosomal DNA templates in a *Drosophila* cell-free system, *Proc. Natl. Acad. Sci. U.S.A.*, 79, 1501, 1982.

49. **Mishima, Y., Financsek, I., Kominami, R., and Muramatsu, M.,** Fractionation and reconstitution of factors required for accurate transcription of mammalian ribosomal RNA genes: identification of a species-dependent initiation factor, *Nucleic Acids Res.*, 10, 6659, 1982.

50. **Wandelt, C. and Grummt, I.,** Formation of stable preinitiation complexes for ribosomal DNA transcription *in vitro, Nucleic Acids Res.*, 11, 3795, 1983.

51. **Learned, R. M., Smale, S. T., Haltiner, M. M., and Tjian, R.,** Regulation of human ribosomal DNA transcription, *Proc. Natl. Acad. Sci. U.S.A.*, 80, 3558, 1983.

52. **Wilkinson, J. and Sollner-Webb, B.,** Transcription of *Xenopus* ribosomal RNA genes by RNA polymerase I *in vitro, J. Biol. Chem.*, 257, 14375, 1982.

53. **Sollne-Webb, B., Wilkinson, J., Roan, J., and Reeder, R. H.,** Nested control regions promote *Xenopus* ribosomal RNA synthesis by RNA polymerase I, *Cell*, 35, 199, 1983.

54. **Cizewski, V. and Sollner-Webb, B.,** A stable transcription complex directs mouse ribosomal RNA synthesis by RNA polymerase I, *Nucleic Acids Res.*, 11, 7043, 1983.

55. **Miesfeld, R. and Arnheim, N.,** Species-specific rDNA transcription is due to promoter-specific binding factors, *Mol. Gen. Biol.*, 4, 221, 1984.

56. **Yamamoto, O., Takakusa, N., Mishima, Y., Kominami, R., and Muramatsu, M.,** Determination of the promoter region of mouse ribosomal RNA gene by an *in vitro* transcription system, *Proc. Natl. Acad. Sci. U.S.A.*, 81, 299, 1984.

57. **Fried, M. G. and Crothers, D. M.,** CAP and RNA polymerase interactions with the lac promoter: binding stoichiometric and long range effects, *Nucleic Acids Res.*, 11, 141, 1983.

58. **Davison, B. L., Egly, J.-M., Mulvihill, E. R., and Chambon, P.,** Formation of stable preinitiation complexes between eukaryotic class B transcription factors and promoter sequences, *Nature (London)*, 301, 680, 1983.

59. **Dynan, W. S. and Tjian, R.,** Isolation of transcription factors that discriminate between different promoters recognized by RNA polymerase II, *Cell*, 32, 669, 1983.

60. **Stark, M. J. R., Gourse, R. L., and Dahlberg, A. E.,** Site-directed mutagenesis of ribosomal RNA. Analysis of ribosomal RNA deletions using maxi cells, *J. Mol. Biol.*, 159, 417, 1982.

61. **Moss, T.,** A transcription function for the repetitive ribosomal spacer in *Xenopus laevis, Nature (London)*, 302, 223, 1983.

62. **Kohorn, B. D. and Rae, P. M. M.,** Localization of DNA sequences promoting RNA polymerase I activity in *Drosophila, Proc. Natl. Acad. Sci. U.S.A.*, 80, 3265, 1983.

63. **Ferris, P. J., Vogt, V. M., and Truitt, C. L.,** Inheritance of extrachromosomal rDNA in *Physarum polycephalum, Mol. Cell. Biol.*, 3, 635, 1983.

64. **Kruger, K., Grabowski, P. J., Zaug, A. J., Sands, J., Gottschling, D. E., and Cech, T. R.,** Self-splicing RNA: auto-excision and auto-cyclization of the ribosomal RNA intervening sequence of *Tetrahymena, Cell,* 31, 147, 1982.
65. **Cech, T. R.,** RNA splicing: three themes with variations, *Cell,* 34, 713, 1983.
66. **Yu, P.-L., Hohn, B., Falk, H., and Drews, G.,** Molecular cloning of the ribosomal RNA genes of the photosynthetic bacterium *Rhodopseudomonas capsulata, Mol. Gen. Genet.,* 398, 392, 1982.
67. **Jordan, B. R.,** Demonstration of intact 26S ribosomal RNA molecules in *Drosophila* cells, *J. Mol. Biol.,* 98, 277, 1975.
68. **Long, E. O. and Dawid, I. B.,** Alternative pathways in the processing of ribosomal RNA precursor in *Drosophila melanogaster, J. Mol. Biol.,* 138, 873, 1980.
69. **Grant, D. M. and Lambowitz, A. M.,** Mitochondrial ribosomal RNA genes, *Cell Nucleus,* 10A, 387, 1982.
70. **Whitfeld, P. R. and Bottomley, W.,** Organization and structure of chloroplast genes, *Ann. Rev. Plant Physiol.,* 34, 279, 1983.
71. **Clark-Walker, G. D. and Azad, A. A.,** Hybridizable sequences between cytoplasmic ribosomal RNA's and 3 micron circular DNA's of *Saccharomyces cerevisiae* and *Torulopsis glabrata, Nucleic Acids Res.,* 8, 1009, 1980.
72. **Weiner, A. M. and Emery, H. S.,** The rDNA of *Dictyostelium discoideum* and *Physarum polycephalum, Cell Nucleus,* 10A, 127, 1982.
73. **Blackburn, E. H.,** Characterization and species differences of rDNA: protozoans, *Cell Nucleus,* 10A, 145, 1982.
74. **Klukas, C.,** Ribosomal gene organization in *Tetrahymena, Nature (London),* 270, 473, 1977.
75. **Meng-Chao, Y. and Gall, J. G.,** A single integrated gene for ribosomal RNA in a eucaryote, *Tetrahymena pyriformis, Cell,* 12, 121, 1977.
76. **Kan, N. C. and Gall, J. G.,** Sequence homology near the center of the extrachromosomal ribosomal DNA palindrome in *Tetrahymena, J. Mol. Biol.,* 153, 1151, 1981.
77. **Miller, O. L. and Beatty, B. R.,** Nucleolar structure and function. *Handbook of Molecular Cytology,* Lima de Faria, A., Ed., North Holland, Amsterdam, 1969, 605.
78. **Thomas, M., White, R. L., and Davis, R. W.,** Hybridization of RNA to double stranded DNA: formation of R-loops, *Proc. Natl. Acad. Sci. U.S.A.,* 73, 2294, 1976.
79. **Franke, W. W., Scheer, U., Spring, H., Trendelenburg, M. F., and Zentgraf, H.,** Organization of nucleolar chromatin, *Cell Nucleus,* 7, 49, 1979.
80. **Zamb, T. J. and Petes, T. D.,** Analysis of the junction between ribosomal RNA genes and single-copy chromosomal sequences in the yeast *Saccharomyces cerevisiae, Cell,* 28, 355, 1982.
81. **Appels, R., Gerlach, W. L., Dennis, E. S., Swift, H., and Peacock, W. J.,** Molecular and chromosomal organization of DNA sequences coding for the ribosomal RNA's in cereals, *Chromosoma,* 78, 293, 1980.
82. **Flavell, R. B. and O'Dell, M.,** Ribosomal RNA genes in homoeologous chromosomes of groups 5 and 6 in hexaploid wheat, *Heredity,* 37, 377, 1976.
83. **Dvorak, J. and Chen, K.-C.,** Distribution of nonstructural variation between wheat cultivars along chromosome arm 6Bp: evidence from the linkage map and physical map of the arm, *Genetics,* 106, 325, 1984.
84. **Flavell, R. B. and Martini, G.,** The genetic control of nucleolus formation with special reference to common breadwheat, in *Nucleolus,* Cullis, C. A. and Jordan, E. G., Eds., Cambridge University Press, London, 1981.
85. **Miller, T. E., Gerlach, W. L., and Flavell, R. B.,** Nucleolus variation in wheat and rye revealed by *in situ* hybridization, *Heredity,* 45, 377, 1980.
86. **Carozza, M. L.,** Number of sites for ribosomal RNA genes in *Triticum durum: in situ* hybridization to mitotic, meiotic and polytene nuclei, *Z. Pflanzenzucht.,* 87, 300, 1981.
87. **Hutchinson, J. and Miller, T. E.,** The nucleolar organisers of tetraploid and hexaploid wheats revealed by *in situ* hybridization, *Theor. Appl. Genet.,* 61, 285, 1982.
88. **Gerlach, W. L., Miller, T. E., and Flavell, R. B.,** The nucleolus organizers of diploid wheats revealed by *in situ* hybridization, *Theor. Appl. Genet.,* 58, 97, 1980.
89. **Mille, T. E., Hutchinson, J., and Reader, S. M.,** The identification of the nucleolus organiser chromosomes of diploid wheat, *Theor. Appl. Genet.,* 65, 145, 1983.
90. **Dvorak, J. and Appels, R.,** Chromosome and nucleotide sequence differentiation in genomes of polyploid *Triticum* species, *Theor. Appl. Genet.,* 63, 349, 1982.
91. **Riley, R., Unrau, J., and Chapman, V.,** Evidence on the origin of the B genome of wheat, *J. Hered.,* 49, 91, 1958.
92. **Dvorak, J.,** personal communication.
93. **Gerlach, W. L. and Bedbrook. J. R.,** Cloning and characterization of ribosomal RNA genes from wheat and barley, *Nucleic Acids Res.,* 7, 1869, 1979.
94. **Appels, R. and Dvorak, J.,** The wheat ribosomal DNA spacer region: its structure and variation in populations and among species, *Theor. Appl. Genet.,* 63, 337, 1982.

95. **Azad, A. A. and Deacon, N. J.**, The 3'-terminal primary structure of five eukaryotic 18S rRNA's determined by the direct chemical method of sequencing. The highly conserved sequences include an invariant region complementary to eukaryotic 5S rRNA, *Nucleic Acids Res.*, 8, 4365, 1980.

96. **Hagenbuchle, O., Santer, M., Steitz, J. A., and Mans, R. J.**, Conservation of the primary structure of the 3' end of 18S rRNA from eukaryotic cells, *Cell*, 13, 551, 1978.

97. **Peacock, W. J., Gerlach, W. L., and Dennis, E. S.**, Molecular aspects of wheat evolution: repeated DNA sequences, in *Wheat Science — Today and Tomorrow*, Evans, L. T. and Peacock, W. J., Eds., Cambridge University Press, London, 1981, 41.

98. **Darvey, N. L. and Driscoll, C. J.**, Nucleolar behaviour in *Triticum*, *Chromosoma*, 36, 131, 1972.

99. **Jordan, E. G., Bennett, M. D., and Smith, J. B.**, Nucleolar organizers and fibrillar centres in *Triticum aestivum* L. cv. Chinese Spring, *Chromosoma*, 87, 447, 1982.

100. **Jordan, E. G., Martini, G., Bennett, M. D., and Flavell, R. B.**, Nucleolar fusion in wheat, *J. Cell Sci.*, 56, 485, 1982.

101. **Longwell, A. C. and Svihla, G.**, Specific chromosomal control of the nucleolus and of the cytoplasm in wheat, *Exp. Cell Res.*, 20, 294, 1960.

102. **Flavell, R. B. and O'Dell, M.**, The genetic control of nucleolus formation in wheat, *Chromosoma*, 71, 135, 1979.

103. **Martini, G., O'Dell, M., and Flavell, R. B.**, Partial inactivation of wheat nucleolus organizers by the nucleolus organizer chromosomes of *Aegilops umbellulata*, *Chromosoma*, 84, 687, 1982.

104. **Cermeno, M. C., Orellana, J., Santos, J. L., and Lacadena, J. R.**, Nucleolar organizer activity in wheat, rye and derivatives analysed by a silver-staining procedure, *Chromosoma*, 89, 370, 1984.

105. **Appels, R.**, Chromosome structure in cereals: the analysis of regions containing repeated sequence DNA and its application to the detection of alien chromosomes introduced into wheat, in *Genetic Engineering in Plants*, Kosuge, T., Meredith, C. P., and Hollaender, A., Eds., Plenum Press, New York, 1983, 229.

106. **Flavell, R.B., O'Dell, M., and Thompson, W. F.**, Cytosine methylation of ribosomal RNA genes and nucleolus organizer activity in wheat, *Kew Chromosome Conference*, Vol. 2, Brandham, P. E. and Bennett, M. D., Eds., Allen & Unwin, Winchester, Mass., 1983, 11.

107. **Cooper, D. N.**, Eukaryotic DNA methylation, *Hum. Genet.* 64, 315, 1983.

108. **Ellis, T. H. N., Goldsbrough, P. B., and Castleton, J. A.** Transcription and methylation of flax rDNA, *Nucleic Acids Res.*, 11, 3047, 1983.

109. **Macleod, D. and Bird, A.**, Transcription in oocytes of highly methylated rDNA from *Xenopus laevis* sperm, *Nature (London)*, 306, 200, 1983.

110. **Pennock, D. G. and Reeder, R. H.**, *In vitro* methylation of Hpa II sites in *Xenopus laevis* rDNA does not affect its transcription in oocytes, *Nucleic Acids Res.*, 12, 2225, 1984.

111. **Ritossa, F.**, The bobbed locus, in *The genetics and Biology of Drosophila*, Vol. 1B, Ashburner, M. and Novitski, E., Eds., Academic Press, New York, 1976, 801.

112. **Hilliker, A. J. and Appels, R.**, Pleiotropic effects associated with the deletion of heterochromatin surrounding rDNA on the X chromosome of *Drosophila*, *Chromosoma (Berlin)*, 86, 469, 1982.

113. **Hilliker, A. J., Appels, R., and Schalet, A.**, The genetic analysis of *Drosophila* heterochromatin. *Cell*, 21, 607, 1980.

114. **Maddern, R. H.**, Exchange between the ribosomal RNA genes of X and Y chromosomes in *Drosophila melanogaster* males, *Genet. Res.*, 38, 1,1981.

115. **McKnight, S. L. and Miller, O. L.**, Ultrastructural patterns of RNA synthesis during early embryogenesis of *Drosophila melanogaster*, *Cell*, 8, 305, 1976.

116. **Glover, D. M. and Hogness, D. S.**, A novel arrangement of the 18S and 28S sequences in a repeating unit of *Drosophila melanogaster* rDNA, *Cell*, 10, 167, 1977.

117. **Wellauer, P. K. and Dawid, I. B.**, The structural organization of ribosomal DNA in *Drosophila melanogaster*, *Cell*, 10, 193, 1977.

118. **Murtif, V. L. and Rae, P. M. M.**, A transcriptional function for repetitive ribosomal spacers in *Xenopus*? *Nature (London)*, 304, 561, 1983.

119. **Kohorn, B. D. and Rae, P. M. M.**, Nontranscribed spacer sequences promote *in vitro* transcription of *Drosophila* ribosomal DNA, *Nucleic Acids Res.*, 10, 6879, 1982.

120. **Breathnack, R. and Chambon, P.**, Organization and expression of eucaryotic split genes coding for proteins, *Ann. Rev. Biochem.*, 50, 349, 1981.

121. **Tartof, K. D. and Dawid, I. B.**, Similarities and differences in the structure of X and Y chromosomal rRNA genes of *Drosophila*, *Nature (London)*, 263, 27, 1976.

122. **Di Nocera, P. P., Digan, M. E., and Dawid, I. B.**, A family of oligo-adenylate-terminated transposable sequences in *Drosophila melanogaster*, *J. Mol. Biol.*, 168, 715, 1983.

123. **Dawid, I. B. and Wellauer, P. K.**, Ribosomal DNA and related sequences in *Drosophila melanogaster*, *Cold Spring Harbor Symp. Quant. Biol.*, 42, 1185, 1977.

124. **Peacock, W. J., Appels, R., Endow, S., and Glover, D.**, Chromosomal distribution of the major insert in *Drosophila melanogaster* 28S rRNA genes, *Genet. Res.*, 37, 209, 1981.

125. **Appels, R. and Hilliker, A. J.**, The cytogenetic boundaries of the rDNA region within the heterochromatin of the X chromosome of *Drosophila melanogaster* and their relation to male meiotic pairing sites, *Genet. Res.*, 39, 149, 1982.

126. **Glover, D. M., Kidd, S. J., Roiha, H. I., Jordan, B. R., Endow, S., and Appels, R.**, *Biochem. Trans.*, 6, 732, 1978.

127. **Lifschytz, E. and Hareven, D.**, Heterochromatin markers: a search for heterochromatin specific middle repetitive sequences in *Drosophila, Chromosoma (Berlin)*, 86, 429, 1982.

128. **deCicco, D. V. and Glover, D. M.**, A DNA segment from *D. melanogaster* which contains five tandemly repeating units homologous to the major rDNA insertion, *Cell*, 19, 103, 1980.

129. **Kidd, S. J. and Glover, D. M.**, A DNA segment from *D. melanogaster* which contains five tandemly repeating units homologous to the major rDNA insertion, *Cell*, 19, 103, 1980.

130. **Roiha, H. and Glover D. M.**, Duplicated rDNA sequences of variable lengths of flanking the short type I insertions in the rDNA of *Drosophila melanogaster, Nucleic Acids Res.*, 9, 5521, 1981.

131. **Pardue, M. L. and Dawid, I. B.**, Chromosomal locations of 2 DNA segments that flank ribosomal insertion-like sequences in *Drosophila.* Flanking sequences are mobile elements, *Chromosoma*, 83, 29, 1981.

132. **Dawid, I. B., Long, E. O., Di Nocera, P. P., and Pardue, M. L.**, Ribosomal insertion-like elements in *Drosophila melanogaster* are interspersed with mobile elements, *Cell*, 25, 399, 1981.

133. **Pellegrini, M., Manning, J., and Davidson, N.**, Sequence arrangement of the rDNA of *Drosophila melanogaster, Cell*, 10, 213, 1977.

134. **Hawley, R. S. and Tartof, K. D.**, The ribosomal DNA of *Drosophila melanogaster* is organized differently from that of *Drosophila hydei, J. Mol. Biol.*, 163, 499, 1983.

135. **Sharp, Z. D., Gandhi, V. V., and Procunier, J. D.**, X chromosome nucleolus organizer mutants which alter major type I repeat multiplicity in *Drosophila melanogaster, Mol. Gen. Genet.*, 190, 438, 1983.

136. **Renkawitz-Pohl, R., Glätzer, K. H., and Kunz, W.**, Ribosomal RNA genes with an intervening sequence are clustered within the X chromosomal ribosomal DNA in *Drosophila hydei, J. Mol. Biol.*, 148, 95, 1981.

137. **Hennig, W., Vogt, P., Jacob, G., and Siegmund, I.**, Nucleolus organizers in *Drosophila* species of the *repleta* group, *Chromosoma (Berlin)*, 87, 279, 1982.

138. **Long, E. O. and Dawid, I. B.**, Expression of ribosomal DNA insertions in *Drosophila melanogaster, Cell*, 18, 1185, 1979.

139. **Jolly, D. J. and Thomas, C. A.**, Nuclear RNA transcripts from *Drosophila melanogaster* ribosomal RNA genes containing introns, *Nucleic Acids Res.*, 8, 67, 1980.

140. **Long, E. O., Rebbert, M. L., and Dawid, I. B.**, Nucleotide sequence of the initiation site for ribosomal RNA transcription in *Drosophila melanogaster*: comparison of genes with and without insertions, *Proc. Natl. Acad. Sci. U.S.A.*, 78, 1513, 1981.

141. **Mandal, R. K. and Dawid, I. B.**, The nucleotide sequence at the transcription termination site of ribosomal DNA in *Drosophila melanogaster, Nucleic Acids Res.*, 9, 1801, 1981.

142. **Beckingham, K.**, Insect rDNA, *Cell Nucleus*, 10A, 205, 1982.

143. **Kidd, S. J. and Glover, D. M.**, *Drosophila melanogaster* ribosomal DNA containing Type II insertions is variably transcribed in different strains and tissues, *J. Mol. Biol.*, 151, 645, 1981.

144. **Glover, D. M.**, The rDNA of *Drosophila melanogaster, Cell*, 26, 297, 1981.

145. **Glover, D. M.**, Cloned segment of *Drosophila melanogaster* rDNA containing new types of sequence insertion, *Proc. Natl. Acad. Sci. U.S.A.*, 74, 4932, 1977.

146. **Dawid, I. B., Wellauer, P. K., and Long, E. O.**, Ribosomal DNA in *Drosophila melanogaster.* 1. Isolation and characterization of cloned fragments, *J. Mol. Biol.*, 126, 749, 1978.

147. **Kunz, W., Petersen, G., Renkazwitz-Pohl, R., Glätzer, K. H., and Schäfer, M.**, Distribution of spacer length classes and the intervening sequence among different nucleolus organizers in *Drosophila hydei, Chromosoma*, 83, 145, 1981.

148. **Rae, P. M. M., Barnett, T., and Murtiff, V. L.**, Nontranscribed spacers in *Drosophila* ribosomal RNA, *Chromosoma*, 82, 637, 1981.

149. **Franz, G. and Kunz, W.**, Intervening sequences in ribosomal RNA genes and bobbed phenotype in *Drosophila hydei, Nature (London)*, 292, 638, 1981.

150. **Endow, S. A. and Glover, D. M.**, Differential replication of ribosomal gene repeats in polytene nuclei of *Drosophila, Cell*, 17, 597, 1979.

151. **Endow, S. A.**, On ribosomal gene compensation in *Drosophila, Cell*, 22, 149, 1980.

152. **Macgregor, H. C.**, Amplification, polytenization and nucleolus organizers, *Nature (London) New Biol.*, 246, 81, 1973.

153. **Endow, S. A.**, Nucleolar dominance in polytene cells of *Drosophila, Proc. Natl. Acad. Sci. U.S.A.*, 80, 4427, 1983.

154. **Franz, G., Kunz, W., and Grimm, C.**, Determination of the region of rDNA replicated in polytene cells of *Drosophila hydei, Mol. Gen. Genet.*, 191, 74, 1983.

155. **Grimm, C., Kunz, W., and Franz, G.,** The rRNA gene number in *Drosophila hydei* is organ-specifically controlled by sex heterochromatin, *Chromosoma*, 89, 48, 1984.

156. **Hawley, R. S. and Tartof, K. D.,** The effect of mei-41 on rDNA redundancy in *Drosophila melanogaster*, *Genetics*, 104, 63, 1983.

157. **Boncinelli, E., Borghese, A., Grazinia, F., Mantia, G. L., Manzi, A., Mariana, C., and Simeone, A.,** Inheritance of the rDNA spacer in *D. melanogaster*, *Mol. Gen. Genet.*, 189, 370, 1983.

158. **Perkowska, E., Macgregor, H. C., and Birnstiel, M. L.,** Gene amplification in the oocyte mucleus of mutant and wild-type *Xenopus laevis*, *Nature (London)*, 217, 649, 1968.

159. **Brown, D. D. and Weber, C. S.,** Gene linkage by RNA-DNA hybridization, *J. Mol. Biol.*, 34, 681, 1968.

160. **Pardue, M. L.,** Localization of repeated DNA sequences in *Xenopus* chromosomes, *Cold Spring Harbor Symp. Quant. Biol.*, 38, 475, 1973.

161. **Elsdale, T. R., Fischberg, M., and Smith, S.,** A mutation that reduces nucleolar number in *Xenopus laevis*, *Exp. Cell Res.*, 14, 642, 1958.

162. **Kahn, J.,** The nucleolar organizer in the mitotic chromosome complement of *Xenopus laevis*, *J. Microsc. Sci.*, 103, 407, 1962.

163. **Wallace, H. and Birnstiel, M. L.,** Ribosomal cistrons and the nucleolar organizer, *Biochim. Biophys. Acta*, 114, 269, 1966.

164. **Knowland, J. and Miller, L.,** Reduction of ribosomal RNA synthesis and ribosomal RNA genes in a mutant of *Xenopus laevis* which organizes only a partial nucleolus, *J. Mol. Biol.*, 53, 321, 1970.

165. **Brown, D. D. and Dawid, I. B.,** Specific gene amplification in oocytes, *Science*, 160, 272, 1968.

166. **Wellauer, P. K., Reeder, R. H., Carroll, D., Brown, D. D., Deutch, A., Higashinakagawa, T., and Dawid, I. B.,** Amplified ribosomal DNA from *Xenopus laevis* has heterogeneous spacer lengths, *Proc. Natl. Acad. Sci. U.S.A.*, 71, 2823, 1974.

167. **Wellauer, P. K., Dawid, I. B., Brown, D. D., and Reeder, R. H.,** The molecular basis for length heterogeneity in ribosomal DNA from *Xenopus laevis*, *J. Mol. Biol.*, 105, 461, 1976.

168. **Stewart, M. A., Hall, L. M. C., and Maden, B. E. H.,** Multiple heterogeneities in the transcribed spacers of ribosomal DNA from *Xenopus laevis*, *Nucleic Acids Res.*, 11, 629, 1983.

169. **Wellauer, P.K., Reeder, R. H., Dawid, I. B., and Brown, D. D.,** The arrangement of length heterogeneity in repeating units of amplified and chromosomal ribosomal DNA from *Xenopus laevis*, *J. Mol. Biol.*, 105, 487, 1976.

170. **Brown, D. D. and Blackler, A. W.,** Gene amplification proceeds by a chromosome copy mechanism, *J. Mol. Biol.*, 63, 75, 1972.

171. **Trendelenburg, M. F.,** Initiations of transcription at ribosomal distinct promoter sites in spacer regions between pre-RNA genes in oocytes in *Xenopus laevis* : an electron microscopic analysis, *Biol. Cell*, 42, 1, 1981.

172. **Hourcade, D., Dressler, D., and Wolfson, J.,** The amplification of ribosomal DNA involves a rolling circle intermediate, *Proc. Natl. Acad. Sci. U.S.A.*, 70, 2926, 1973.

173. **Dawid, I. B., Brown, D. D., and Reeder, R. H.,** Composition and structure of chromosomal and amplified ribosomal DNA's of *Xenopus laevis*, *J. Mol. Biol.*, 51, 341, 1970.

174. **Boseley, P., Moss, T., Machler, R., Portmann, R., and Birnstiel, M. L.,** Sequence organization of the spacer DNA in a ribosomal gene unit of *Xenopus laevis*, *Cell*, 17, 19, 1979.

175. **Dawid, I. B. and Wellauer, P. C.,** A reinvestigation of the 5'-3' polarity in 40S ribosomal RNA precursor of *Xenopus laevis*, *Cell*, 8, 443, 1976.

176. **Hershfield, V., Boyer, H. W., Yanofsky, C., Lovett, M. A., and Helinsky, D. R.,** Plasmid Col El as a molecular vehicle for cloning and amplification of DNA, *Proc. Natl. Acad. Sci. U.S.A.*, 71, 3455, 1974.

177. **Botchan, P. M., Reeder, R. A., and Dawid, I. B.,** Restriction analysis of the nontranscribed spacers of *Xenopus laevis* ribosomal DNA, *Cell*, 11, 599, 1977.

178. **Reeder, R. H., Brown, D. D., Wellauer, P. K., and Dawid, I. B.,** Patterns of ribosomal DNA spacer lengths are inherited, *J. Mol. Biol.*, 105, 507, 1976.

179. **Buongiorno-Nardelli, M., Amaldi, F., Beccari, E., and Junakovic, N.,** Size of ribosomal DNA repeating units in *Xenopus laevis*: limited individual heterogeneity and extensive population polymorphism, *J. Mol. Biol.*, 110, 105, 1977.

180. **Sollner-Webb, B. and Reeder, R. H.,** The nucleotide sequence of the initiation and termination sites for ribosomal RNA transcription in *X. laevis*, *Cell*, 18, 485, 1979.

181. **Moss, T. and Birnstiel, M. L.,** The putative promoter of a *Xenopus laevis* ribosomal gene is reduplicated, *Nucleic Acids Res.*, 6, 3733, 1979.

182. **Moss, T., Boseley, P. G., and Birnstiel, M. L.,** More ribosomal spacer sequences from *Xenopus laevis*, *Nucleic Acids Res.*, 8, 467, 1980.

183. **Bakken, A., Morgan, G., Sollner-Webb, B., Ruan, J., Busby, S., and Reeder, R. A.,** Mapping of transcription initiation and termination signals on *Xenopus laevis* ribosomal DNA, *Proc. Natl. Acad. Sci. U.S.A.*, 79, 56, 1982.

184. **Trendelenburg, M. F.,** Chromatin structure of *Xenopus* rDNA transcription termination sites. Evidence for a two-step process of transcription termination, *Chromosoma,* 86, 703, 1982.
185. **Franke, W. W., Scheer, U., Spring, H., Trendelenburg, M. F., and Krohne, G.,** Evidence for transcription in apparent spacer intercepts and cleavages in the elongating nascent RNA, *Exp. Cell. Res.,* 100, 233, 1976.
186. **Scheer, U., Trendelenburg, M. F., Krohne, G., and Franke, W. W.,** Lengths and patterns of transcription units in the amplified nucleoli of oocytes of *Xenopus laevis, Chromosoma,* 60, 147, 1977.
187. **Rungger, D., Crippa, M., Trendelenburg, M. F., Scheer, U., and Franke, W. W.,** Visualization of ribosomal DNA spacer transcription in *Xenopus* oocytes treated with flouro-uridine, *Exp. Cell Res.,* 116, 481, 1978.
188. **Mueller, K., Oebbecke, C., and Forster, G.,** Capacity of ribosomal RNA promoters of *E. coli* to bind RNA polymerase, *Cell,* 10, 121, 1977.
189. **Morgan, G. T., Bakken, A. H., and Reeder, R. H.,** Initiation of transcription in ribosomal gene spacers of *Xenopus* oocytes, *J. Cell Biol.,* 91, 365, 1981.
190. **Morgan, G. T., Reeder, R. H., and Bakken, A. H.,** Transcription in cloned spacers of *Xenopus laevis* rDNA, *Proc. Natl. Acad. Sci. U.S.A.,* 80, 6490, 1983.
191. **Reeder, R. H., Roan, J. G., and Dunaway, M.,** Spacer regulation of *Xenopus* ribosomal gene transcription: competition in oocytes, *Cell,* 35, 449, 1983.
192. **Henderson, A. S., Eicher, E. M., Yu, M. T., and Atwood, K. C.,** The chromosomal location of ribosomal DNA sites in the mouse, *Chromosoma,* 49, 155, 1974.
193. **Henderson, A. S., Eicher, E. M., Yu, M. T., and Atwood, K. C.,** Variation in ribosomal RNA gene number in mouse chromosomes, *Cytogen. Cell. Genet.,* 17, 307, 1976.
194. **Elsevier, S. M. and Ruddle, F. H.,** Localization of genes coding for 18S and 28S ribosomal RNA within the genome of *Mus musculus, Chromosoma,* 52, 219, 1975.
195. **Dev, V. G., Tantravahi, R., Miller, D. A., and Miller, O. J.,** Nucleolus organizers in *Mus musculus* subspecies in the RAG mouse cell line, *Genetics,* 86, 389, 1977.
196. **Arnheim, N. and Kuehn, M.,** The genetic behaviour of a cloned mouse ribosomal DNA segment mimics mouse ribosomal gene evolution, *J. Mol. Biol.,* 134, 743, 1979.
197. **Arnheim, N., Treco, D., Taylor, B., and Eicher, E. M.,** Distribution of ribosomal gene length variants among mouse chromosomes, *Proc. Natl. Acad. Sci. U.S.A.,* 79, 4677, 1982.
198. **Arnheim, N. and Southern, E. M.,** Heterogeneity of the ribosomal genes in mice and men, *Cell,* 11, 363, 1977.
199. **Cory, S. and Adams, J. M.,** A very large repeating unit of mouse DNA containing the 18S, 28S, 5.8S rRNA genes, *Cell,* 11, 795, 1977.
200. **Bachellerie, J.-P., Michot, B., and Raynal, F.,** Recognition signals for mouse pre-rRNA processing. A potential role for U3 nucleolar RNA, *Mol. Biol. Rep.,* 1983.
201. **Michot, B., Bachellerie, J.-P., and Raynal, F.,** Structure of mouse rRNA precursors. Complete sequence and potential folding of the spacer regions between 18S and 28S rRNA, *Nucleic Acids Res.,* 11, 3375, 1983.
202. **Kominami, R., Urano, Y., Mishima, Y., Muramatsu, M., Moriwaki, K., and Yoshikura, H.,** Novel repetitive sequence families showing size and frequency polymorphism in the genomes of mice, *J. Mol. Biol.,* 165, 209, 1983.
203. **Kominami, R., Mishima, Y., Urano, Y., Sakai, M., and Muramatsu, M.,** Cloning and determination of the transcription termination site of ribosomal RNA gene of the mouse, *Nucleic Acids Res.,* 10, 1963, 1982.
204. **Mishima, Y., Sakai, M., Muramatsu, M., Kataoka, T., and Honjo, T.,** Purification and cloning of a ribosomal RNA gene fragment from mouse DNA, *Proc. Jpn. Acad.,* B54, 657, 1978.
205. **Arnheim, N.,** Characterization of mouse ribosomal gene fragments purified by molecular cloning, *Gene,* 7, 83, 1979.
206. **Grummt, I., Soellner, C., and Scholz, I.,** Characterization of a cloned ribosomal fragment from mouse which contains the 18S coding region and adjacent spacer sequences, *Nucleic Acids Res.,* 6, 1351, 1979.
207. **Arnheim, N. and Southern, E. M.,** Heterogeneity of the ribosomal genes in mice and men, *Cell,* 11, 363, 1977.
208. **Grummt, I. and Gross, H. J.,** Structural organization of mouse rDNA. Comparison of transcribed and non-transcribed regions, *Mol. Gen. Genet.,* 177, 23, 1980.
209. **Kuehn, M. and Arnheim, N.,** Nucleotide sequence of the genetically labile repeated elements 5′ to the origin of mouse rRNA transcription, *Nucleic Acids Res.* 11, 211, 1983.
210. **Mishima, Y., Yamamoto, O., Kominami, R., and Muramatsu, M.,** *In vitro* transcription of a cloned mouse ribosomal RNA gene, *Nucleic Acids Res.,* 9, 6773, 1981.
211. **Miller, K. G. and Sollner-Webb, B.,** Transcription of mouse rRNA genes by RNA polymerase I: *in vitro* and *in vivo* initiation and processing, *Cell,* 27, 165, 1981.

212. **Bach, R., Grummt, I., and Allet, B.,** The nucleotide sequence of the initiation region of the ribosomal transcription unit from mouse, *Nucleic Acids Res.,* 9, 1559, 1981.

213. **Urano, Y., Kominami, R., Mishima, Y., and Muramatsu, M.,** The nucleotide sequence of the putative transcription initiation site of a cloned ribosomal RNA gene of the mouse, *Nucleic Acids Res.,* 8, 6043, 1980.

214. **Reichel, R., Monstein, H.-J., Jansen, H.-W., Philipson, L., and Benecke, B.-J.,** Small nuclear RNA species are encoded in the nontranscribed region of ribosomal spacer DNA, *Proc. Natl. Acad. Sci. U.S.A.,* 79, 3106, 1982.

215. **Eliceiri, G. L. and Green, H.,** Ribosomal RNA synthesis in human-mouse hybrid cells, *J. Mol. Biol.,* 41, 253, 1969.

216. **Croce, C. M., Talavera, A., Basilico, C., and Miller, O. J.,** Suppression of production of mouse 28S ribosomal RNA in mouse-human hybrids segregating mouse chromosomes, *Proc. Natl. Acad. Sci. U.S.A.,* 74, 694, 1977.

217. **Soprano, K. J., Dev, V. G., Croce, C. M., and Baserga, R.,** Reactivation of silent rRNA genes by simian virus 40 in human-mouse hybrid cells, *Proc. Natl. Acad. Sci. U.S.A.,* 76, 3885, 1979.

218. **Southern, E. M.,** Detection of specific sequences among DNA fragments separated by gel electrophoresis, *J. Mol. Biol.,* 98, 503, 1975.

219. **Coen, E. S., Thoday, J. M., and Dover G.,** Rate of turnover of structural variants in the rDNA gene family of *D. melanogaster, Nature (London),* 295, 564, 1982.

220. **Coen, E. S., Strachan, T., and Dover, G.,** Dynamics of concerted evolution of ribosomal DNA and histone gene families in the melanogaster species subgroup of *Drosophila. J. Mol. Biol.,* 158, 17, 1982.

221. **Kossel, H., Edwards, K., Fritzsche, E., Koch, W., and Schwarz, Z.,** Phylogenetic significance of nucleotide sequence analysis, in *Protein and Nucleic Acids in Plant Systematics,* Jensen, U. and Fairbrothers, D. E., Eds., Springer-Verlag, Basel, 1983.

222. **Klipper-Bälz, R. and Schleifer, K. H.,** DNA-rRNA hybridization studies among staphylococci and some other gram-positive bacteria, *FEMS Microbiol. Lett.,* 10, 357, 1981.

223. **Mordarski, M., Kacz, A., Goodfellow, M., Pulverer, G., Peters, G., and Schumacher-Perdreau, F.,** Ribosomal RNA similarities in the classification of *Staphylococcus, FEMS Microbiol Lett.,* 11, 159, 1981.

224. **Stackebrandt, E., Wunner-Fuessl, B., Fowler, V. J., and Schleifer, K.-H.,** DNA homologies and ribosomal RNA similarities among spore forming members of the actinomycetale, *Int. J. Syst. Bacteriol.,* 31, 420, 1981.

225. **Brown, D. D., Wensink, P. C., and Jordan, E.,** A comparison of the ribosomal DNA's of *Xenopus laevis* and *Xenopus mulleri:* the evolution of tandem genes, *J. Mol. Biol.,* 63, 57, 1972.

226. **Bach, R., Allet, B., and Crippa, M.,** Sequence organization of the spacer in the ribosomal genes of *Xenopus clivii* and *Xenopus borealis, Nucleic Acids Res.,* 9, 5311, 1981.

227. **Appels, R. and Dvorak, J.,** Relative rates of divergence of spacer and gene sequences within the rDNA region of species in the *Triticeae:* implications for the maintenance of homogeneity of a repeated gene family, *Theor. Appl. Genet.,* 63, 361, 1982.

228. **Arnold, M. L.,** Ph.D. thesis, Australian National University, Canberra, Australia.

229. **Qu, L. H., Michot, B., and Bachellerie, J.-P.,** Improved methods for structure probing in large RNA's: a rapid "heterologous" sequencing approach is coupled to the direct mapping of nuclease accessible sites. Application to the 5' terminal domain of eukaryotic 28S rRNA, *Nucleic Acids Res.,* 11, 5903, 1983.

230. **Church, G. M. and Gilbert, W.,** Genomic sequencing, *Proc. Natl. Acad. Sci. U.S.A.,* 81, 1991, 1984.

231. **Maxam, A. M. and Gilbert, W.,** Sequencing end-labelled DNA with base-specific chemical cleavages, *Meth. Enzymol.,* 65, 499, 1980.

232. **Hemleben, V., Grierson, D., and Dertmann, H.,** The use of equilibrium centrifugation of actinomycin-D/cesium chloride for the purification of ribosomal DNA, *Plant Sci. Lett.,* 9, 129, 1977.

233. **Warburton, D., Atwood, K. C., and Henderson, A. S.,** Variation in the number of genes for rRNA among human acrocentric chromosomes: correlation with frequency of satellite association, *Cytogen. Cell. Genet.,* 17, 221, 1976.

234. **Miller, D. A., Breg, W. R., Warburton, D., Dev, V. G., and Miller, O. J.,** Regulation of rRNA gene expression in a human familial 14 pt marker chromosome, *Hum. Genet.,* 43, 289, 1978.

235. **Krystal, M., Eustachio, P. D., Ruddle, F. H., and Arnheim, N.,** Human nucleolus organisers on non-homologous chromosomes can share the same ribosomal gene variants, *Proc. Natl. Acad. Sci. U.S.A.,* 78, 5744, 1981.

236. **White, M. J. D., Dennis, E. S., Honeycutt, R. L., Contreras, N., and Peacock, W. J.,** Cytogenetics of the parthenogenetic grasshopper *Warramaba virgo* and its bisexual relatives, *Chromosoma,* 85, 181, 1982.

237. **Schmidt, E. R. and Godwin, E. A.,** The nucleotide sequence of an unusual nontranscribed spacer and its ancestor in the rDNA of *Chironomus thummi, EMBO J.,* 2, 1177, 1983.

238. **Israelewski, N. and Schmidt, E. R.**, Spacer size heterogeneity in ribosomal DNA of *Chironomus thummi* is due to a 120 bp repeat homologous to a predominantly centromeric repeated sequence, *Nucleic Acids Res.*, 10, 7689, 1982.

239. **Schmidt, E. R., Godwin, E. A., Keyl, H.-G., and Israelewski, N.**, Cloning and analysis of ribosomal DNA from *Chironomus thummi piger* and *Chironomus thummi thummi*, *Chromosoma*, 87, 389, 1982.

240. **Rae, P. M. M., Kohorn, B. D., and Wade, R. P.**, The 10 kb *Drosophila virilis* 28S rDNA intervening sequence is flanked by a direct repeat of 14 base pairs of coding sequence, *Nucleic Acids Res.*, 8, 3491, 1980.

241. **Higuchi, R., Stang, H. D., Browne, J. K., Martin, M. O., Huot, M., Lipeles, J., and Salser, W.**, Human ribosomal RNA gene spacer sequences are found interspersed elsewhere in the genome, *Gene*, 15, 177, 1981.

242. **Arnheim, N., Seperack, P., Banerji, J., Lang, R. B., Miesfeld, R., and Marcu, K. B.**, Mouse rDNA nontranscribed spacer sequences are found flanking immunoglobulin CH genes and elsewhere throughout the genome, *Cell*, 22, 179, 1980.

243. **Junakovic, N., Poretti, A., Amaldi, F., and Buongiorno-Nardelli, M.**, Differently sized rDNA repeating units of *Xenopus laevis* are arranged as internally homogeneous clusters along the nucleolar organizer, *Nucleic Acids Res.*, 5, 1335, 1978.

244. **Berger, S. and Schweiger, H.-G.**, Ana apparent lack of non-transcribed spacers in rDNA of a green alga, *Mol. Gen. Genet.*, 139, 269, 1975.

245. **Appels, R. and Moran, L. B.**, Molecular analysis of alien chromatin introduced into wheat, in *16th Stadler Symposium*, Gustafson, J. P., Ed., Plenum Press, New York, 1984, 529.

246. **Dvorak, J.**, personal communication.

247. **Naylor, S. L., Sakaguchi, A. Y., Schmickel, R. D., Woodworth-Gutai, M., and Shows, T. B.** Organization of rDNA spacer fragment variants among human acrocentric chromosomes in somatic cell hybrids, *J. Mol. Appl. Genet.*, 2, 137, 1983.

248. **Indik, Z. K. and Tartof, K. D.**, Long spacers among ribosomal genes of *Drosophila melanogaster*, *Nature (London)*, 284, 477, 1980.

249. **Tartof, K. D.**, Evolution of transcribed and spacer sequences in the ribosomal RNA Genes of *Drosophila*, *Cell*, 17, 607, 1979.

250. **Palumbo, G., Caizzi, R., and Ritossa, F.**, Relative orientation with respect to the centromere of ribosomal RNA genes of the X and Y chromosomes of *Drosophila melanogaster*, *Proc. Natl. Acad. Sci. U.S.A.*, 70, 1883, 1973.

251. **Coen, E. S. and Dover, G.**, Phenotype and genetic consequences of unequal molecular exchanges between the X and Y chromosomal rDNA arrays in *D. melanogaster*, *Cell*, 33, 849, 1983.

252. **Wellauer, P. K., Dawid, I. B., and Tartof, K. D.**, X and Y chromosomal ribosomal DNA of *Drosophila*. comparison of spacers and insertions, *Cell*, 14, 269, 1978.

253. **Rae, P. M. M.**, Unequal crossing-over accounts for the organization of *Drosophila virilis* rDNA insertions and the integrity of flanking 28S gene, *Nature (London)*, 296, 579, 1982.

254. **Long, E. O. and Dawid, I. B.**, Restriction analysis of spacers in ribosomal DNA of *Drosophila melanogaster*, *Nucleic Acids Res.*, 7, 205, 1979.

255. **Coen, C. S. and Dover, G. H.**, Multiple Pol I initiation sequences in rDNA spacers of *Drosophila melanogaster*, *Nucleic Acids Res.*, 10, 7017, 1982.

256. **French, C. K., Fouts, D. L., and Manning, J. E.**, Sequence arrangement of the rRNA genes of the dipteran *Sarcophaga bullata*, *Nucleic Acids Res.*, 9, 2563, 1981.

257. **Schäfer, M., Wyman, A. R., and White, R.**, Length variation in the NTS of *Calliphora erythrocephala* ribosomal DNA is due to a 350 base-pair repeat, *J. Mol. Biol.*, 146, 179, 1981.

258. **Krystal, M. and Arnheim, N.**, Length heterogeneity in a region of the human ribosomal gene spacer is not accompanied by extensive population polymorphism, *J. Mol. Biol.*, 126, 91, 1978.

259. **Schmickel, R. D., Waterson, J. R., Knoller, M., Szura, L. L., and Wilson, G. N.**, HeLa cell identification by analysis of ribosomal DNA segment patterns generated by endonuclease restriction, *Am. J. Hum. Genet.*, 32, 890, 1980.

260. **Erickson, J. M., Rushford, C. L., Dorney, D. J., Wilson, G. N., and Schmickel, R. D.**, Structure and variation of human ribosomal DNA: molecular analysis of cloned fragments, *Gene*, 16, 1, 1981.

261. **Wilson, G.**, The structure and organization of human ribosomal genes, *Cell Nucleus*, 10B, 287, 1982.

262. **Arnheim, N., Krystal, M., Schmickel, R., Wilson, G., Ryder, O., and Zimmer, E.**, Molecular evidence for genetic exchanges among ribosomal genes on nonhomologous chromosomes in man and apes, *Proc. Natl. Acad. Sci. U.S.A.*, 77, 7323, 1980.

263. **Arnheim, N.**, Concerted evolution of multigene families, in *Evolution of Genes and Proteins*, Koehn, R. and Nei, M., Eds., Sinaner Assoc., Sunderland, Mass., 1983.

264. **Petes, T. D.**, Unequal meiotic recombination within tandem arrays of yeast ribosomal DNA genes, *Cell*, 19, 765, 1980.

265. **Szostak, J. W., and Wu, R.,** Unequal crossing over in the ribosomal DNA of *Saccharomyces cerevisiae, Nature (London),* 284, 426, 1980.

266. **Maden, B. E. H., Moss, M., and Salim, M.,** Nucleotide sequence of an external transcribed spacer in *Xenopus laevis* rDNA: sequences flanking the 5′ and 3′ ends of 18S rRNA are non-complementary, *Nucleic Acids Res.,* 10, 2387, 1982.

267. **Furlong, J. C. and Maden, B. E. H.,** Patterns of major divergence between the internal transcribed spacers of ribosomal DNA in *Xenopus borealis* and *Xenopus laevis,* and of minimal divergence with ribosomal coding regions, *EMBO J.,* 2, 443, 1983.

268. **Gourse, R. L. and Gerbi, S. A.,** Sequences that flank intervening sequences in ribosomal DNA are highly conserved in evolution, *Eur. J. Cell Biol.,* 22, 10, 1980.

269. **Triezenberg, S. J., Rushford, C., Hart, R. P., Berkner, K. L., and Folk, W. R.,** Structure of the Syrian hamster ribosomal DNA repeat and identification of homologous and nonhomologous regions shared by human and hamster ribosomal DNA's, *J. Biol. Chem.,* 257, 7826, 1982.

270. **Gourse, R. L. and Gerbi, S. A.,** Fine structure of ribosomal RNA. III. Location of evolutionarily conserved regions within ribosomal DNA, *J. Mol. Biol.,* 140, 321, 1980.

271. **Michot, B., Bachellerie, J.-P., Raynal, F., and Renalier, M.-H.,** Homology of the 5′-terminal sequence of 28S rRNA of mouse with yeast and *Xenopus.* Implications for the secondary structure of the 5.8S-28S RNA complex, *FEBS Lett.,* 140, 193, 1982.

272. **Rubin, G. M.,** The nucleotide sequence of *Saccharomyces cerevisiae* 5.8S ribosomal nucleic acid, *J. Biol. Chem.,* 248, 3860, 1973.

273. **Khan, M. S. N. and Maden, B. E. H.,** Nucleotide sequence relationships between vertebrate 5.8S ribosomal RNA's, *Nucleic Acids Res.,* 4, 2495, 1977.

274. **Hoshikawa, Y., Iida, Y., and Iwabuchi, M.,** Nucleotide sequence of the transcriptional initiation region of *Dictyostelium discoideum* rRNA gene and comparison of the initiation regions of three lower eukaryotes' genes, *Nucleic Acids Res.,* 11, 1725, 1983.

275. **Financsek, I., Mizumoto, K., and Muramatsu, M.,** Nucleotide sequence of the transcription initiation region of a rat ribosomal RNA gene, *Gene,* 18, 115, 1982.

276. **Treco, D., Brownell, E., and Arnheim, N.,** The ribosomal gene non-transcribed spacer, *Cell Nucleus,* 12C, 101, 1982.

277. **Barnett, T. and Rae, P. M. M.,** A 9.6 kb intervening sequence in *D. virilis* rDNA and sequence homology in rDNA interruptions of diverse species of *Drosophila* and other Diptera, *Cell,,* 16, 763, 1979.

278. **Sears, E. R.,** The origin and future of wheat, in *Crop Resources,* Academic Press, New York, 1977, 193.

279. **Wilson, G. N., Knoller, M., Szura, L. L., and Schmickel, R. D.,** Individual and evolutionary variation of primate ribosomal DNA transcription initiation regions, *Mol. Biol. Evol.,* 1, 221, 1984.

280. **Nelkin, B., Strayer, D., and Vogelstein, B.,** Divergence of primate ribosomal RNA genes as assayed by restriction enzyme analysis, *Gene,* 11, 89, 1980.

281. **Marco, Y. and Rochaix, J.-D.,** Comparison of the nuclear ribosomal units of five *Chlamydomonas* species, *Chromosoma (Berlin),* 81, 629, 1981.

282. **Din, N. and Engberg, J.,** Extrachromosomal rRNA genes in *Tetrahymena.* Structure and evolution, *J. Mol. Biol.,* 134, 555, 1979.

283. **Swanton, M. T., McCarroll, R. M., and Spear, B. B.,** The organization of macronuclear rDNA molecule of four hypotrichous ciliated protozoans, *Chromosoma,* 85, 1, 1982.

284. **Renkawitz-Pohl, R., Glätzer, K. H., and Kunz, W.,** Characterization of cloned ribosomal DNA from *Drosophila hydei, Nucleic Acids Res.,* 8, 4593, 1980.

285. **Dover, G.,** Molecular drive: a cohesive mode of species evolution, *Nature (London),* 229, 111, 1982.

286. **Smith, G. P.,** Unequal cross-over and the evolution of multigene families, *Cold Spring Harbor Symp. Quant. Biol.,* 38, 507, 1973.

287. **Smith, G. P.,** Evolution of repeated DNA sequences by unequal cross-over, *Science,* 191, 528, 1976.

288. **Birky, C. W. Jr. and Skavaril, R. V.,** Maintenance of genetic homogeneity in systems with multiple genomes, *Genet. Res. (Cambridge),* 27, 249, 1976.

289. **Ohta, T.,** On the gene conversion model as a mechanism for maintenance of homogeneity in systems with multiple genomes, *Genet. Res. (Cambridge),* 30, 89, 1977.

290. **Ohta, T.,** Evolution and variation of multigene families. Lecture notes, *Biomathmatics,* and Springer-Verlag, New York, 1980, 37.

291. **Amikam, D., Razin, S., and Glaser, G.,** Ribosomal RNA genes in *Mycoplasma, Nucleic Acids Res.,* 10, 4215, 1982.

292. **Tomioka, N., Shinozaki, K., and Sugiura, M.,** Molecular cloning and characterization of ribosomal RNA genes from a blue-green alga, *Anacystis nidulans, Mol. Gen. Genet.,* 184, 359, 1981.

293. **Williamson, S. E. and Doolittle, W. F.,** Genes for tRNA^{Ile} and tRNA^{Ala} in the spacer between the 16S and 23S rRNA genes of a blue-green alga: strong homology to chloroplast tRNA genes and tRNA genes of the *E. coli* rrnD gene cluster, *Nucleic Acids Res.,* 11, 225, 1983.

294. **Morgan, C. P. and Bott, K. F.**, Restriction enzyme analysis of *Bacillus subtilis* ribosomal ribonucleic acid genes, *J. Bacteriol*, 140, 99, 1979.

295. **Loughney, K., Lund, E., and Dahlbert, J. E.**, tRNA genes are found between the 16S and 23S rRNA genes in *Bacillus subtilis, Nucleic Acids Res.*, 10, 1607, 1982.

296. **Ogasawara, N., Seiki, M., and Yoshikawa, H.**, Replication origin region of *Bacillus subtilis* chromosome contains two rRNA operons, *J. Bacteriol.*, 154, 50, 1983.

297. **Klier, A., Kunst, F., and Rapoport, G.**, Structure of cloned ribosomal DNA cistrons from *Bacillus thuringiensis, Nucleic Acids Res.*, 7, 997, 1979.

298. **Ohta, N. and Newton, A.**, Isolation and mapping of ribosomal RNA genes of *Caulobacter crescentus, J. Mol. Biol.*, 153, 291, 1981.

299. **Jarsch, M., Altenbuchner, J., and Böck, A.**, Physical organization of the genes for ribosomal RNA in *Methanococcus vannielii, Mol. Gen. Genet.*, 189, 41, 1983.

300. **Jarsch, M. and Böck, A.**, DNA sequence of the 16S rRNA/23S rRNA intercistronic spacer of two rDNA operons of the archaebacterium *Methanococcus vanniellii, Nucleic Acids Res.*, 11, 7537, 1983.

301. **Sawada, S., Osawa, S., Kobayashi, H., Hori, H., and Muto, A.**, The number of ribosomal RNA genes in *Mycoplasma capricolum, Mol. Gen. Genet.*, 182, 502, 1981.

302. **Hofman, J. E., Lau, R. H., and Doolittle, W. F.**, The number, physical organization and transcription of ribosomal RNA cistrons in an archaebacterium *Halobacterium halobium, Nucleic Acids Res.*, 7, 1321, 1979.

303. **Ulbrich, N., Kumagai, I., Erdmann, V. A.**, The number of ribosomal RNA genes in *Thermus thermophilus* HB8, *Nucleic Acids Res.*, 12, 2055, 1984.

304. **Trendelenburg, M. F.**, Morphology of ribosomal RNA cistrons in oocytes of the water beetle *Dytiscus marginalis* L., *Chromosoma*, 48, 119, 1974.

305. **Spring, H., Krohne, G., Franke, W. W., Scheer, U., and Trendelenburg, M. F.**, Homogeneity and heterogeneity of sizes of transcriptional units and spacer regions in nucleolar genes of *Acetabularia, J. Microsc. Biol. Cell*, 25, 107, 1976.

306. **Berger, S., Zellmer, D. M., Kloppstech, K., Richter, G., Dillar, W. L., and Schweiger, H.-G.**, Alternating polarity in rRNA Genes, *Cell Biol. Int. Rep.*, 2, 41, 1978.

307. **D'Alessio, J. M., Harris, G. H., Perna, P. J., and Paule, M. R.**, Ribosomal ribonucleic acid repeat unit of *Acanthamoeba castellanii* : cloning and restriction map, *Biochemistray*, 20, 3822, 1981.

308. **Steele, R. E. and Rae, P. M. M.**, Comparison of DNAs of *Crypthecodinium cohnii*-like Dinoflagellates from widespread geographic locations, *J. Protozool.*, 27, 479, 1980.

309. **Curtis, S. E. and Rawson, J. R. Y.**, Characterization of the nuclear ribosomal DNA of *Euglena gracilis, Gene*, 15, 237, 1981.

310. **Katzen, A. L., Cann, G. M., and Blackburn, E. H.**, Sequence-specific fragmentation of macronuclear DNA in a Holotrichous ciliate, *Cell*, 24, 313, 1981.

311. **Leon, W., Fouts, D. L., and Manning, J.**, Sequence arrangement of the 16S and 26S rRNA genes in the pathogenic haemoflagellate *Lesihmania donovani, Nucleic Acids, Res.*, 5, 491, 1978.

312. **Findley, R. C. and Gall, J. G.**, Organization of ribosomal genes in *Paramecium tetraurelia, J. Cell Biol.*, 84, 547, 1980.

313. **Lipps, H. L. and Steinbruck, G.**, Free genes for rRNA's in the macronuclear genome of the ciliate *Stylonychia mytilus, Chromosoma*, 69, 21, 1982.

314. **Wild, M. A. and Sommer, R.**, Sequence of a ribosomal RNA gene intron from *Tetrahymena, Nature (London)*, 283, 693, 1980.

315. **Niles, E. G., Cunningham, K., and Jain, R.**, Structure of the *Tetrahymena pyriformis* ribosomal RNA gene nucleotide sequence of the transcription termination region, *J. Biol. Chem.*, 256, 12857, 1981.

316. **Wild, M. A. and Gall, J. G.**, An intervening sequence in the gene coding for 25S ribosomal RNA of *Tetrahymena pigmentosa, Cell*, 16, 565, 1979.

317. **Hasan, G., Turner, M. J., and Cordingley, J. S.**, Ribosomal RNA genes of *Trypanosoma brucei*. Cloning of a rRNA gene containing a mobile element, *Nucleic Acids Res.*, 10, 6747, 1982.

318. **Rozek, C. E. and Timberlake, W. E.**, Restrictions endonuclease mapping by crossed contact hybridization: the ribosomal RNA genes of *Achlya ambisexualis, Nucleic Acids Res.*, 7, 1567, 1979.

319. **Borsuk, P. A., Nagiec, M. M., Stephien, P. P., and Bartnik, E.**, Organization of the rRNA gene cluster in *Aspergillus nidulans, Gene*, 17, 147, 1982.

320. **Cockburn, A. F., Nonkirk, M. J., and Firtel, R. A.**, Organization of the ribosomal RNA genes of *Dictyostelium discoideum*: mapping of the nontranscribed spacer regions, *Cell*, 9, 605, 1976.

321. **Cihlar, R. L. and Sypherd, P. S.**, The organization of the ribosomal RNA genes in the fungus *Mucor racemosus, Nucleic Acids Res.*, 8, 793, 1980.

322. **Hall, L. and Braun, R,** The organization of genes for transfer RNA and ribosomal RNA in amoebae and plasmodia of *Physarum polycephalum, Eur. J. Biochem.*, 76, 165, 1977.

323. **Campbell, G. R., Littau, V. C., Melera, P. W., Allfrey, V. G., and Johnson, E. M.,** Unique sequence arrangement of ribosomal genes in the palidromic rDNA molecule of *Physarum polycephalum, Nucleic Acids Res.,* 6, 1433, 1979.

324. **Ferris, P. J. and Vogt, V. M.,** Structure of the central spacer region of extrachromosomal ribosomal DNA in *Physarum polycephalum, J. Mol. Biol.,* 159, 359, 1982.

325. **Nath, K. and Bollon, A. P.,** Organization of the yeast ribosomal RNA gene cluster via cloning and restriction analysis, *J. Biol. Chem.,* 253, 6562, 1977.

326. **Bollon, A. P.,** Organization of fungal ribosomal RNA genes, *Cell Nucleus,* 10A, 68, 1982.

327. **Barnitz, J. T., Cramer, J. H., Rownd, R. H., Cooley, L., and Söll, D.,** Arrangement of the ribosomal RNA genes in *Schizosaccharomyces pombe, FEBS Lett.,* 143, 129, 1982.

328. **Russell, P. J.,** Personal communication.

329. **Tabata, S.,** Structure of the 5S ribosomal RNA gene and its adjacent regions in *Torulopsis utilis, Eur. J. Biochem.,* 110, 107, 1980.

330. **Kavanagh, T. A. and Timmis, J. N.,** personal communication.

331. **Fodor, I. and Beridze, T.,** Structural organization of plant ribosomal DNA, *Biochem. Int.,* 1, 493, 1980.

332. **Doyle, J. J., Beachy, R. N., and Lewis, W. H.,** personal communication.

333. **Leara, G. H.,** personal communication.

334. **Jorgensen, R. A.,** personal communication.

335. **Kato, A., Yakura, K., and Tanifuji, S.,** Organization of ribosomal DNA in the carrot, *Plant Cell Physiol.,* 23, 151, 1982.

336. **Appels, R.,** unpublished data.

337. **Schaal, B.,** personal communication.

338. **Friedrich, H., Hemleben, V., Meagher, R. B., and Key, J. L.,** Purification and restriction endonuclease mapping of soybean, 18S and 25S ribosomal RNA gene, *Planta,* 146, 467, 1979.

339. **Doyle, J. J. and Beachy, R. N.,** Personal communication.

340. **von Kalm, L. and Smyth, D. R.,** Variation in the ribosomal RNA genes of *Lilium henryi,* in *Manipulation and Expression of Genes in Eukaryotes,* Nagley, P., Linnane, A. W., Peacock, W. J., and Pateman, J. A., Ed., Academic Press, New York, 1983, 239.

341. **von Kalm, L.,** personal communication.

342. **Goldsbrough, P. D. and Cullis, C. A.,** Characterization of the genes for ribosomal RNA in flax, *Nucleic Acids Res.,* 9, 1301, 1981.

343. **Goldsbrough, P. B., Ellis, T. H. N., and Cullis, C. A.,** Organization of the 5S RNA genes in flax, *Nucleic Acids Res.,* 9, 5895, 1981.

344. **Sytsma, K. J., Schaal, B. A., and Raven, P. H.,** personal communication.

345. **Jorgensen, R. A., Cuellar, R. E., and Thompson, W. F.,** Modes and tempos in the evolution of nuclear encoded ribosomal RNA genes in legumes, *Carnegie Institution of Washington Year Book,* Vol 80, Washington, D.C., 1982.

346. **Rafalski, J. A., Wiewiorowski, M., and Söll, D.,** Organization of ribosomal DNA in yellow lupine (*Lupinus luteus*) and sequence of the 5.8S rRNA gene, *FEBS Lett.,* 152, 241, 1983.

347. **Uchimiya, H., Ohgawara, T., Kato, H., Akiyama, T., Harada, H.,and Sugiura, M.,** Detection of two different nuclear genomes in parasexual hybrids by ribosomal RNA gene analysis, *Theor. Appl. Genet.,* 64, 117, 1983.

348. **Oono, K. and Suguira, M.,** Heterogeneity of the ribosomal RNA gene clusters in rice, *Chromosoma,* 76, 85, 1980.

349. **Tanifuji, S., Yakura, K., and Kato, A.,** Structural organization of ribosomal DNA in four *Trillium* species and *Paris verticillata, Plant Cell Physiol.,* 24, 1231, 1983.

350. **Waldron, J., Dunsmuir, P., and Bedbrook, J.,** Characterization of the rDNA repeat units in the Mitchell *Petunia* genome, *Plant Mol. Biol.,* 2, 57, 1983.

351. **Delseny, M., Aspart, L., Cooke, R., Grellet, F., and Penon, P.,** Restriction analysis of radish nuclear genes coding for rRNA: evidence for heterogeneity, *Biochem. Biophys. Res. Commun.,* 91, 540, 1979.

352. **Delseny, M., Aspart, L., Cooke, R., and Got, A.,** Nuclear genes coding for radish ribosomal RNA, *Physiol. Veg.,* 18, 373, 1981.

353. **Timmis, J. N. and Scott, N. S.** personal communication.

354. **Zimmer, E. and Walbot, V.,** personal communication.

355. **Yakura, K. and Tanifuji, S.,** The organization of rRNA genes in *Vicia faba, Plant Cell Physiol.,* 22, 1105, 1981.

356. **Yakura, K. and Tanifuji, S.,** Molecular cloning and restriction analysis of EcoRI fragments of *Vicia faba* rDNA, *Plant Cell Physiol.,* 24, 1327, 1983.

357. **Yakura, K., Kato, A., and Tanifuji, S.,** Length heterogeneity of the large spacer of *Vicia faba* rDNA is due to the differing number of a 325 bp repetitive sequence elements, *Mol. Gen. Genet.,* in press.

358. **Rivin, C. I., Zimmer, E. A., Cullis, C. A., Walbot, V., Huynh, T., and Davis, R. W.,** Evaluation of genomic variability at the nucleic acid level, *Plant Mol. Biol. Rep.,* 1, 9, 1983.

359. **Files, J. G. and Hirsch, D.**, Ribosomal DNA of *Caenorhabditis elegans, J. Mol. Biol.* 149, 223, 1981.
360. **Cave, M. D.**, Length heterogeneity of amplified circular rDNA molecules in oocytes of the house cricket *Acheta domesticus* (Orthoptera:Gryllidae), *Chromosoma*, 71, 15, 1979.
361. **Trendelenburg, M. F., Scheer, W., Zentgraf, H., and Franke, W. W.**, Heterogeneity of space lengths in circles of amplified ribosomal DNA of 2 insect species *Dytiscus marginalis* and *Acheta domesticus, J. Mol. Biol.*, 108, 453, 1976.
362. **Vaughn, J. C., Whitman, D. J., Bagshaw, J. C., and Helder, J. C.**, Molecular cloning and characterization of ribosomal RNA genes from the brine shrimp, *Biochim. Biophys. Acta*, 697, 156, 1982.
363. **Sheng, Z., Qian, X., Chu, M., Zhang, A., and Li, Z.**, The restriction map of ribosomal RNA gene in silkworm *Attacus rieini, Acta Genet. Sin.*, 8, 203, 1981.
364. **Manning, R. F., Samols, D. R., and Gage, L. P.**, The genes for 18S, 5.8S and 28S ribosomal RNA of *Bombyx mori* are organized into tandem repeats of uniform length, *Gene*, 4, 153, 1978.
365. **Beckingham, K. and White, R.**, The ribosomal DNA of *Calliphora erythrocephala*: an analysis of hybrid plasmids containing ribosomal DNA, *J. Mol. Biol.*, 137, 349, 1980.
366. **Beckingham, K.**, Ribosomal DNA of *Calliphora erythrocephala* cistron classes of total genomic DNA, *J. Mol. Biol.*, 149, 141, 1981.
367. **Gall, J. G. and Rochaix, J. D.**, The amplified ribosomal DNA of *Dytiscid* beetles, *Proc. Natl. Acad. Sci. U.S.A.*, 71, 1819, 1974.
368. **Degelmann, A., Royer, H.-D., and Hollenberg, C. P.**, The organization of the ribosomal RNA genes of *Chironomus tentans* and some closely related species, *Chromosoma*, 71, 263, 1979.
369. **DeSalle, R.**, personal communication.
370. **Schaaäfer, M. and Kunz, W.**, personal communication.
371. **Foe, V. E., Wilkinson, L. E., and Laird, C. D.**, Comparative organization of active transcription units in *Oncopeltus fasciatus, Cell*, 9, 131, 1976.
372. **Israelewski, N.**, personal communication.
373. **Zaha, A., Leoncini, O., Hollenberg, C. P., and Lara, F. J. S.**, Cloning and characterization of the ribosomal RNA genes of *Rhynchosciara americana, Chromosoma*, 87, 103, 1982.
374. **Renkawitz-Pohl, R., Matsumoto, L., and Gerbi, S. A.**, Two distinct intervening sequences in different ribosomal DNA repeat units of *Sciara coprophila, Nucleic Acids Res.*, 9, 3747, 1981.
375. **Amabis, J. M. and Nair, K. K.**, Ultrastructure of gene transcription in spermatocytes of *Trichosia pubescens* Morgante 1969 (Diptera: *Sciaridae*), *Z. Naturforsch.*, C32, 186, 1976.
376. **Blin, N., Sperraza, J. M., Wilson, F. E., Bieber, D. G., Mickel, F. S., and Stafford, D. W.**, Organization of the ribosomal RNA gene cluster in *Lytechinus variegatus, J. Biol. Chem.*, 254, 2716, 1979.
377. **Botchan, P. M. and Dayton, A. I.**, A specific replication origin in the chromosomal rDNA of *Lytechinus variegatus, Nature (London)*, 299, 453, 1982.
378. **Passananti, C., Felsani, A., Giordano, R., Metafora, S., and Spadafora, C.**, Cloning and characterization of the ribosomal genes of the sea-urchin *Paracentrotus lividus, Eur. J. Biochem.*, 137, 233, 1983.
379. **Kuprijanova, N., Popenko, V., Eisner, G., Vengerov, J. U., Timofeeva, M., Tiknonenko, A., Skryabin, K., and Bayev, A.**, Organization of loach *Misgurnus fossilis* ribosomal genes, *Mol. Biol. Rep.*, 8, 143, 1982.
380. **Schwab, M.**, personal communication.
381. **Trendelenburg, M. F.**, As quoted in Reference 79, 1977.
382. **Jordan, B. R., Latil-Damotte, M., and Jourdan, R.**, Coding and spacer sequences in the 5.8S-2S region of *Sciara coprophila* ribosomal DNA, *Nucleic Acids Res.*, 8, 3565, 1980.
383. **Miller, O. L. and Beatty, B. R.**, Nucleolar structure and function, in *Handbook of Molecular Cytology*, Lima de Faria, A., Ed., North Holland, Amsterdam, 1969, 605.
384. **Angelier, N. and Lacrioix, J. C.**, Complexes de transcription de'orgines nucleolaire et chromosomique d'ovocytes de *Pleurodeles waltlii* et *P. poipeti, Chromosoma*, 51, 323, 1975.
385. **Trendelenburg, M. F. and McKinnell, R. G.**, Transcriptionally active and inactive regions of nucleolar chromatin in amplified nucleoli of fully grown oocytes of hibernating frogs, *Rana pipiens* (Amphibia, Anura), *Differentiation*, 15, 73, 1979.
386. **Nardi, I.**, personal communication.
387. **Nardi, I., Barsacchi-Pilone, G., Batistoni, R., and Andronico, F.**, Chromosome location of the ribosomal RNA genes in *Triturus vulgaris meridionalis* (Amphibia, Urodela). II. Intraspecific variability in number and position of the chromosomal loci for 18S and 28S rRNA, *Chromosoma (Berlin)*, 64, 67, 1977.
388. **McClements, W. and Skalka, A. M.**, Analysis of chicken ribosomal RNA genes and construction of lambda hybrids containing gene fragments, *Science*, 196, 195, 1977.
389. **Blin, N., Stephenson, E. C., and Stafford, D. W.**, Isolation and some properties of a mammalian ribosomal DNA, *Chromosoma (Berlin)*, 58, 41, 1976.
390. **Stambrook, P. J.**, Heterogeneity in Chinese Hamster ribosomal DNA, *Chromosoma (Berlin)*, 65, 153, 1978.

391. **Stumph, W. E., Wu, J. R., and Bonner, J.,** Determination of the size of rat ribosomal DNA repeating units by electron microscopy, *Biochemistry,* 18, 2864, 1979.

392. **Neumann, H., Gierl, A., Tu, J., Leibrock, J., Staiger, D., and Zillig, W.,** Organization of the genes for ribosomal RNA in archaebacteria, *Mol. Gen. Genet.,* 192, 66, 1983.

393. **Lecanidou, R., Eickbush, T. H., and Kafatos, F. C.,** Ribosomal DNA genes of *Bombyx mori:* a minor fraction of the repeating units contains insertions, *Nucleic Acids Res.,* 12, 4702, 1984.

394. **Wilson, G. N., Szura, L. L., Rushford, C., Jackson, D., and Erickson, J.,** Structure and variation of human ribosomal DNA: the external spacer and adjacent regions, *Am. J. Hum. Genet.,* 34, 32, 1982.

395. **Hattori, M., Ljljana, A., and Sakaki, Y.,** Direct repeats surrounding the ribosomal RNA genes of *Physarum polycephalum, Nucleic Acids Res.,* 12, 2047, 1984.

396. **Trendelenburg, M. F., Spring, H., Scheer, U., and Franke, W. W.,** Morphology of nucleolar cistrons in a plant cell, *Acetabularia mediterranea, Proc. Natl. Acad. Sci. U.S.A.,* 71, 3626, 1974.

397. **McKay, R. M., Spencer, D. F., Doolittle, W. F., and Gray, M. W.,** Nucleotide sequences of wheat embryo cytosol 5S and 5.8S ribosomal ribonucleic acids, *Eur. J. Biochem.,* 112, 561, 1980.

398. **Gilbert, S. F., de Boer, H. A., and Nomura, M.,** Identification of initiation sites for the *in vitro* transcription of rRNA operons rrnE and rrnA in *E. coli, Cell,* 17, 211, 1979.

399. **Glaser, G. and Cashel, M.,** *In vitro* transcripts from the rrnB ribosomal RNA cistron originate from two tandem promoters, *Cell,* 16, 111, 1979.

400. **Maden, B. E. H. and Tartof, K. D.,** Nature of the ribosomal RNA transcribed from the X and Y chromosomes of *Drosophila melanogaster, J. Mol. Biol.,* 90, 51, 1974.

401. **Young, R. A. and Steitz, J. A.,** Tandem promoters direct *E. coli* RNA synthesis, *Cell,* 17, 225, 1979.

402. **Rae, P. M. M.,** Coding region deletions associated with the major form of rDNA interruption in *Drosophila melanogaster, Nucleic Acids Res.,* 9, 4997, 1981.

403. **Dawid, I. B. and Rebbert, M.,** Nucleotide sequences at the boundaries between gene and insertion regions in the rDNA of *Drosophila melanogaster, Nucleic Acids Res.,* 9, 5011, 1981.

404. **Simeone, A., deFalco, A., Macino, G., and Boncinelli, E.,** Sequence organization of the ribosomal spacer of *D. melanogaster, Nucleic Acids Res.,* 10, 8263, 1982.

405. **deBoer, H. H., Gilbert, S. F., and Nomura, M.,** DNA sequences of promoter regions for rRNA operons rrnE and rrnA in *E. coli, Cell,* 17, 201, 1979.

406. **Miller, R. J., Hayward, D. C., and Glover, D. M.,** Transcription of the "non-transcribed" spacer of *Drosophila melanogaster* rDNA, *Nucleic Acids Res.,* 11, 11, 1983.

407. **Kominami, R., Urano, Y., Mishima,Y., and Muramatsu, M.,** Organization of ribosomal RNA gene repeats of the mouse, *Nucleic Acids Res.,* 9, 3219, 1981.

408. **Bieber, D., Blin, N., and Stafford, D. W.,** The region of transcription initiation in *Lytechinus variegatus* ribosomal RNA gene, *Biochim. Biophys. Acta,* 655, 366, 1981.

409. **Berger, S. and Schweiger, H.-G.,** Characterization and species differences of rDNA in algae, *Cell Nucleus,* 10A, 31, 1983.

410. **Cech, T. R., Zaug, A. J., Grabowski, P. J., and Brehm, S. L.,** Transcription and splicing of the ribosomal RNA precursor of *Tetrahymena, Cell Nucleus,* 10A, 171, 1982.

411. **Chisholm, R.,** Gene amplification during development, *Trends Biochem. Sci.,* 7, 161, 1982.

412. **Din, N., Engberg, J., and Gall, J.,** The nucleotide sequence at the transcription termination site of the rRNA gene in *Tetrahymena thermophila, Nucleic Acids Res.,* 10, 1503, 1982.

413. **Emery, H. S. and Weiner, A. M.,** An irregular satellite sequence is found at the termini of the linear extrachromosomal ribosomal DNA in *Dictyostelium discoideum, Cell,* 26, 411, 1981.

414. **Engberg, J., Din, N., Eckert, W. A., Kaffenberger, W., and Pearlman, R. E.,** Detailed transcription map of the extrachromosomal ribosomal RNA genes in *Tetrahymena thermophila, J. Mol. Biol.,* 142, 289, 1980.

415. **Frankel, G., Cockburn, A. F., Kindle, K. L., and Firtel, R. A.,** Organization of the ribosomal RNA genes of *Dictyostelium discoideum:* mapping of the transcribed region, *J. Mol. Biol.,* 109, 539, 1977.

416. **Frankham, R., Briscoe, D. A., and Nurthen, R. K.,** Unequal crossing over at the rRNA tandon as a source of quantitative genetic variation in *Drosophila, Genetics,* 95, 727, 1980.

417. **Gourse, R. L., Stark, M. J. R., and Dahlberg, A. E.,** Site directed mutagenesis of ribosomal RNA: construction and characterization of deletion mutants, *J. Mol. Biol.,* 159, 397, 1982.

418. **Grummt, I.,** Nucleotide sequence requirements for specific initiation of transcription by RNA polymerase I., *Proc. Natl. Acad. Sci. U.S.A.,* 79, 6908, 1982.

419. **Grimm, C. and Kunz, W.,** Disproportionate rDNA replication does occur in diploid tissue in *Drosophila hydei, Mol. Gen. Genet.,* 180, 23, 1980.

420. **Gupta, R., Lanther, J. M., and Woese, C. R.,** Sequence of the 16S ribosomal RNA from *Halobacterium volcanii,* an archaebacterium, *Science,* 221, 656, 1983.

421. **Jordan, B. R. and Glover, D. M.,** 5.8S and 2S ribosomal DNA is located in the transcribed spacer region between the 18S and 26S ribosomal RNA genes in *Drosophila melanogaster, FEBS Lett.,* 78, 271, 1977.

422. **Kohorn, B. D. and Rae, P. M. M.,** A component of the *Drosophila* RNA polymerase I promoter lies within the rRNA transcription unit, *Nature (London),* 304, 179, 1983.

423. **Kukita, T., Sakaki, Y., Nomiyama, H., Otsuka, T., Kuhara, S., and Takagi, Y.,** Structure around the 3′ terminus of the 26S ribosomal RNA gene of *Physarum polycephalum, Gene,* 16, 309, 1981.

424. **Laird, C. D. and Chooi, W. Y.,** Morphology of transcription units in *Drosophila melanogaster, Chromosoma,* 58, 193, 1976.

425. **Larionov, V. L., Grishin, A. V., Kraev, A. S., Skryabin, K. G., and Bayev, A. A.,** Comparison of the extrachromosomal and chromosomal ribosomal DNA in the yeast *Saccharomyces cerevisiae, Genetika,* 18, 191, 1982.

426. **Nath, K. and Bollon, A. P.,** Restriction analysis of tandemly repeated yeast ribosomal RNA genes, *Mol. Gen. Genet.,* 160, 235, 1978.

427. **Naylor, S. L., Sakaguchi, A. Y., Schmickel, R. D., Gutai, M. W., and Shows, T. B.,** Homogeneous arrangement of ribosomal DNA variants on individual acrocentric chromosomes of somatic cell hybrids, *Am. J. Hum. Genet.,* 33, 112A, 1981.

428. **Nomiyama, H., Sakaki, Y., and Takagi, Y.,** Nucleotide sequence of a ribosomal RNA gene intron from slime mold *Physarum polycephalum, Proc. Natl. Acad. Sci. U.S.A.,* 78, 1376, 1981.

429. **Perkowska, E., Macgregor, H. C., and Birnstiel, M. L.,** Gene amplification in the oocyte nucleus of mutant and wild-type *Xenopus laevis, Nature (London),* 217, 649, 1968.

430. **Sakaki, Y., Nakamura, M., Nomiyama, H., and Takagi, Y.,** Cloning and characterization of ribosomal RNA genes of *Physarum polycephalum, J. Biochem.,* 89, 1693, 1981.

431. **Spear, B. B.,** Isolation and mapping of the rRNA genes in the macronucleus of *Oxytricha fallax, Chromosoma,* 77, 193, 1980.

432. **Stewart, G. C., Wilson, F. E., and Bott, K. F.,** Detailed physical map of the ribosomal RNA genes of *Bacillus subtilis, Gene,* 19, 153, 1982.

433. **Swanton, M. T., Greslin, A. F., and Prescott, D. M.,** Arrangement of coding and non-coding sequences in the DNA molecules coding for rRNA's in *Oxytricha* sp., *Chromosoma,* 77, 203, 1980.

434. **Torczynski, R., Bollon, A. P., and Fuke, M.,** Nucleotide sequence of the 3′-terminal region of rat 18S ribosomal DNA, *Mol. Gen. Genet.,* 184, 557, 1981.

435. **Varsany-Breiner, A., Busella, J. F., Keys, C., Housman, D. E., Sullivan, D., Brisson, N., and Verma, D. P. S.,** The organization of a nuclear DNA sequence from a higher plant: molecular cloning and characterization of soybean ribosomal DNA, *Gene,* 7, 317, 1979.

436. **Wellauer, P. R. and Dawid, I. B.,** Isolation and sequence organization of human ribosomal DNA, *J. Mol. Biol,* 128, 289, 1979.

437. **Wilson, F. E., Blin, N., and Stafford, D. W.,** Arrangement of the ribosomal RNA sequences in the ribosomal DNA of *Lytechinus variegatus, Chromosoma,* 65, 373, 1978.

438. **Liang, G. H., Wang, A. S., and Phillips, R. L.,** Control of ribosomal RNA gene multiplicity in wheat, *Can. J. Genet. Cytol.,* 19, 425, 1978.

439. **Brownell, E., Krystal, M., and Arnheim, N.,** Structure and evolution of human and african ape rDNA pseudogenes, *Mol. Biol. Evol.,* 1, 29, 1983.

440. **Roiha, H., Miller, R. J., Woods, L. C., and Glover, D. M.,** Arrangements and rearrangements of sequences flanking the two types of rDNA insertion in *D. melanogaster, Nature (London),* 290, 749, 1981.

441. **Chan, Y.-L., Endo, Y., and Wool, I. G.,** The sequence of the nucleotides at the α-Sarcin cleavage site in rat 28S ribosomal RNA, *J. Biol. Chem.,* 258, 12768, 1983.

442. **Godwin, E. A. and Schmidt, E. R.,** personal communication.

Chapter 6

23S rRNA-DERIVED SMALL RIBOSOMAL RNAs: THEIR STRUCTURE AND EVOLUTION WITH REFERENCES TO PLANT PHYLOGENY

A. V. Troitsky and V. K. Bobrova

TABLE OF CONTENTS

I. INTRODUCTION

Phylogenetic relations between plants are less well known than those between animals. As a result, there is a great variety of plant taxonomic systems suggested. These taxonomies differ in the way families are grouped into orders and orders are united by the degree of relatedness. Due to the general progress of botany (owing both to the accumulation of new data in the old fields of research and to the use of new methods and approaches), the modern macrosystems of flowering plants have many more features in common than the ones suggested at the turn of the century.[1] However, too many questions remain unanswered and there are few groups of flowering plants studied sufficiently well to enable us to make reliable phylogenic conclusions.[1,2] There are several reasons for this situation. First, paleobotanic data are much more scarce than paleozoological, due to a weaker preservation of plant remnants compared to those of animals.[3-5] Fossils of some taxa are hard to find; for others, only fragments of organs or tissues are available and this makes it extremely difficult to reconstruct the overall pattern of a plant. Thus, the analysis of phylogenic relations has to be based mainly on a comparative study of living forms. However, there is another obstacle here, namely, numerous cases of parallel and convergent evolution of morphological characters in plants. In addition, taxonomic studies involve the problem of the weighing of phenetic features, which is hard to resolve due to heterobatmy,[1,6] or "mosaic evolution";[7] i.e., the difference in the evolutionary state of various characters in a particular taxon, and also the question about the criteria of their relative evolutionary advancement.[8]

Nor is there unanimity in approaches to the interrelationships between such large taxons as classes and divisions of archegoniates and algae. It is not clear what organisms gave birth to land plants.[5] Meyen[9] pointed to the futility of hypothesizing on this subject without new data, however no definite data are available at present. In recent years, numerous fossil plant remnants have been found dating back to the early steps of land plant evolution.[4,5] The data obtained testify that diverse terrestrial flora existed in the Lower Silurian and possibly earlier in the Upper Ordovican.[4,5] But many questions remain unsolved.

How can the molecular-evolutionary approach help in elucidating interrelationships between major large plant phyla and macrotaxonomy? It is known that a comparison of nucleotide sequences of total DNA or unique and repeated sequences from various plant species by means of DNA-DNA hybridization is possible only for representatives of a single or closely related families of flowering plants. For more distantly related species, the hybridization level is so low that it cannot be registered by the available methods.[10,11] Hybridization of chloroplast DNA makes it possible to compare less similar species from diverse angiosperm orders.[12-14]

For macrotaxonomy of plants, use should evidently be made of individual genes or gene products which represent highly conservative parts of the genome. For each individual marker, it is not clear *a priori* how closely we can approach the roots of the phylogenetic tree, since each type of macromolecule has its own rate of evolution,[15] and apparently its own limit of evolutionary variability determined by functional constraints.

The pronounced evolutionary stability of ribosomal RNA has been demonstrated in rRNA-DNA hybridization experiments for more than 10 years. As a result the existence of homologous regions in rRNA of even highly diverged species has been established, and the degree of rRNA divergence in various phyletic lines has been estimated.[16-24] Progress in the development of nucleic acid sequencing methods has made it possible to compare nucleotide sequences of individual rRNA and their genes.

In this review, we shall present and discuss the available data on the structure and evolution of low molecular weight rRNA, which we designate as 23S rRNA-derived; it includes 5.8S rRNA from eukaryote cytosol and 4.5S rRNA from chloroplast ribosomes. The validity of such denotation will be substantiated below. We shall try to show what opportunities are offered by the studies of these rRNAs for phylogenetic analysis and systematics.

It should also be mentioned that the molecular-evolutionary studies have two aspects. The data obtained are used on the one hand to establish relationships between species, and on the other, as a basis for a comparative study of the structure and mode of macromolecule functioning.

II. SPECIES OF rRNA AND THE PECULIARITY OF THEIR SET IN A PLANT CELL

Each of the two ribosomal subunits contains a copy of high molecular weight rRNAs differing in size. The large subunit contains a large size rRNA (L-rRNA), and the small subunit contains a small size rRNA (S-rRNA). The molecular weights and the sedimentation coefficients of these rRNAs are different in prokaryotes and cytoplasmic ribosomes of lower and higher eukaryotes, as well as in ribosomes of cell organelles, chloroplasts, and mitochondria. In addition to L-rRNA, the large ribosomal subunit contains a copy of each low molecular-weight rRNA in prokaryotes, 5S rRNA; in eukaryotes, 5S and 5.8S rRNA.

A plant cell has a more complex genetic organization than cells of other organisms. The plant genome is represented by three genetic compartments localized in the nucleus, mitochondria, and chloroplasts. Cytoplasmic ribosomes encoded by the nuclear genome are ribosomes of eukaryotic type and contain two low molecular weight rRNAs, 5.8S and 5S rRNA. Ribosomes of plant mitochondria and chloroplasts are quite close to those of bacteria; they contain 5S rRNA and are free of 5.8S rRNA.[25,26] Chloroplast ribosomes also possess a component which is designated 4.5S rRNA; it has been observed thus far only in higher plants (see below). According to the widely accepted endosymbiotic hypothesis,[27-30] chloroplasts and mitochondria are prokaryote-symbiont secondary intruders of a protoeukaryotic cell. This endosymbiosis, however, is very ancient; it must date back to the appearance of primary eukaryotic organisms. The organelle genome later evolved as the part of the eukaryotic total genetic system. A parallel analysis of macromolecule evolution from organelle and cytoplasm allows one to make more precise phylogenetic analyses and to specify the evolution of individual genetic compartments.

III. GENE ORGANIZATION AND PROCESSING OF 23S rRNA-DERIVED SMALL RIBOSOMAL RNAs

A. Cytosol 5.8S rRNA

In large subunits of eukaryotic ribosomes, 5.8S rRNA is specifically bound to L-rRNA by noncovalent interactions. The 5.8S rRNA-L-rRNA complex may be isolated from ribosomes; it dissociates in denaturing conditions, and may be reconstituted in vitro.[31-37] The gene of 5.8S rRNA is an integral part of an operon, which also includes genes of S-rRNA and L-rRNA. This gene is present in hundreds or thousands of copies per genome.[38,39] The organization of the ribosomal operon has been studied in dozens of eukaryotic species. In various species, they may differ in number, in arrangement within the genome, and in details of their inner organization, first of all in the size of intergenic spacers. The general, strictly obeyed rule is the 5′-S-rRNA-5.8S rRNA-L-rRNA-3′ order of genes in the direction of transcription. These three genes are read off as a single transcript, which is then processed in several steps.[40-44] The first step is its splitting into the precursor of S-rRNA and the precursor of 5.8S rRNA + L-rRNA.

Another low molecular weight rRNA constituent of a large ribosomal subunit, 5S rRNA, is usually coded in eukaryotes in a separate region of the genome. On the contrary, in prokaryotes, 5S rRNA is originally synthesized within a single transcript, including 16S and 23S rRNA.[40,41] The comparison of the position of genes in pro- and eukaryotic rRNA initially prompted a suggestion that 5.8S rRNA is homologous with 5S rRNA of prokaryotes and that these two low molecular weight RNAs have similar functions in pro- and eukaryotic ribosomes.[45,46] However, later comparisons of nucleotide sequences of 5.8S and 5S rRNA of prokaryotes showed that they are diverse molecular species. It is 5S rRNAs of pro- and eukaryotes that are homologous.[47-52]

In 1980—1981, several researchers demonstrated that 5.8S rRNA is homologous with the 5' end of prokaryotic 23S rRNA.[53-55] As new sequences became known, this conclusion was further substantiated. At present, it may be rightfully concluded that in the course of evolution, 5.8S rRNA originated from the 5' end sequence of prokaryotic L-rRNA as a result of incorporation of a noncoding sequence. In the eukaryotic ribosomal RNA operon this sequence is represented by the internal transcribed spacer ITS-2 between the 3' end of 5.8S rRNA and the 5' end of L-rRNA excised from the primary transcript upon processing. The formation of 5.8S rRNA as a discrete component may thus be regarded as alteration of the normal splicing of the split L-rRNA gene. The region of *Escherichia coli* 23S rRNA, which is homologous with 5.8S rRNA, is part of its sequence between nucleotide residues 10 to 13 and 170 to 173 from the 5' end of 23S rRNA. The degree of homology between this region and the 5.8S rRNA of several species of vertebrates and *Neurospora* is about 50%.[53-55] This level of homology is rather high, the same as that between 5S rRNA of pro- and eukaryotes. None of the other regions of the transcriptional unit of *E. coli* rRNA genes (>5000 nucleotide residues) is as homologous with 5.8S rRNA.[55] The distribution of identical residues over the zone of homology between 5.8S rRNA and 23S rRNA is not uniform. The 5' end region of the homology zone contains a larger proportion of identical residues (> 50%).[53,55] Comparison of nucleotide sequences of 5.8S rRNA from various sources also indicates a stronger conservation of the 5' end half of the 5.8S rRNA molecules.

The above scheme of formation, in the course of evolution, of 5.8S rRNA from the 5' end of prokaryotic L-rRNA is supported by the fact that the region comprising nucleotide residues 1 to 170 of *E. coli* 23S rRNA has no counterparts within the 5' end region of eukaryotic L-rRNAs. However, it is followed in 23S rRNA by the area of considerable homology with the 5' end of eukaryotic L-rRNA.[54-57] It is of interest that in mammalian mitochondria with a compact genome[58,59] L-rRNA has no 5' end segment corresponding to 5.8S rRNA.[55,60-62] In these organelles, L-rRNA does not seem to have an equivalent 5.8S rRNA region, nor is it found in the filamentous fungus *Aspergillus nidulans* mitochondrial L-rRNA, although the rest of the molecule can be folded into a secondary structure almost similar to that of *E. coli* 23S rRNA.[63] The flanking sequence also has no region corresponding to the 1 to 164 nucleotide residues of *E. coli* 23S rRNA.[63] On the other hand, in *Saccharomyces cerevisiae*, mitochondria with a much larger genome, residues 1 to 160 of the 21S rRNA are similar to the 5'-terminal region of the *E. coli* 23S rRNA and homologous with 5.8S rRNA.[64]

B. 4.5S rRNA of Chloroplasts

If the 5'-terminal region of prokaryotic L-rRNA evolved into eukaryotic 5.8S rRNA, the analogous modification of the normal processing of the L-rRNA precursor at the 3' end evidently caused the appearance of 4.5S rRNA. This type of rRNA was originally found in flowering plant chloroplasts.[65-67] 4.5S rRNA is a component which is unique for the large ribosomal subunit of chloroplasts. On circular restriction maps of chloroplast DNA from several angiosperm species, 4.5S rRNA genes localize in the inverted repeat region together with the other rRNA genes.[68-75] The organization of chloroplast rRNA genes in all angiosperms studied thus far is the same (5'-16S-23S-4.5S-5S-3').

The data on the mode of transcription and processing of chloroplast rRNA are rather scarce. There is evidence that in spinach chloroplast 4.5S rRNA is present in a direct precursor of 23S rRNA (1.05×10^6 daltons) having a mol wt of 1.28×10^6 daltons and originating, in its turn, from pre-rRNA with a mol wt of 2.7×10^6 daltons.[41,76,77]

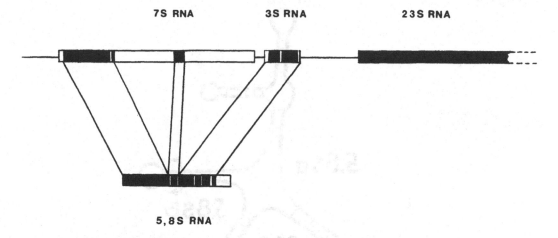

FIGURE 1. Part of the chloroplast ribosomal RNA unit of *Chlamydomonas reinhardii* and sequence homologies between chloroplast 7S and 3S RNAs and cytoplasmic 5.8S rRNA. Nucleotides which do not have counterparts are indicated by open spaces.[85]

MacKay[78] and Edwards et al.[72] were the first investigators to notice that chloroplast 4.5S rRNA is homologous with the 3'-terminal region of prokayotic 23S rRNA. The degree of homology of the 3'-terminal segment of *E. coli* 23S rRNA with the maize and tobacco chloroplast 4.5S rRNAs is about 70%. New sequencing data supported the existence of an essential homology between chloroplast 4.5S rRNA and the 3'-terminal region of prokaryotic L-rRNA.[73,79-81] It was also found that chloroplast 4.5S rRNAs of higher plants reveal homology with the 3' end of *Chlamydomonas reinhardii* chloroplast 23S rRNA.[82] The spacer, 101 nucleotide residues long, between the genes of tobacco chloroplast 23S and 4.5S rRNA is not homologous with any of the *E. coli* 23S rRNA regions.[80] Thus, in this case, as in the case of 5.8S rRNA, we deal with the insertion of an alien sequence near one of the ends of the prokaryotic type L-rRNA gene; this insertion produces the new discrete type of a low molecular weight rRNA. The excision of this segment upon the precursor processing entails no ligation of the ends. This scheme is supported by the fact that the 5' end of chloroplast 4.5S rRNA is not phosphorylated,[65,67,83] and splicing is known to occur between the 3'-phosphoryl and 5'-hydroxyl ends of RNA chains.

C. Other Cases of 23S rRNA Splicing Modification

Besides the above-mentioned cases of the disturbance of normal splicing during L-rRNA maturation, resulting in the appearance of new components and evolutionally established in large phylogenetic lines, similar situations have also been observed only in individual species.

1. Chloroplasts of Chlamydomonas reinhardii

In the region of the *Ch. reinhardii* chloroplast genome, between the 3' end of the 16S rRNA gene and the 5' end of the 23S rRNA gene, two small rRNAs, 7S and 3S rRNA (282 and 47 nucleotide residues long, respectively), are encoded.[84,85] Genes of 7S and 3S rRNA are separated by an AT-rich spacer containing 23 pairs of nucleotide residues. The nucleotide sequences of these rRNA are homologous with the 5' end of 23S rRNA from prokaryotes and chloroplasts of higher plants. It was also established that 7S and 3S rRNAs are homologous with the 5' and 3' end halves of the eukaryotic 5.8S rRNA molecule, respectively. 7S and 3S rRNA unlike 5.8S rRNA, are weakly bound to L-rRNA.[84] The *Ch. reinhardii* chloroplast rRNA gene organization and the correspondence between 7S and 3S rRNA genes and a 5.8S rRNA gene are presented in Figure 1.

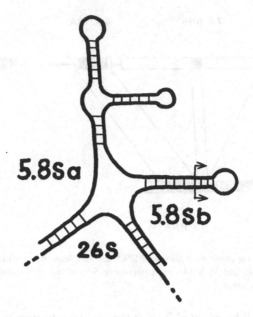

FIGURE 2.   5.8Sa-5.8Sb-26S rRNAs complex of *Sciara* and *Drosophila*.
The cleavage points in precursor rRNA which generate 5.8Sa and 5.8Sb
RNA are shown by arrows.[89]

2. Insects

In the two *Dyptera* species, *Sciara coprophila* and *Drosophila melanogaster*, 5.8S rRNA
is present in ribosomes as two discrete components designated as 5.8Sa and 2S rRNA (or
5.8Sa and 5.8Sb).[86-89] The genes of these two low molecular weight rRNA are separated
by a small region, which can be excised from rRNA during its processing, with the termini
of the resultant 5.8Sa and 5.8Sb rRNA remaining nonligated. This does not prevent them
from forming a complex with 28S rRNA, which is very similar in structure to complexes
formed by "normal" 5.8S rRNA (Figure 2). Two "pieces" of 5.8S rRNA are bound by
an intermolecular helix and each of the "pieces" is hydrogen bonded to a specific region
of 28S rRNA. In three other investigated insects, butterflies and aphid, and in the Crustacean
Artemia salina, 5.8S rRNA has a usual structure.[90-93]

3. Protozoan Crithidia fasciculata

In *Crithidia fasciculata*, a trypanosomatid protozoan, the large ribosomal subunit contains,
in addition to 5S and 5.8S rRNA, 4 low molecular weight rRNAs composed of 212, 183,
135 to 136, and 72 to 73 nucleotide residues.[94] These rRNAs have unique sequences and
obviously are not products of L-rRNA degradation during the isolation procedure. They are
monophosphorylated at the 5′ end and have a free hydroxyl group at the 3′ end. The
biosynthetic origin and functions of these RNAs have not been elucidated so far. Several
small rRNAs have also been found in *Leishmania tarentole*, *Trypanosoma brucei*, and
Euglena gracilis.[94-96]

4. Breaks and Insertions in L-rRNA

L-rRNAs of most, but not all, protostomia and protozoa contain breaks.[97-101] These breaks
were called "hidden" because L-rRNA pieces remain in the complex due to complementary
basepairing. Even closely related species may differ by the presence or absence of the nick
in L-rRNA.[102] Among insects, there are species with broken and unbroken L-rRNA.[90] The
nick locates approximately at the center of the L-rRNA chain or lies off-center. In *Tetra-*

hymena thermophila, introduction of the hidden break in L-rRNA occurs in the cytoplasm as a last step of the processing.[44] In *Drosophila melanogaster*, there is a small region of approximately 120 nucleotide residues specifically removed from the rRNA precursor at the point of hidden break introduction and not presented in mature L-rRNA.[87,103-106] No ligation of ends follows thereafter.

Introns have been found in L-rRNA genes of some lower eukaryotes and their organelles.[57,63,64,85,107-111] The same genes of higher eukaryotes do not contain any introns. The intervening sequences which separate the mature L-rRNA coding region do not coincide with hidden breaks as it was shown for L-rRNA *D. melanogaster*[105] and *Tetrahymena pigmentosa*.[107] Noller et al.[62] and Branlant et al.[112] have studied the order of intron arrangement in the L-rRNA genes. It has been found that introns seemed to localize in functionally essential regions rather than split structural domains in the L-rRNA secondary structure models. The nonexcised intron will probably have a tangible effect on the functioning of L-rRNA. The genes of eukaryotic L-rRNA also contain insertions that are not excised upon L-rRNA processing; these insertions make eukaryotic L-rRNAs longer than prokaryotic.[54,57,113] Although the length of the inserted sequences varies, they are found in the same relative positions in yeast 26S, *Physarum* 26S, and *Xenopus* 28S rDNA. The comparison of nucleotide sequences in pro- and eukaryotic L-rRNA reveals the alternation of evolutionarily conservative and variable segments.

Thus, the above facts indicate a significant fluidity of L-rRNA genes in the course of evolution. In various phyletic lines, they may be subjected to diverse specific rearrangements, with the functional activity of the resulting products remaining retained. The concrete features of these rearrangements may serve as quality markers for the distinction of various groups of organisms. The events occurring in L-rRNA and their genes in the course of evolution are outlined in Figure 3. The present-day variants probably reflect only a small part of the options in the course of evolution. It is noteworthy that evolution "handled" mainly L-rRNA and not S-rRNA. The latter is much more conservative; its sequence[22,114] and length[100,101] were altered to a lesser degree during the volution. S-rRNAs have no introns — the single exception found to date is the 17S rRNA from malaria parasite *Plasmodium lophurae*.[115]

IV. STRUCTURE OF 5.8S rRNA

A. Primary Structure

A number of nucleotide sequences (31) of 5.8S rRNA are known to date (Table 1), and the list is increasing, although not as rapidly as in the case of 5S rRNA. For plants, the 5.8S rRNA sequences of only two species of angiosperm dicots (broad bean and lupine) and one species of monocots (wheat) have been published.

Recently, we sequenced 5.8S rRNA of species from the evolutionarily more distant group of higher plants, the moss *Mnium rugicum*. Also known is the 5.8S rRNA sequence of green flagellate *Chlamydomonas reinhardii*.[116] The lists of known nucleotide sequences were published periodically in the journal *Nucleic Acids Research*. In early 1983 the list included 20 nucleotide sequences.[117] Most of them have been determined by new rapid methods, but some (from turtle and rainbow trout), were determined only by oligonucleotide analysis. Since they may contain errors, they are excluded from subsequent consideration. Several sequences determined by the new methods also proved erroneous and were corrected later. It should be noted that single errors have a negligible effect on phylogenetic trees inferred from these sequences, although they may bear upon an analysis of secondary structure models.

Most of the 5.8S rRNA molecules consist of 156 to 167 nucleotide residues. Variations in length come from insertions and the presence or absence of additional nucleotide residues at the 5' and/or 3' ends. In some species, the 5.8S rRNA population is found to be heter-

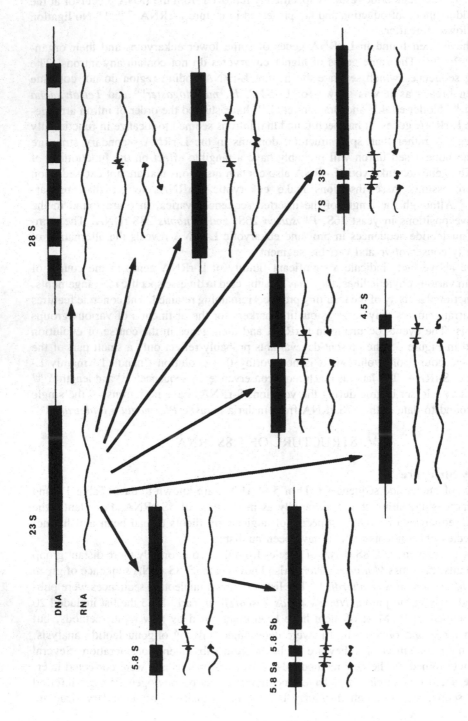

FIGURE 3.   Rearrangements of L-RNA and its genes in the course of evolution. Boxes represent rDNA coding regions. Open areas in boxes denote insertions in the coding region. Horizontal arrows indicate ends of RNA after endonucleolytic cleavages.

Table 1
SEQUENCED 5.8S rRNAs

Species	No. of residues	Ref.
Protozoa		
Acanthamoeba castellanii	161	190
Crithidia fasciculata	170—171	191
Crypthecodinium cohnii	156	170
Tetrahymena pyriformis	154	90
Myxomycetes		
Dictyostelium discoideum	162	144
Physarum polycephalum	155	192[a]
Fungi		
Neurospora crassa	158	193[a], 139[b]
Thermomyces lanuginosus	157	124
Saccharomyces cerevisiae	158	143[a], 194
Schizosaccharomyces pombe	158—165	195[a]
Chlorophyta		
Chlamydomonas reinhardii	156	116
Higher plants		
Mnium rugicum	158	[c]
Lupinus luteus	164	196[a]
Vicia faba	164	145[b], 197
Triticum vulgare (aestivum)[b]	162	125[b], 198
Porifera		
Hymeniacidon sanguinea	156	136
Mollusca		
Arion rufus	157	136
Arthropoda		
Artemia salina	159—162	93
Sciara coprophila	123	89[a]
Drosophila melanogaster	123	88
Acyrthosiphon magnoliae	161	90
Bombyx mori	167	91
Philosamia cynthia ricini	169	92
Vertebrata		
Salmo gairdneri	162	199
Xenopus laevis	161	56,[a] 137,[a] 200, 201
Xenopus borealis	161	200, 201
Terrapene carolina	159	202
Gallus gallus	159	146[b], 200
Mus musculus	159	126,[b] 140,[b] 203
Rattus rattus	158	35, 203
Homo sapiens	159	200, 203

[a]   Inferred from DNA sequence.
[b]   Correction of the sequence.
[c]   Our data.

ogenous at the ends. Individual components differ by the presence or absence of one or several nucleotide residues. The largest number of components is found in the yeast *Schizosaccharomyces pombe*. There are 8 species of 5.8S rRNA in them, 158 to 165 nucleotide residues long. Two of them, consisting of 164 and 159 nucleotide residues are the main species. This heterogeneity is the result of the presence of additional residues at the 5′ end.

The large majority of 5.8S rRNA studied in this respect thus far contains 2 types of modified nucleotides, pseudouridylic acid residues and 2′-*O*-methyl nucleotides. The sole exception is the 5.8S rRNA *Dictyostelium discoideum*. The total number of modified nucleotides in different rRNA varies from 2 to 5. There are no distinct regularities in their location. It was shown that methylation may induce conformational changes in 5.8S rRNA.[118]

B. Secondary Structure

5.8S rRNA, like any other macromolecules, carries out its functions in the folded state. In the course of evolution, selection pressure affects the primary structure indirectly via higher-order structures, secondary and tertiary. Therefore, the knowledge of the spatial organization of macromolecules and the changes it undergoes in evolution may be of great importance for molecular-phylogenetic studies. The use of this approach is limited by the difficulty of quantitative interpretation of such kind of data and by insufficient information.

There are several approaches to RNA secondary structure models, and all of them have certain limitations.

For theoretical analysis, it is essential to search for potentially complementary sites in molecules and to find a combination which could provide for a free energy minimum of the structures obtained. These calculations are also used to gauge the effect of nucleotide substitutions on RNA stability. As a rule, a number of mutually excluding variants of complementary basepairing can be found in RNA molecules. The thermodynamic stabilities of the resulting structures might not differ much. The free energy values for basepair doublets for model compounds obtained by Tinoco et al.[119] and usually employed in calculations as well as empirical rules for RNA secondary structure predictions[120-123] are evidently a certain approximation. Furthermore, it is not obvious that rRNAs have a minimal energy conformation within a functioning ribosome in vivo.

The study of the accessibility of various nucleotide residues in RNA to specific modifying reagents and nucleases is of great use in distinguishing between single-stranded and double-helical regions. The results obtained by various authors for 5.8S rRNA[34,35,124-129] do not always coincide in full. The mobility of RNA structure, sterical hindrances caused by spatial structure, changes in the accessibility of some sites in the course of a reaction — all pose difficulties for the interpretation.

The study of native RNAs and their denaturation by various spectroscopy methods[130-134] makes it possible to estimate the amount of nucleotide residues in single-stranded and double-helical regions, the nucleotide composition, and the number of these sites, etc. As a rule, only very general features may be deduced in this manner.

The comparative-evolutionary analysis of the secondary structure is based on the postulate that homologous RNAs fullfil the same or very similar functions in the cell. This approach is realized by finding the best conformity between the secondary structure of the molecules and localization of the evolutionally conservative nucleotide residues. Such "phylogenetic proving" is widely used now, however, for this, one must be sure that structural requirements for a molecule as a whole and its constituent parts do not change in evolution. It will be shown below that this is not always the rule.

RNA molecules certainly contain many sets of sites potentially capable of complementary pairing. RNA molecules are flexible systems, the various metastable states of which may be in dynamic equilibrium brought about by the nucleotide sequence of potentially complementary sites and by their possible interaction with other sites of the same molecule, i.e., tertiary interactions, or by other macromolecules, proteins, and nucleic acids. It should be emphasized that the generally used methods of secondary structure calculation ignore tertiary interactions which may be significant for both the statics and the dynamics of RNA. This is not a very optimistic point of view in regard to structural modeling. Here we might just as well indicate that for the intensively studied 5S rRNA, over a dozen various secondary structure models have already been suggested.[135] For 5.8S rRNA, there are fewer models so far (Figure 4). None of them are in full agreement with all the data obtained.

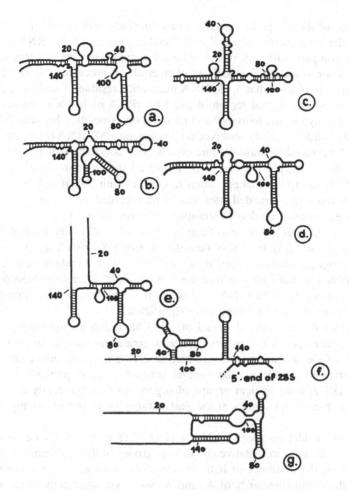

FIGURE 4.   Secondary structure models of 5.8S rRNA proposed by:(a,b) Ford and Mathieson.[201] (c) Luoma and Marschall.[130] (d) Nazar.[35] (e) Pace.[34] (f) Walker et al.[126] (g) Ursi et al.[93]

Nevertheless the Nazar "burp-gun" model[35] and its modifications[34,93,126,136] are the best approximations so far available for the conformation of 5.8S rRNA.

The basic difference between the "burp-gun" model and its variant proposed by Pace et al.[34] ("burp-gun with a wide-open muzzle") is in the state of the 5' and 3' end regions on the molecule. As mentioned above, in the ribosome 5.8S rRNA forms a complex with L-rRNA. The 5' and 3' end regions of 5.8S rRNA, each about 20 nucleotide residues long, are involved in the formation of the complex.[34,37,89,126,137-139] These regions are basepaired with the immediate 5' end and a region 300 to 400 nucleotide residues from the 5' end terminus of 28S rRNA.[62,126,138,140-143] There is indirect evidence that the complex of 28S rRNA with 20 nucleotide residues from the 3'-terminus of 5.8S rRNA is stabilized by so-called "GC-rich" helix of 5.8S rRNA due to the coaxial helix stacking.[34,138]

As noted above, the comparison of nucleotide sequences showed the existence of homology between the 5.8S rRNA and about 150 nucleotide residues from the 5' end terminus of prokaryotic 23S rRNA. According to the secondary structure models suggested for *E. coli* 23S rRNA, the 5' end of the 23S rRNA can be folded into a structure very similar to the supposed complex of 5.8S rRNA with 164 to 270 nucleotide residues of eukaryotic L-rRNA,[62,112] the conservative residues localizing in single-stranded regions. The 5' end of 23S rRNA from maize chloroplasts can also form a similar, although more distorted structure.[112]

The same is true of the 5' end of L-rRNA yeast *Saccharomyces cerevisiae* mitochondria.[64]

The data on the participation of the 5' and 3' end segments of 5.8S rRNA in the formation of a molecular complex with 28S rRNA were the main reason for constructing the "burp-gun with a wide-open muzzle" model. Walker et al.,[126] proceeding from their own data, have come to the conclusion that 5.8S rRNA nucleotide residues 1 to 35 can form a hairpin of their own without the 3' end region of the 5.8S rRNA molecule being involved. It was suggested that this hypothetic hairpin may unloop upon association between 5.8S rRNA and 28S rRNA. This hairpin is hardly observed on comparing 5.8S rRNA from various species.[144] Walker et al.[126] hesitated to draw definite conclusions about the structure of 20 nucleotide residues from the 3' end terminus of 5.8S rRNA; all the more so since according to their data, 5.8S rRNA undergoes changes when in contact with 28S rRNA. In their secondary structure model the single-stranded sites should be regarded as having a yet unknown secondary structure, whereas the double-stranded are certainly appointed.

Thus, Nazar's model in its original form is apparently valid only for free 5.8S rRNA in solution. There are strongly indicative data that in free 5.8S rRNA the 5'- and 3'-terminal regions are hydrogen bonded to a certain extent.[35,124,127,145-147] In addition, it should be noted that the 5.8S rRNA is transcribed before the 28S rRNA.[148] Therefore, basepairing between the 5' and 3' ends of the 5.8S rRNA may occur in vivo. At any rate, complementarity of the terminal segments must be biologically significant.

Construction of the generalized model of the 5.8S rRNA encompassing all the known nucleotide sequences poses difficulties. When a greater number of sequences is studied, some elements of the secondary structure can hardly be revealed, while others have to be modified significantly to fit into the general scheme. This is particularly obvious upon studying 5.8S rRNA from ancient groups of organisms that apparently diverged from the line, leading to higher eukaryotes at the early stages of evolution — myxomycetes and protozoans.

In terms of the model proposed by Nazar et al.,[35] (Figure 5 A,C) we shall consider its basic elements as far as representatives of various groups of living organisms are concerned.

The question of the existence of helix A was discussed earlier in the chapter. It should be added that the complementarity of A' and A" well expressed in the 5.8S rRNA of yeast and higher eukaryotes (Figure 6), disappears in the myxomycetes *Dictyostelium discoideum* (class Acrasiomycetes).[144] Neither can a good scheme of the base pairing between the 5' and 3' ends of the protozoan *Acanthamoeba castellani* 5.8S rRNA be suggested. Satisfactory pairing is observed in 5.8S rRNA of other protists; in myxomycetes *Physarum polycephalum* it is rather good.

Arm D-III is a very conservative structural element in the course of evolution (Figures 7 and 8). Usually helix D includes 4 to 6 complementary basepairs. In the aphid *Acyrthosiphon magnoliae*, this hairpin is longer and contains 8 bp. In higher plants, yeasts, and *A. magnoliae*, but not other insects, an alternative basepairing is quite possible with formation of a rather good helix. This entails changes in the nucleotide sequence and size of loops II and III. The size of loop III varies from four nucleotide residues in most of the studied insects and vertebrates to eight nucleotide residues in *Artemia salina* and *Drosophila melanogaster*. Thus, the sizes of helix D and loops II and III do not prove absolutely conservative in evolution. Areas with identical secondary structure formed by homologous nucleotide sequences are revealed only in specific groups of living organisms.

Arm E-IV, the so-called "AU-rich" hairpin is also a conservative structural element (Figures 7 and 8). In animals, loop IV is longer and contains up to 10 unpaired nucleotide residues, whereas in yeasts and plants it consists of only 4 residues. It is remarkable that in the 5.8S rRNA of vertebrates the basepairing pattern in helix E is different from that in other higher eukaryotes and yeasts; i.e., the conservatism of the secondary structure is maintained by involvement of nonhomologous nucleotide sequence elements. In *E. coli*, the

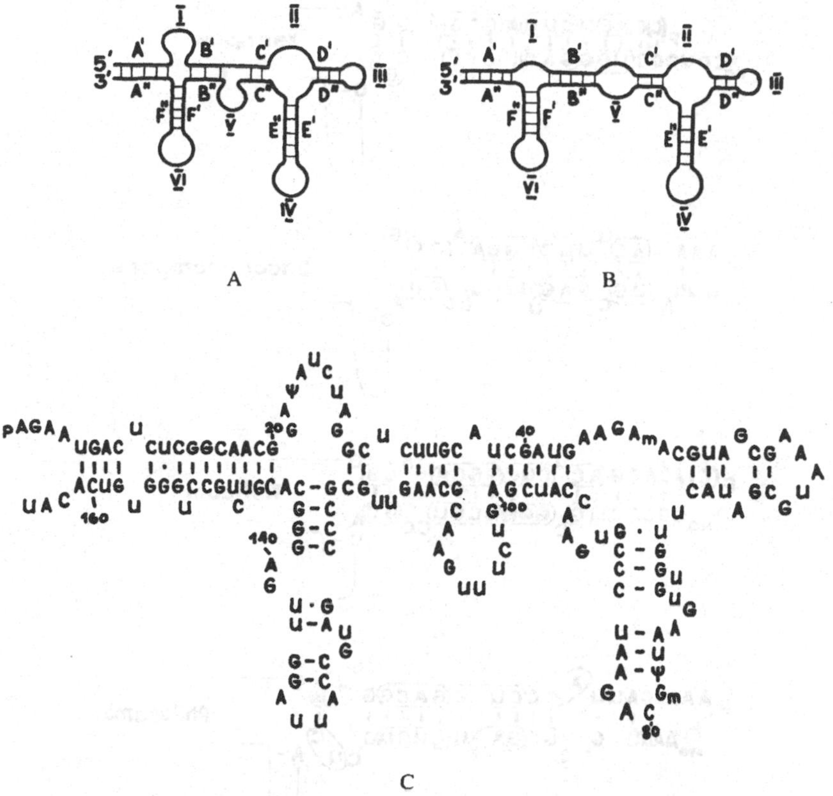

FIGURE 5.   5.8S rRNA secondary structure. (A) Scheme of basepairing in Nazar's model.[35] (B) Scheme of basepairing in Ursi et al. model.[93] (C) 5.8S rRNA of *Vicia faba* folded according to Nazar's "burp-gun" model.

basepairing scheme in helix E is also different. In protists, there is a broad range of helix E stability; its formation is doubtful in 5.8S rRNA *Acanthamoeba castellanii*, although in 5.8S rRNA *Crithidia fasciculata* the pairing in this region is rather good. Structural defects in helix E are seen in 5.8S rRNA of all the studied organisms, except for vertebrates, dipterans, and the snail.

Helix C is seen in all the known 5.8S rRNA and consists of five to eight complementary basepairs. The comparison of the secondary structure model with aligned nucleotide sequences shows that there exists a helical "nucleus". This is formed, in various species, by homologous nucleotide residues. The ends of the helix in various species may shift from both sides of the nucleus, so that the corresponding homologous residues may in some species be contained in the helix, and in the others may remain in the unpaired state. In the *E. coli* 23S rRNA, the folding of a corresponding region into a helix is impossible. Based on structural mapping data of mammalian[35,126,127] and fungal *Thermomyces lanuginosus*[124] 5.8S rRNA, Olsen and Sogin[144] suggested that helix C was not present in vivo. Neither is the state of the nucleotide residues corresponding to chain B' and the 3' end of loop I determined unequivocally. According to the model of Walker et al.,[126] this region in the free 5.8S rRNA is single-stranded, and in Nazar's model[35] B' is included in the helical region. Helix B may be formed as an alternative to the "burp-gun" model pairing, with the 3' end segment of loop I being involved (Figures 5 and 9). For *Artemia salina* 5.8S rRNA, a fit structure may be built only by this second method.[93] The variant of the generalized secondary structure model proposed by Ursi et al.[93,136] differs from Nazar's model[35] by the substitution of inner loop for bulge (Figure 5). Ursi et al.[93] calculated the free energy of

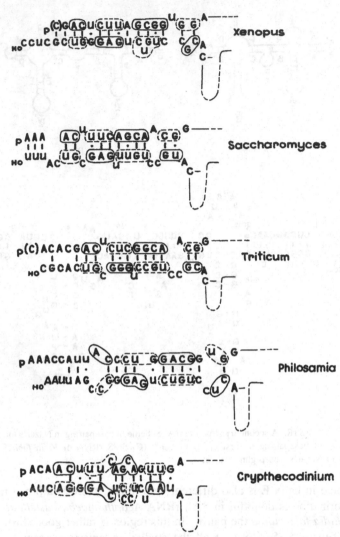

FIGURE 6.   The structures of helix A in 5.8S rRNAs of different species.
Homologous nucleotides are outlined by solid or dashed lines.

5.8S rRNA secondary structure formation for their own model and that of Nazar (Table 2). It should be noted that Nazar's model has an evident advantage for higher plant 5.8S rRNA and the model of Ursi et al. for protozoan 5.8S rRNA. For the *Xenopus* and yeast 5.8S rRNAs, both variants are almost energetically equivalent. For 5.8S rRNA *Chlamydomonas reinhardii* the energy of the secondary structure formation is positive in both cases, however, the Ursi variant is somewhat preferable. Arm F-VI, the so-called "GC-rich" hairpin, is revealed in all 5.8S rRNA, as well as in the homologous region of the *E. coli* 23S rRNA (Figure 10). The paradox consists in that this most universal structural element is at the same time the most variable region of the molecule both in the size of the helix and in the nucleotide sequence. Helix F contains, in various species, 7 to 11 bp. In fungi, vertebrates, several invertebrates, protozoans, and *E. coli*, helix has no defects; in other species it contains several looped-out bases. In the *D. discoideum* 5.8S rRNA, helix F is elongated through extending of pairing into chains A″ and B″. In the protozoan *Crithidia fasciculata*, this helix is somewhat longer due to insertion. In insects with a nicked 5.8S rRNA *(Drosophila melanogaster* and *Sciara coprophila)*, helix F forms due to intermolecular interaction between 5.8Sa and 5.8Sb rRNA[88,89] (Figure 2).

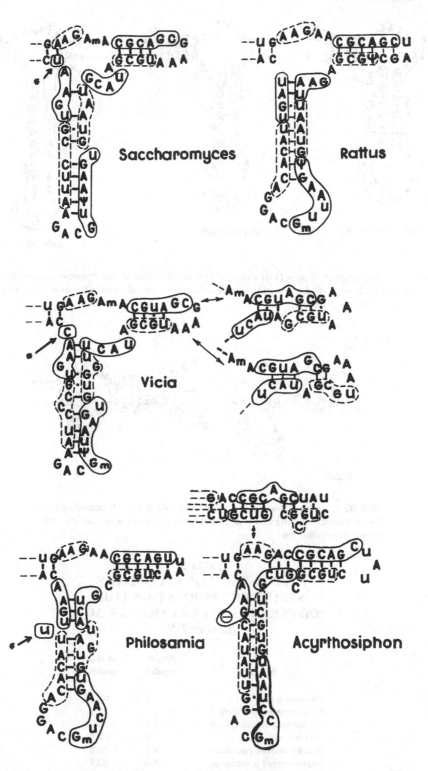

FIGURE 7. The structure of arms D-III and E-IV in 5.8S rRNAs of several multicellular species. Homologous nucleotides are outlined by solid or dashed lines. Inserted nucleotides are indicated by arrows with asterisks. Deleted nucleotide is indicated by circle with minus.

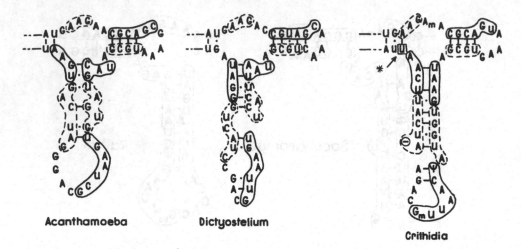

Acanthamoeba   **Dictyostelium**   **Crithidia**

FIGURE 8.   The structure of arms D-III and E-IV in 5.8S rRNAs of several *Protozoa* species. Homologous nucleotides are outlined by solid or dashed lines. Inserted nucleotide is indicated by the arrow. Deleted nucleotide is indicated by circle with minus.

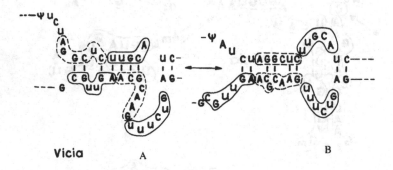

Vicia   A   B

FIGURE 9.   The folding of *Vicia faba* 5.8S rRNA helix B according to: (A) Nazar's model[35] and (B) Ursi et al. model.[93] Homologous nucleotides are outlined by solid or dashed lines.

Table 2
FREE ENERGY OF SECONDARY STRUCTURE FORMATION FOR DIFFERENT 5.8S rRNA MODELS ΔG (kcal/mol)[93]

Species	Nazar model	Ursi et al. model
Xenopus laevis	− 67.4	− 65.3
Crypthecodinium cohnii	+ 3.5	− 9.4
Acanthamoeba castellanii	− 3.3	− 8.0
Neurospora crassa	− 17.9	− 21.8
Saccharomyces cerevisiae	− 20.8	− 26.0
Thermomyces lanuginosus	− 14.8	− 20.9
Triticum aestivum	− 30.2	− 21.1
Vicia faba	− 28.0	− 9.9
Chlamydomonas reinhardii	+ 11.8	+ 2.7

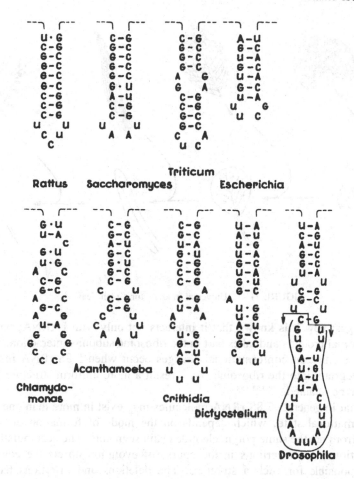

FIGURE 10.   The structure of arm F-VI in 5.8S rRNA of several species. Homologous nucleotides are outlined by solid or dashed lines. The excised region from the precursor of the 5.8Sa and 5.8Sb rRNAs of *Drosophila* is indicated by arrows.

Consideration of 5.8S rRNAs secondary structure suggests certain conclusions. First, in a number of cases, nonhomologous nucleotide residues may occupy structurally equivalent positions. Second, for some regions of the 5.8S rRNA molecule in certain groups of organisms, alternative modes of helix forming are possible. We believe it would be wrong to ignore these variants in an attempt to build a unified 5.8S rRNA secondary structure model. The existence of such energetically close variants of 5.8S rRNA structure in solution or in the ribosome is not at variance with the experimental data. In trying to build a generalized model, we run the risk of depriving it of the essential structural features which may be different in various phylogenetic groups and come to a bare scheme devoid of any functional meaning. In their evolutionary analysis of secondary structure of 9 5.8S rRNA, Olsen and Sogin[144] came to the conclusion that "it portrays 5.8S rRNA as devoid of the secondary structure with one or at most two exceptions", arms F-VI and D-III. In fact, discarding all nonuniversal elements, we may have none at all, as shown in Figure 11. This illustrates the results of our experiment on building a universal model for a plant leaf. We carried it out together with our son who has not yet studied botany at school.

Actually, we know next to nothing about the role of 5.8S rRNA in the ribosome and in the cell. 5.8S rRNA is only a constituent part of higher rank functional complexes. In the course of evolution, not only 5.8S rRNA itself but all the elements associated with it have

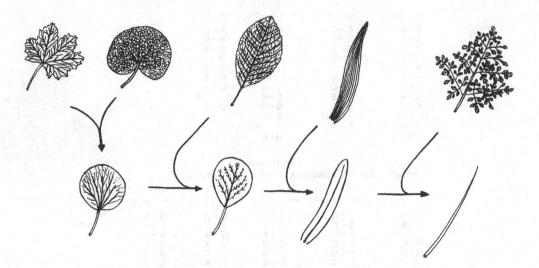

FIGURE 11.   "Universal model" for a plant leaf.

undergone changes; now it is known that it interacts not only with L-rRNA, but also with tRNA and ribosomal proteins and takes part in the ribosome subunits interaction.[149-152] There is evidence that significant conformational changes occur when 5.8S rRNA interacts with L-rRNA and integrates into the ribosome. As a result a more uniform structure for various 5.8S rRNA may be attained.[125,153,154]

We assume that in general, 5.8S rRNA molecules may exist in more than one potentially possible conformational state, which depends on the mode of formation of functionally similar regions from not the same polynucleotide chain segments. The accumulation of point mutations, deletions, and insertions in the course of evolution upsets the equilibrium of interactions responsible for such a structure. The deletions and insertions have a more deleterious effect, since it is doubtful that their consequences can be corrected by single compensatory point mutations. As a result, an alternative way of basepairing, involving nonhomologous regions of the polynucleotide chain, may hold greater advantages. The former type of base pairing may be seen sometimes as a relic. The negative selection pressure (whereby the molecule retains its basic functional properties) ensures the conservation in the evolution of the main functionally important structure elements. The structurally equivalent parts of molecules, helixes, or single-stranded regions between them, formed by nonhomologous nucleotides should be called analogous. In this case, the principal features maintained by selection are the spatial structure elements rather than a concrete nucleotide sequence. This switching process is phenomenologically similar to the one in which the functions of organs are changed and functionally identical organs are formed from genetically nonhomologous structures (analogous organs) a not frequent phenomenon in the evolution of organisms.

The constant rate of macromolecule evolution is determined by the invariability of its functions. If functions alter, the change in the set of tolerable and advantageous mutational states of the gene takes place, with a resultant increase in the rate of mutational replacement. This inconstancy of molecular evolution rate hampers the inference of phylogeny from sequence data. Such phyletic lines, with the evolution rate deviating from the average, may be revealed upon studying the peculiarities of the 5.8S rRNA secondary structure, and also upon comparing the phylogenetic trees built by different procedures and for different macromolecules. On the other hand, the "comparative-morphological" analysis of rRNA may prove quite useful in molecular-evolutionary studies. As Goodman[155] states, despite the perfection of the methods for phylogenetic reconstruction from sequence data there are cases of inconsistency between trees and strongly supported traditional views on the species phylogeny. In these cases, additional valuable information may be provided by the study of such qualitative molecular characters as the presence of certain deletions or insertions and the spatial structure peculiarities.

C. Evolution of 5.8S rRNA

In constructing the phylogenetic trees, two basic approaches are usually employed. The first is based on computing a matrix of differences between nucleotide sequences and building the corresponding dendrogram by clustering methods. The second approach consists of the reconstitution of ancestral sequences at each node of the tree and in constructing the phylogenetic tree of minimal length. Various methods of phylogenetic tree construction and the problems associated with them have been discussed.[155-163] Here we must point out that methods based on the use of dissimiliarity (distance) matrixes may yield incorrect topologies of trees for the macromolecules that evolved with different rates in different lineages; however, Klotz and Blanken[164] suggested a method abolishing this limitation. We should also stress the advantage of methods that operate with sequences, rather than difference matrixes, since even intuitively one can see that converting sequence data into the difference matrix results in the loss of information because events occurring at concrete positions of the sequences cannot be taken into account.

The first step in phylogenetic tree construction is the alignment of nucleotide sequences, with the number of differences between nucleotide sequences at homologous positions and the number of gaps being minimal. The alignment of 5.8S rRNA sequences is somewhat difficult due to a high variability of the "GC-rich" hairpin and adjacent region. As a result of nucleotide substitutions, deletions, and insertions, unambiguous alignment of all known 5.8S rRNA sequences simultaneously in this part of the molecule is hardly achieved. Therefore, to calculate the difference matrix, we used only regions between residues 3 to 155, excluding several 5′ end residues because of 5.8S rRNA variability in length.

The phenogram for 25 sequences of 5.8S rRNA and the homologous 5′-terminal part of *E. coli* 23S rRNA molecule was constructed by the use of a simple clustering procedure (Figure 12). A gap vs. nucleotide was counted as one nucleotide substitution regardless of the size of a gap. The root was naturally introduced between eukaryotic and prokaryotic lineages.

A large conservation of 5.8S rRNA can be seen from the matrix and the phenogram. The identity between compared parts of 5.8S rRNA from rodents and man is 100%; from mammals and chicken, 97%; and mammals, chicken, and amphibia, 90%. The compared regions of 5.8S rRNA from two angiosperm classes, Monocotyledoneae and Dicotyledoneae are 97% identical and 99% from *Vicia faba* and *Lupinus luteus* of the same dicot family Leguminosae. The number of known higher plant 5.8S rRNA sequences is not large thus far. The already-available data allow one to conclude that the degree of 5.8S rRNA variability is not sufficiently high for the elucidation of evolutionary relations between orders and families of angiosperms. The addition of more variable 3′ end regions of 5.8S rRNA for sequence comparison does not improve the statistical significance of differences between angiosperm 5.8S rRNA sequences. In this case, the identity of 5.8S rRNA from two dicots is 95% and from dicots and monocots, 93%. The comparison of 5.8S rRNA nucleotide sequences may help in determining the degree of affinity between the higher taxa, classes, and divisions. Mosses (Bryophyta) are in the independent line of land plant evolution which has diverged from the branch leading to angiosperms in Lower Devonian or Upper Silurian.[5,165-169] The dominant phase in this line is the gametophyte, whereas the lines leading to ferns and to angiosperms are due to the reduction of gametophyte and the increase in the role of sporophyte came over. Thus, two lines, gametophytic and sporophytic, split at the

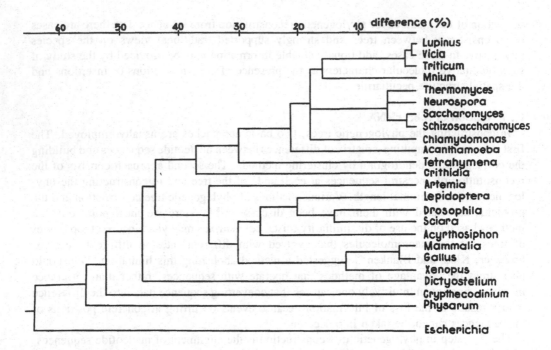

FIGURE 12.   Phenogram for 5.8S rRNA sequences. For references see Table 1.

ancient time and evolved independently thereafter. A comparison of 5.8S rRNA nucleotide sequences confirms this conclusion. The moss *Mnium rugicum* 5.8S rRNA is almost equidistant from the 5.8S rRNA of angiosperms and fungi (84 to 85 and 82 to 85% similiarities, respectively.)

In the preceding paragraph, it was suggested on the basis of the secondary structure consideration that the rate of 5.8S rRNA evolution varies significantly in different phyletic lineages. This may interfere in elucidating evolutionary relationships from sequence data. Therefore, we build the phylogenetic tree for 5.8S rRNA by the "present-day ancestor" method,[164] which is not susceptible to rate differences. The yeast sequences were used as a "present-day ancestor". The topologies of the phenogram (Figure 12) and the tree constructed by a later method (Figure 13) are different in several parts. These differences are indicative of inconstancy of 5.8S rRNA evolution rates in different lineages. Two dendrogram comparisons reveal in them some common elements; therefore, by assuming that 5.8S rRNA phylogeny reflects the evolution of species, several conclusions may be considered:

1.   Fungi are more closely related to plants than to multicellular animals. The divergence of fungi and plants occurred after the branching-off of the Metazoan line. These three kingdoms form three distinct clusters on both dendrograms, the connection between which, as stated above, is traced with good resolution. The above-mentioned comparison of the secondary structures is also evidence that yeast 5.8S rRNAs are closer to plant 5.8S rRNAs than to those of animals. Olsen and Sogin[144] came to a similar conclusion by analyzing the 5.8S rRNA from eight species and the homologous 23S rRNA region. The method for phylogenetic tree construction used by them was different. Hinnebusch et al.,[170] considering data on six 5.8S rRNAs, concluded that there might be two alternative interpretations of the results, according to which either fungi had diverged from the line leading to plants after the divergence of animals and plants; or animals, plants, and fungi had diverged almost at the same time. Comparison of T_1 oligonucleotide catalogs for S-rRNAs also indicates that the radiation of plants

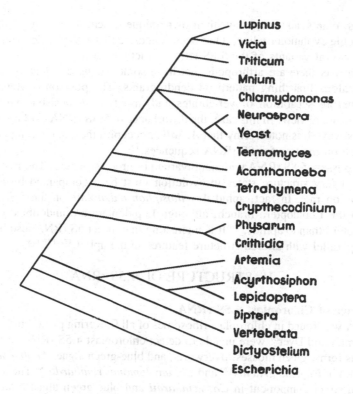

FIGURE 13. Topology of phylogenetic tree for 5.8S rRNA sequences constructed by "present-day ancestor" method of Klotz and Blanken.[161]

occurred at the time of animal-fungal dichotomy.[171] On the other hand, 5S rRNA[52,170,172] and tRNA[173] sequence data indicate that fungi are closer to Metazoa or are isolated into an individual branch prior to the divergence of animals and plants.

2. The green flagellate *Chlamydomonas* is more closely related to plants than to non-chlorophyll flagellates *Crithidia fasciculata* (Zoomastigina) and *Crypthecodinium cohnii* (Dinoflagellata). *Chlamydomonas*, plants, and fungi diverged from the common ancestral at nearly the same time and approximately equidistant.

3. Protists are a diverse paraphyletic group, no more related to Metazoa than to plants and fungi. Protists do not form a single cluster on dendrograms. This is in accordance with contemporary views on single-cellular eukaryotes as a very diversified polyphyletic group. Recently, protists have been divided into several different kingdoms, the relations between which remain obscure.[174,175] The data on 5.8S rRNA confirm that these groups are very ancient and have existed as several independent lines for an indefinite time.

4. The divergence of *Dictyostelium discoideum* (Acrasyomycetes, Myxomyceta) from the mainstream of eukaryotic descent proceeded early in evolution. This inference is in full coincidence with the conclusions that have been drawn by Olsen and Sogin.[144] Other candidates for ancient affinity to prokaryotes are *Physarum* (Myxogasteromycetes, Myxomyceta) and *Crypthecodinium* (Dinoflagellata). The 5.8S rRNA sequences of these three protists are most similar to the 5.8S rRNA-like sequence of *E. coli* 23S rRNA.

The dendrograms derived from 5.8S rRNA do not show great resemblance to those for 5S rRNA in the branching positions of different protist lines.[52,172] 5.8S rRNAs or protozoans are the most variable both in nucleotide sequence and in secondary structure, whereas those of vertebrates, plants, and fungi have their own unique structural elements. Since protozoans are not the single evolutionary line, it has been suggested that at the earliest steps of eukaryote emergence, several variants of the 5.8S rRNA structure existed.

Besides protists there are arthropods that have some "unusual" features of 5.8S rRNA and an anomalous branching pattern on dendrograms. The position of *Artemia salina* on phenogram before separation of vertebrates and insects is inconsistent with the strongly supported traditional view. In this case, the disturbance of 5.8S rRNA evolution rate occurred in an obvious way. It is noteworthy that *A. salina* occupies the same wrong position among other Metazoa on the tree for 5S rRNA sequences.[172]

Insects do possess 5.8S rRNA with noninvariant in-group structure. The switching between different secondary structure states in evolution must be accompanied by changes of the mutation fixation rate. In fact, aphid *Acyrthosiphon magnoliae* on the 5.8S rRNA tree is connected to the Lepidoptera branch, although Lepidoptera are undoubtedly more closely related to Diptera than to aphids.[176] It is interesting that insect 5S rRNA also has unexpected affinities in parallel with altered structure features in the aphid.[172,177,178]

V. STRUCTURE OF 4.5S rRNA

A. Occurrence of Chloroplast 4.5S rRNA

4.5S rRNA was found in chloroplast ribosomes of all flowering plants studied (see Section III.B). Bowman and Dyer[67] were unable to detect chloroplast 4.5S rRNA in more primitive plants such as ferns, green mosses, liverworts, and blue-green algae (*Anabaena sp.*). Neither was it revealed in *Euglena gracilis*[179] and *Chlamydomonas reinhardii*.[84] The absence of 4.5S rRNA as a distinct component in *Ch. reinhardii* and blue-green algae *Anacystis nidulans* chloroplasts is evidenced by regions at the 3' end of its 23S rRNAs homologous to the 4.5S rRNA of higher plant chloroplasts.[82,180] However, the question about the presence of chloroplast 4.5S rRNA in various groups of plants and algae has not been elucidated. Recently, its presence has been revealed in the fern *Dryopteris acuminata*.[181] We found 4.5S rRNA in several fern species, in lycopodium, green mosses, and liverwort *Marchantia polymorpha*. Ohyama et al.[182] detected 4.5S rRNA gene on the circular chloroplast DNA from this liverwort. Thus, 4.5S rRNA is evidently an integral component of all higher plant chloroplast ribosomes. We could not detect 4.5S rRNA in the only multicellular green algae investigated thus far: *Cladophora* sp.

B. Primary Structure

By now the primary structures of chloroplast 4.5S rRNA from two Bryophyta species (*Mnium rugicum* and *Marchantia polymorpha*), one fern species (*Dryopteris acuminata*),[181] five angiosperms, two dicots (spinach[183] and tobacco[69,83]), and three monocots (wheat,[184] maize,[72,73] and duckweed, *Spirodela oligorhiza*[185]) *have been determined. All the sequences were obtained by the direct sequencing of 4.5S rRNA or corresponding chloroplast gene. In addition, for 4.5S rRNA of duckweed Lemna minor*, broad bean *Vicia faba*, and dwarf bean *Phaseolus vulgaris* catalogues of RNase T₁ oligonucleotides have been determined.[67] The molecules are 102 to 103 nucleotide residues long, with deletion of 7 nucleotide residue pieces in the 4.5S rRNA of wheat and maize, and with three additional nucleotide residues at the 5' end in spinach 4.5S rRNA. It is noteworthy that the same trinucleotide precedes the 4.5S rRNA gene in tobacco chloroplasts.[69,83] This may testify to the differences in the rRNA processing mechanism in chloroplasts of these species. About 10% of spinach 4.5S rRNA molecules have no residue C at the 3' end. It was pointed out that in some angiosperms 4.5S rRNA molecule may contain less than 70 nucleotide residues.[67]

C. Secondary Structure

Four models for the secondary structure of chloroplast 4.5S rRNA have been proposed

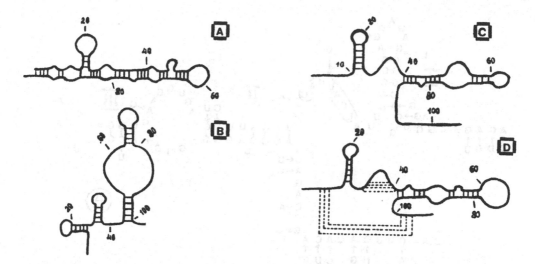

FIGURE 14.   Models of chloroplast 4.5S rRNA secondary structure proposed by: (A) Wildeman and Nazar.[184] (B) Takaiwa and Sugiura.[83] (C) Machatt et al.[79] (D) Kumagai et al.[183,186]

(Figure 14) based on the data from wheat 4.5S rRNA structural mapping by RNases,[184] on spinach 4.5S rRNA mapping by nucleases and diethylpyrocarbonate,[183,186] on comparison of tobacco and wheat 4.5S rRNA with the 3′ end sequences of prokaryotic 23S rRNAs and mapping of these regions by nucleases and dimethylsulfate,[79] and on the comparison of possible modes of tobacco 4.5S rRNA folding.[83] The common feature for the last three models is the presence of evolutionary conservative hairpin I, stable for nucleases and not accessible to diethylpyrocarbonate. It is followed by a single-stranded region, which seems to be capable of forming, under favorable conditions, a short hairpin. This sequence region is absent in cereal 4.5S rRNAs and *E. coli* 23S rRNA. The results of structural mapping make it possible to give preference to the Kumagai et al. model[183,186] over the Machatt et al. model.[79] ΔG for helixes II and III in the model of Machatt et al. is equal to −9.8 kcal/mol and in the model of Kumagai et al. to −10.6 kcal/mol; i.e., the later model is thermodynamically more advantageous.[186] The former is more stable in the evolutionary sense, however; nucleotide substitutions in 4.5S rRNAs from various plant species do not break the basepairing scheme (Figure 15). For the 3′ end part of 23S rRNA *E. coli* homologous with 4.5S rRNA, the Kumagai et al. model shortens helix III down to 4 bp and for 4.5S rRNA of monocots, fern, moss, and liverwort breaks helix II.

The presence of Mg^{2+} makes some regions of 4.5S rRNA more stable for nucleases; this is particularly true for the 5′ and 3′ end segments, and also for the residues U31 and C32.[183] Within ribosomes or their 50S subunits among several adenine residues, which are accessible to diethylpyrocarbonate, only the A33 residue retains accessibility, and its reactivity becomes much higher in this case.[186] Thus, 4.5S rRNA conformation in solution and within the ribosome may be different. Significantly, the A33 residue of the spinach 4.5S rRNA locates in the region that is absent in the wheat and maize 4.5S rRNA.

D. Evolution of Chloroplast 4.5S rRNA

It is not difficult to align 4.5S rRNA nucleotide sequences, since they are highly conservative (Table 3). Only in 3 regions are gaps introduced for a better sequence match. Nucleotide substitutions are located primarily in the 5′ end region (nucleotide residues 1 to 18) and in the 3′ end region (residues 85 to 100). The 3′ end region is more variable.

For distance matrix calculation (Table 4), a gap vs. nucleotide(s) was counted as one base substitution no mean the size of the gap. The difference between the 4.5S rRNA of different

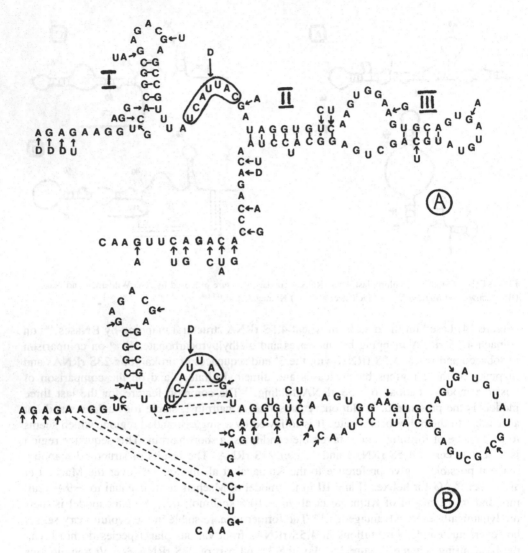

FIGURE 15. 4.5S rRNA of spinach folded according to (A) Machatt et al. model[79] and (B) Kumagai et al. model.[183,186] Dashed lines denote possible additional basepairing. Arrows indicate bases replaced in any other 4.5S rRNAs, and letters D denote deletions. The region deleted in *Cereales* 4.5S rRNA is boxed.

representatives of angiosperms varies from 1% for two cereal species to 13% for species from the classes of monocotyledons and dicotyledons. The nucleotide sequences of angiosperm 4.5S rRNAs differ from those of the fern 4.5S by 9 to 16%, and by 9 to 14% from the Bryophyta 4.5S rRNAs. The fern 4.5S rRNA is near equidistant from the 4.5S rRNA of angiosperms and Bryophyta; the differences between sequences are 9 to 16 and 8 to 11%, respectively. The 4.5S rRNA of the representatives of two Bryophyta classes, Hepaticae and Musci, differs only in 4% of nucleotide residues, despite the fact that both groups are quite ancient and emerged evidently soon after the gametophyte line had separated from the sporophyte line.[165-169] Thus, the evolution of Bryophyta 4.5S rRNA was much slower than that of the angiosperm. It is remarkable that the anatomomorphological evolution of Bryophyta also proceeded at a low rate; the most ancient fossils Hepaticae, are included in the same genera or families as extant species.[165-169]

From a distance matrix, the phenogram for 4.5S rRNA was constructed by the simple cluster procedure (Figure 16). Its topology coincides with those of trees derived by the

Table 3
ALIGNMENT OF CHLOROPLAST 4.5S rRNA SEQUENCES

Ref.		
— [a]	*Mnium rugicum*	Mn.
— [a]	*Marchantia polimorpha*	Mr.
181	*Dryopteris acuminata*	Dr.
183	*Spinacia oleracea*	Sn.
69,83	*Nicotiana tabacum*	Nc.
185,188	*Spirodela oligorhisa*	Sr.
184	*Triticum aestivum*	Tr.
72,73	*Zea mays*	Zea
189	*Escherichia coli* [b]	Esh.

```
                  10        20        30        40        50
                   |         |         |         |         |
      UAAGGU-GACGGCAAGACUAGCCGUUUAUCAUCACGAUAGGUGCCAAGUGG
Mn.
Mr.
Dr.
Sn.   AGAG       C          G      UU U      C         U
Nc.   G          C          G         U         U       U
Sr.              C          U         U         U       U
Tr.   GAG        G          G      -----A    -----A    U
Zea   AG         G          G      -----A    -----A    U
Esh.  G    --A UUG A  G C              ------     CCGGGU U
                          A
                    80
```

```
                  60        70        80        90        100
                   |         |         |         |         |
      AAGUGCAGUAAUGUAUGCAGCUGAGGCAUCCUAACAGACCGAGAGAUUUGAAAC  3'
Mn.
Mr.
Dr.   G             U                    U            G
Sn.   G                           C C    U-    G       G
Nc.   G                           GU     C             G
Sr.   G                                  U-            G
Tr.   G                           A AC   -  A AC       G
Zea   G                           A AC   -  A AC       G
Esh.  C    A      U --   CG UG  CG     UGA     U  GC -  CUU
           CC
```

Note: Bars denote gaps.

[a] Our data.

[b] 3' end of 23S rRNA.

Table 4
MATRIX OF NUCLEOTIDE DIFFERENCES BETWEEN
CHLOROPLAST 4.5S rRNA SEQUENCES (IN %)

	Mn.	Mr.	Dr.	Sn.	Nc.	Sr.	Tr.	Zea
Mnium rugicum		5	8	12	11	9	14	13
Marchantia polymorpha			11	13	12	10	14	13
Dryopteris acuminata	8	11		14	13	9	16	14
Spinacia oleracea	12	13	14		4	8	13	12
Nicotiana tabacum	11	12	13	4		7	12	11
Spirodela oligorhisa	9	10	9	8	7		10	9
Triticum aestivum	14	14	16	13	12	10		1
Zea mays	13	13	14	12	11	9	1	

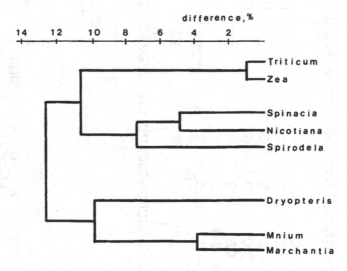

FIGURE 16.   Phenogram for 4.5S rRNA sequences. For references, see Table 3.

"present-day ancestor" method of Klotz and Blanken,[164] with *Mnium rugicum* or *Triticum aestivum* chosen as an ancestor. The root in the dendrogram may be introduced in a manner which seemed natural — between the gametophyte and sporophyte lines.

Both on the trees and the phenogram, the duckweed *Spirodela oligorhiza* (Lemnaceae), traditionally believed to be a monocot, is more closely related to dicots. This is in parallel with the absence of a 7 nucleotides long gap in 4.5S rRNA of the dicotyledon species and *S. oligorhiza*, but not of cereals. According to Takhtajan,[1] the order Arales to which Lemnaceae belongs includes Arecidae, one of the three Monocotyledoneae subclasses, whereas cereals are included in another subclass, Liliidae. It is postulated that all three subclasses (Liliidae, Arecidae, and Alismatidae) have a common origin from a hypothetical extinct herbaceous group of Magnoliidae. However, in the opinion of other investigators Arecidae may be more distant from typical Monocotyledoneae and may be related to Piperales with which they may share a common ancestor.[187] There is other molecular evidence of Arales' affiliation to Dicotyledoneae. The homology between the chloroplast 23S and 4.5S rRNA genes of *S. oligorhiza* is 87% compared with *Nicotiana* and 77% compared with *Zea*.[188] On the phylogenetic tree based on 5S rRNA sequences, duckweed *Lemna* branched off before other monocots and dicots.[52] It is of interest that in the *E. coli*[189] and *Anacystis nidulans*[180] 23S rRNA, the regions homologous with 4.5S rRNA have deletions of 9 bases exactly at the same position where 7 bases are deleted in 4.5S rRNA of cereals. It is unlikely that nearly the same sequences were inserted independently in the angiosperms, except for cereals, in the ferns, and in Byrophyta. It must be concluded that in ancestors of present-day prokaryotes, on the one hand, and cereals on the other, deletions of this region occurred independently. It is not obviously essential for functioning.

It seems from the comparison of the small number of chloroplast 4.5S rRNA sequences known at present that this RNA may be used for phylogenetic reconstruction studies in the plant kingdom.

VI. CONCLUSIONS

5.8S and 4.5S rRNAs derived from 23S rRNA in the course of evolution. Like other rRNAs, they are highly conservative in primary structure and can be used for implying phylogenetic affinities between taxons of higher rank.

The relatively small size of these RNAs seems to be advantageous, as it makes possible the rapid accumulation of sequence data. On the other hand, the statistical significance of inferences is reduced because of small absolute number of differences between sequences. For overcoming this obstacle more sequences must be used for analysis, and several different macromolecules must be considered in parallel.

The 23S rRNA derived small ribonucleic acids evolved with unequal rates in different phyletic lineages. This phenomenon is more pronounced for 5.8S rRNA participating in complicated intraribosomal interactions. The parts of the 5.8S rRNA molecule changed their job in the course of evolution and this change led to alterations of mutation fixation rates and patterns of nucleotide replacement. These irregularities in tempo and mode of 5.8S rRNA evolution call for more sophisticated approaches to phylogenetic reconstruction.

It must be emphasized that secondary structural peculiarities and gap positions must be considered. In addition, the gross features of rRNA operons and L-rRNA genes in separate phyletic lines should be taken into account.

The thorough comparisons of such characters may help not only in elucidation of phylogeny, but also in producing an insight into rRNA structure-function relationships.

REFERENCES

1. **Takhtajan, A. L.**, Outline of the classification of flowering plants (Magnoliophyta), *Bot. Rev.*, 46, 225, 1980.
2. **Cronquist, A.**, *The Evolution and Classification of Flowering Plants*, Nelson, London, 1968.
3. **Knoll, A. H. and Rothwell, G. W.**, Paleobotany: perspectives in 1980, *Paleobiology*, 7, 7, 1981.
4. **Taylor, T. N.**, *Paleobotany: An Introduction to Fossil Plant Biology*, McGraw-Hill, New York, 1981.
5. **Taylor, T. N.**, The origin of land plants: a paleobotanical perspective, *Taxon*, 31, 155, 1982.
6. **Takhtajan, A. L.**, *Flowering Plants: Origin and Dispersal*, Oliver & Boyd, Edinburgh, 1969.
7. **Stebbins, G. L.**, Mosaic evolution: an integrating principle for the modern synthesis, *Experientia*, 39, 823, 1983.
8. **Doyle, J. A.**, Origin of angiosperms, *Annu. Rev. Ecol. Syst.*, 9, 365, 1978.
9. **Meyen, S. V.**, *Sledy Trav Indejskih*, Misl, Moscow, 1981 (in Russian).
10. **Valiejo-Roman, K. M., Antonov, A. S., and Kamaletdinova, M. A.**, An analysis of phylogenetic interrelatedness of some Umbelliferae genera by means of DNA hybridization, *Dokl. Acad. Nauk SSSR*, 262, 749, 1982.
11. **Dührssen, E., Saavedra, E., and Neumann, K.-H.**, DNA reassociation kinetics and hybridization in different angiosperms, *Plant Syst. Evol.*, 136, 267, 1980.
12. **Lamppa, G. K. and Bendich, A. J.**, Chloroplast DNA sequence homologies among vascular plants, *Plant Physiol.*, 63, 660, 1979.

13. **Bisaro, D. and Siegel, A.,** Sequence homology between chloroplast DNAs from several higher plants, *Plant Physiol.,* 65, 234, 1980.

14. **Bobrova, V. K. and Troitsky, A. V.,** Higher plants chloroplast DNA homologies. II. Nucleotide sequence divergence of angiosperms chloroplast DNA, *Biol. Nauki,* 6, 22, 1982.

15. **Dickerson, R. E.,** The structure of cytochrome C and the rates of molecular evolution, *J. Mol. Evol.,* 1, 26, 1971.

16. **Matsuda, K. and Siegel, A.,** Hybridization of plant ribosomal RNA to DNA. The isolation of a DNA component rich in ribosomal RNA cistrons, *Proc. Natl. Acad. Sci. U.S.A.,* 58, 673, 1967.

17. **Trewavas, A. J. and Gibson, I.,** Ribosomal RNA nucleotide sequence homologies in plants, *Plant Physiol.,* 43, 445, 1968.

18. **Sinclair, J. H. and Brown, D. D.,** Retention of common nucleotide sequences in the ribosomal deoxyribonucleic acid of eukaryotes and some of their physical characteristics, *Biochemistry,* 10, 2761, 1972.

19. **Vodkin, M. and Katterman, F. R. H.,** Divergence of ribosomal RNA sequences within angiospermae, *Genetics,* 69, 435, 1971.

20. **Bendich, A. J. and McCarthy, B. J.,** Ribosomal RNA homologies among distantly related organisms, *Proc. Natl. Acad. Sci. U.S.A.,* 65, 349, 1979.

21. **Maggini, F.,** Homologies of ribosomal RNA nucleotide sequences in monocots, *J. Mol. Evol.,* 4, 317, 1975.

22. **Gerbi, S. A.,** Fine structure of ribosomal RNA. I. Conservation of homologous regions within ribosomal RNA of eukaryotes, *J. Mol. Biol.,* 106, 791, 1976.

23. **Gourse, R. L. and Gerbi, S. A.,** Fine structure of ribosomal RNA. III. Location of evolutionary conserved regions within ribosomal DNA, *J. Mol. Biol.,* 140, 321, 1980.

24. **Petrov, N. B., Poltaraus, A. B., and Antonov, A. S.,** Determination of the degree of ribosomal genes conservativity in some invertebrate phylums, *Biokhimiya,* 45, 165, 1980.

25. **Leaver, C. J. and Gray, M. W.,** Mitochondrial genome organization and expression in higher plants, *Annu. Rev. Plant Physiol.,* 33, 373, 1982.

26. **Dyer, T. A.,** RNA sequences, in *Nucleic Acids and Proteins in Plants II. Structure, Biochemistry and Physiology of Nucleic acids,* Parthier, B. and Boulter, D., Eds., Springer-Verlag, Berlin, 1982, 171.

27. **Taylor, D. L.,** Chloroplasts as symbiotic organelles, *Int. Rev. Cytol.,* 27, 29, 1970.

28. **Margulis, L.,** Simbiotic theory of the origin of eukaryotic organelles: criteria for proof, *Symp. Soc. Exp. Biol.,* 29, 21, 1975.

29. **Margulis, L.,** *Symbiosis in Cell Evolution,* W. H. Freeman, San Francisco, 1981.

30. **Schwartz, R. M. and Dayhoff, M. O.,** Origins of prokaryotes, eukaryotes, mitochondria and chloroplasts, *Science,* 199, 395, 1978.

31. **Pene, J. J., Knight, E., Jr., and Darnell, J. E., Jr.,** Characterization of a new low molecular weight RNA in HeLa cell ribosomes, *J. Mol. Biol.,* 33, 609, 1968.

32. **Weinberg, R. A. and Penman, S.,** Small molecular weight monodisperse nuclear RNA, *J. Mol. Biol.,* 38, 289, 1968.

33. **Oakden, K. M. and Lane, B. G.,** Chain termini of the satellite RNA from yeast ribosomes, *Can. J. Biochem.,* 51, 520, 1973.

34. **Pace, N. R., Walker, T. A., and Schroeder, E.,** Structure of the 5.8S RNA component of the 5.8S-28S ribosomal RNA junction complex, *Biochemistry,* 16, 5321, 1977.

35. **Nazar, R. N., Sitz, T. O., and Busch, H.,** Structural analysis of mammalian ribosomal ribonucleic acids and its precursors. Nucleotide sequence of ribosomal 5.8S ribonucleic acid, *J. Biol. Chem.,* 250, 8591, 1975.

36. **Nazar, R. N.,** The release and reassociation of 5.8S rRNA with yeast ribosomes, *J. Biol. Chem.,* 253, 4505, 1978.

37. **Nazar, R. N. and Sitz, T. O.,** Role of the 5'-terminal sequence in the RNA binding site of yeast 5.8S rRNA, *FEBS Lett.,* 115, 71, 1980.

38. **Long, E. O. and Dawid, I. B.,** Repeated genes in eukaryotes, *Annu. Rev. Biochem.,* 49, 727, 1980.

39. **Nosikov, V. V. and Braga, E. A.,** Ribosomal RNA genes, in *Itogi Nauki, i Tekniki, Molecular Biology,* Vol. 18, Kisselev, L. L., Ed., VINITI, Moscow, 1982.

40. **Hadjiolov, A. A.,** Biogenesis of ribosomes in eukaryotes, in *Subcellular Biochemistry,* Vol. 7, Roodyn, D. B., Ed., Plenum Press, New York, 1980, 1.

41. **Grierson, D.,** RNA processing and other posttranscriptional modifications, in *Nucleic Acids and Proteins in Plants II,* Parthier, B. and Boutler, D., Eds., Springer-Verlag, Berlin, 1982, 192.

42. **Cech, T. R., Zaug, A. J., Grabowski, P. J., and Brehm, S. L.,** Transcription and splicing on the ribosomal RNA precursor of *Tetrahymena,* in *The Cell Nucleus,* Vol. 10, Busch, H. and Rothblum, L., Eds., Academic Press, New York, 1982, 171.

43. **Ellis, T. H. N., Goldsbrough, P. B., and Castleton, J. A.,** Transcription and methylation of flax rDNA, *Nucleic Acids Res.,* 11, 3047, 1983.

44. **Kister, K.-P., Müller, B., and Eckert, W. A.,** Complex endonucleolytic cleavage pattern during early events in the processing of pre-rRNA in the lower eukaryote. *Tetrahymena thermophila, Nucleic Acids Res.*, 11, 3487, 1983.

45. **Doolittle, W. F. and Pace, N. R.,** Transcriptional organization of the ribosomal RNA cistrons in *Escherichia coli, Proc. Natl. Acad. Sci. U.S.A.*, 68, 1786, 1971.

46. **Wrede, P. and Erdmann, V. A.,** *Escherichia coli* 5S RNA binding proteins L18 and L25 interact with 5.8S RNA but not with 5S RNA from yeast ribosomes, *Proc. Natl. Acad. Sci. U.S.A.*, 74, 2706, 1977.

47. **Cedergren, R. J. and Sankoff, D.,** Evolutionary origin of 5.8S ribosomal RNA, *Nature (London)*, 260, 74, 1976.

48. **Luehrsen, K. R. and Fox, G. E.,** Secondary structure of eukaryotic cytoplasmic 5S ribosomal RNA, *Proc. Natl. Acad. Sci. U.S.A.*, 78, 2150, 1981.

49. **Böhm, S., Fabian, H., and Welfle, H.,** Universal secondary structures of prokaryotic and eukaryotic ribosomal 5S RNA derived from comparative analysis of their sequences, *Acta Biol. Med. Germ.*, 40, K19, 1981.

50. **Delihas, N. and Andersen, J.,** Generalized structures of the 5S ribosomal RNAs, *Nucleic Acids Res.*, 10, 7323, 1982.

51. **De Wachter, R., Chen, M.-W., and Vanderberghe, A.,** Conservation of secondary structure in 5S ribosomal RNA: a uniform model for eukaryotic, eubacterial, archebacterial and organelle sequences is energetically favourable, *Biochimie*, 64, 311, 1982.

52. **Küntzel, H., Piechulla, B., and Hahn, U.,** Consensus structure and evolution of 5S rRNA, *Nucleic Acids Res.*, 11, 893, 1983.

53. **Nazar, R. N.,** A 5.8S rRNA-like sequence in prokaryotic 23S rRNA, *FEBS Lett.*, 119, 212, 1980.

54. **Cox, R. A. and Kelly, J. M.,** Mature 23S rRNA of prokaryotes appears homologous with the precursor of 25-28 rRNA of eukaryotes. Comments on the evolution of 23-28 rRNA, *FEBS Lett.*, 130, 1, 1981.

55. **Jacq, B.,** Sequence homologies between eukaryotic 5.8S rRNA and the 5'-end of prokaryotic 23S rRNA: evidences for a common evolutionary origin, *Nucleic Acids Res.*, 9, 2913, 1981.

56. **Hall, L. M. C. and Maden, B. E. H.,** Nucleotide sequence through the 18S-28S intergene region of a vertebrate ribosomal transcription unit, *Nucleic Acids Res.*, 8, 5993, 1980.

57. **Otsuka, T., Nomizama, H., Yoshida, H., Kukita, T., Kuhara, S., and Sakaki, Y.,** Complete nucleotide sequence of the 26S rRNA gene of *Physarum polycephalum*: its significance in gene evolution, *Proc. Natl. Acad. Sci. U.S.A.*, 80, 3163, 1983.

58. **Bibb, M. J., Van Etten, R. A., Wright, C. T., Walberg, M. W., and Clayton, D. A.,** Sequence and gene organization of mouse mitochondrial DNA, *Cell*, 26, 167, 1981.

59. **Anderson, S., Bankier, A. T., Barrell, B. G., de Bruijn, M. H. L., Coulson, A. R., Drouin, J., Eperon, I. C., Nierlich, D. P., Roe, B. A., Sanger, F., Schreier, P. H., Smith, A. J. H., Staden, R., and Young, I. G.,** Sequence and organization of the human mitochondrial genome, *Nature (London)*, 290, 457, 1981.

60. **Eperon, I. C., Anderson, S., and Nierlich, D. P.,** Distinctive sequence of human mitochondrial ribosomal RNA genes, *Nature (London)*, 286, 460, 1980.

61. **Van Etten, R. A., Walberg, M. W., and Clayton, D. A.,** Precise localization and nucleotide sequence of the two mouse mitochondrial rRNA genes and three immediately adjacent novel tRNA genes, *Cell*, 22, 157, 1980.

62. **Noller, H. F., Kop, J. A., Wheaton, V., Brosius, J., Gutell, R. R., Kopylov, A. M., Dohme, F., Herr, W., Stahl, D. A., Gupta, R., and Woese, C. R.,** Secondary structure model for 23S ribosomal RNA, *Nucleic Acids Res.*, 9, 6167, 1981.

63. **Köchel, H. G. and Küntzel, H.,** Mitochondrial L-rRNA from *Aspergillus nidulans*: potential secondary structure and evolution, *Nucleic Acids Res.*, 10, 4795, 1982.

64. **Sor, F. and Fukuhara, H.,** Complete DNA sequence coding for the large ribosomal RNA of yeast mitochondria, *Nucleic Acids Res.*, 11, 339, 1983.

65. **Dyer, T. A. and Bowman, C. M.,** A sequence analysis of low-molecular weight rRNA from chloroplasts of flowering plants, in *Genetics and Biogenesis of Chloroplasts and Mitochondria*, Bucher, Th., Neupert, W., Sebald, W., and Werner, S., Eds., North-Holland, Amsterdam, 1976, 645.

66. **Whitfeld, P. R., Leaver, C. J., Bottomley, W., and Atchison, B. A.,** Low-molecular-weight (4.5S) ribonucleic acid in higher plant chloroplast ribosomes, *Biochem. J.*, 175, 1103, 1978.

67. **Bowman, C. M. and Dyer, T. A.,** 4.5S ribonucleic acid, a novel ribosome component in the chloroplasts of flowering plants, *Biochem. J.*, 183, 605, 1979.

68. **Bohnert, H. J., Gordon, K., Driesel, A. J., Crouse, E. J., and Herrmann, R. G.,** Mapping of genes on the restriction endonuclease site map of *Spinacia oleracea* chloroplast DNA, in *Chloroplast Development*, Akoyunoglou, G. and Argyroudi-Akoyunoglou, J. H., Eds., North-Holland, Amsterdam, 1978, 569.

69. **Takaiwa, F. and Sugiura, M.,** Nucleotide sequences of the 4.5S and 5S ribosomal RNA genes from tobacco chloroplasts, *Mol. Gen. Genet.*, 180, 1, 1980.

70. **Takaiwa, F. and Sugiura, M.,** Cloning and characterization of 4.5S and 5S RNA genes in tobacco chloroplasts, *Gene,* 10, 95, 1980.

71. **Kusuda, J., Shinozaki, K., Takaiwa, F., and Sugiura, M.,** Characterization of the cloned ribosomal DNA of tobacco chloroplasts, *Mol. Gen. Genet.,* 178, 1, 1980.

72. **Edwards, K., Bedbrook, J., Dyer, T., and Kössel, H.,** 4.5S rRNA from *Zea mays* chloroplasts shows structural homology with the 3'-end of procaryotic 23S rRNA, *Biochem. Int.,* 2, 533, 1981.

73. **Edwards, K. and Kössel, H.,** The rRNA operon from *Zea mays* chloroplasts: nucleotide sequence of 23S rDNA and its homology with *E. coli* 23S rDNA, *Nucleic Acids Res.,* 9, 2853, 1981.

74. **Keus, R. J. A., Roovers, D. J., Van Heerikhuizen, H., and Groot, G. S. P.,** Molecular cloning and characterization of the chloroplast ribosomal RNA genes from *Spirodela oligorhisa, Curr. Genet.,* 7, 7, 1983.

75. **Sun, Ch.-R., Endo, T., Kusuda, M., and Sugiura, M.,** Molecular cloning of the genes for ribosomal DNAs from broad bean chloroplast DNA, *Jpn. J. Genet.,* 57, 397, 1982.

76. **Hartley, M. R. and Head, C.,** The synthesis of chloroplast high-molecular-weight ribonucleic acid in spinach, *Eur. J. Biochem.,* 96, 301, 1979.

77. **Hartley, M. R.,** The synthesis and origin of chloroplast low-molecular-weight ribosomal ribonucleic acid in spinach, *Eur. J. Biochem.,* 96, 311, 1979.

78. **MacKay, R. M.,** The origin of plant chloroplast 4.5S ribosomal RNA, *FEBS Lett.,* 123, 17, 1981.

79. **Machatt, M. A., Ebel, J.-P., and Branlant, C.,** The 3'-terminal region of bacterial 23S ribosomal RNA: structure and homology with the 3'-terminal region of eukaryotic 28S rRNA and with chloroplast 4.5S rRNA, *Nucleic Acids Res.,* 9, 1533, 1981.

80. **Takaiwa, F. and Sugiura, M.,** The complete nucleotide sequence of a 23S rRNA gene from tobacco chloroplasts, *Eur. J. Biochem.,* 124, 13, 1982.

81. **Takeishi, K. and Gotoh, O.,** Computer analysis of the sequence relationships among 4.5S RNA molecular species from various sources, *J. Biochem.,* 92, 1173, 1982.

82. **Dron, M., Rahire, M., and Rochaix, J.-D.,** Sequence of the chloroplast 16S rRNA gene and its surrounding regions of *Chlamydomonas reinhardii, Nucleic Acids Res.,* 10, 7609, 1982.

83. **Takaiwa, F. and Sugiura, M.,** The nucleotide sequence of 4.5S ribosomal RNA from tobacco chloroplasts, *Nucleic Acids Res.,* 8, 4125, 1980.

84. **Rochaix, J.-D. and Malnoe, P.,** Anatomy of the chloroplast ribosomal DNA of *Chlamydomonas reinhardii, Cell,* 15, 661, 1978.

85. **Rochaix, J.-D. and Darlix, J.-L.,** Composite structure of the chloroplast 23S ribosomal RNA genes of *Chlamydomonas reinhardii.* Evolutionary and functional implications, *J. Mol. Biol.,* 159, 383, 1982.

86. **Jordan, B. R., Jourdan, R., and Jacq, B.,** Late steps in the maturation of *Drosophila* 26S ribosomal RNA: generation of 5.8S and 2S by cleavage occuring in the cytoplasm, *J. Mol. Biol.,* 101, 85, 1976.

87. **Jordan, B. R. and Glover, D. M.,** 5.8S and 2S is located in the "transcribed spacer" region between the 18S and 26S rRNA genes in *Drosophila melanogaster, FEBS Lett.,* 78, 271, 1977.

88. **Pavlakis, G. N., Jordan, B. R., Wurst, R. M., and Vournakis, J. N.,** Sequence and secondary structure of *Drosophila melanogaster* 5.8S and 2S rRNAs and of the processing site between them, *Nucleic Acids Res.,* 7, 2213, 1979.

89. **Jordan, B. R., Latil-Damotte, M., and Jourdan, R.,** Coding and spacer sequences in the 5.8S-2S region of *Sciara coprophila* ribosomal DNA, *Nucleic Acids Res.,* 8, 3565, 1980.

90. **Fujiwara, H. and Ishikawa, H.,** Primary and secondary structures of *Tetrahymena* and aphid 5.8S rRNAs: structural features of 5.8S rRNA which interacts with the 28S rRNA containing the hidden break, *Nucleic Acids Res.,* 10, 5173, 1982.

91. **Fujiwara, H., Kawata, Y., and Ishikawa, H.,** Primary and secondary structure of 5.8S rRNA from the silkgland of *Bombyx mori, Nucleic Acids Res.,* 10, 2415, 1982.

92. **Feng, Y.-X., Krupp, G., and Gross, H. J.,** The nucleotide sequence of 5.8S rRNA from the posterior silk gland of the silkworm *Philosamia cynthia ricini, Nucleic Acids Res.,* 10, 6383, 1982.

93. **Ursi, D., Vandenberghe, A., and De Wachter, R.,** The sequence of the 5.8S ribosomal RNA of the crustacean *Artemia salina* with a proposal for a general secondary structure model for 5.8S ribosomal RNA, *Nucleic Acids Res.,* 10, 3517, 1982.

94. **Schnare, M. N., Spencer, D. F., and Gray, M. W.,** Primary structures of four novel small ribosomal RNAs from *Crithidia fasciculata, Can. J. Biochem. Cell Biol.,* 61, 38, 1983.

95. **Simpson, L. and Simpson, A. M.,** Kinetoplast RNA of *Leischmania tarentolae, Cell,* 14, 169, 1978.

96. **Delihas, N., Anderson, J., Andersini, W., Kaufman, L., and Lyman, H.,** The 5S ribosomal RNA of *Euglena gracilis* cytoplasmic ribosomes is closely homologous to the 5S RNA of the trypanosomatid protosoa, *Nucleic Acids Res.,* 9, 6627, 1981.

97. **Ishikawa, H.,** Comparative studies on the thermal stability of animal ribosomal RNAs, *Comp. Biochem. Physiol,* 46B, 217, 1973.

98. **Ishikawa, H.,** Arthropod ribosomes: integrity of ribosomal ribonucleic acids from aphids and water-fleas, *Biochim. Biophys. Acta,* 435, 258, 1976.

99. **Ishikawa, H.,** Evolution of ribosomal RNA, *Comp. Biochem. Physiol.,* 58B, 1, 1977.

100. **Londei, P., Cammarano, P., Mazzei, F., and Romeo, A.,** Size heterogeneity of ribosomal RNA in eukaryote evolution. I. rRNA molecular weights in species containing intact large ribosomal subunit RNA, *Comp. Biochem. Physiol.,* 73B, 423, 1982.

101. **Cammarano, P., Londei, P., Mazzei, F., and Biagini, R.,** Size heterogeneity of ribosomal RNA in eukaryote evolution. II. rRNA molecular weights in species containing discontinuous large ribosomal subunit RNA, *Comp. Biochem. Physiol.,* 73B, 435, 1982.

102. **Hyde, J. E., Zolg, J. W., and Scaife, J. G.,** Isolation and characterization of ribosomal RNA from the human malaria parasite *Plasmodium falciparum, Mol. Biochem. Parasitol.,* 4, 283, 1981.

103. **Glover, D. M. and Hogness, D. S.,** A novel arrangement of the 18S and 28S sequences in a repeating unit of *Drosophila melanogaster* rDNA, *Cell,* 10, 167, 1977.

104. **White, R. L. and Hogness, D. S.,** R-loop mapping of the 18S and 28S sequences in the long and short repeating units of *Drosophila melanogaster* rDNA, *Cell,* 10, 177, 1977.

105. **Wellauer, P. K. and Dawid, I. B.,** The structural organization of ribosomal DNA in *Drosophila melanogaster, Cell,* 10, 193, 1977.

106. **Pellegrini, M., Manning, J., and Davidson, N.,** Sequence arrangement of the rDNA of *Drosophila melanogaster, Cell,* 10, 213, 1977.

107. **Wild, M. A. and Gall, J. G.,** An intervening sequence in the gene coding for 25S ribosomal RNA of *Tetrahymena pigmentosa, Cell,* 16, 565, 1979.

108. **Rae, R. M. M., Kohorn, B. D., and Wade, R. P.,** The 10 kb *Drosophila virilis* 28S rDNA intervening sequence is flanked by a direct repeat of 14-base pairs of coding sequence, *Nucleic Acids Res.,* 8, 3491, 1980.

109. **Beckingham, K.,** The ribosomal DNA of *Calliphora erythrocephala.* The cistron classes of total genomic DNA, *J. Mol. Biol.,* 149, 141, 1981.

110. **Kan, N. C. and Gall, J. G.,** The intervening sequence of the ribosomal RNA gene is highly conserved between two *Tetrahymena* species, *Nucleic Acids Res.,* 10, 2809, 1982.

111. **Burke, J. M. and Raj Bhandary, U. L.,** Intron within the large rRNA gene of *Neurospora crassa* mitochondria: a long open reading frame and a consensus sequence possibly important in splicing, *Cell,* 31, 509, 1982.

112. **Branlant, C., Krol, A., Machatt, M. A., Pouyet, J., Ebel, J.-P., Edwards, K., and Kössel, H.,** Primary and secondary structures of *Escherichia coli* MRE 600 23S ribosomal RNA. Comparison with models of secondary structure for maize chloroplast 23S rRNA and for large portions of mouse and human 16S mitochondrial rRNAs, *Nucleic Acids Res.,* 9, 4303, 1981.

113. **Ware, V. C., Tague, B. W., Clark, C. G., Gourse, R. L., Brand, R. C., and Gerbi, S. A.,** Sequence analysis of 28S ribosomal DNA from the amphibian *Xenopus laevis, Nucleic Acids Res.,* 11, 7795, 1983.

114. **Torczynsky, R., Bollon, A. P., and Fuke, M.,** The complete nucleotide sequence of the rat 18S ribosomal RNA gene and comparison with the respective yeast and frog gene, *Nucleic Acids Res.,* 11, 4879, 1983.

115. **Unnasch, T. R. and Wirth, D. F.,** The cloned rRNA genes of *Plasmodium lophurae*: a novel rDNA structure, *Nucleic Acids Res.,* 11, 8461, 1983.

116. **Darlix, J.-L. and Rochaix, J.-D.,** Nucleotide sequence and structure of cytoplasmic 5S RNA and 5.8S RNA of *Chlamydomonas reinhardii, Nucleic Acids Res.,* 9, 1291, 1981.

117. **Erdmann, V. A., Huysmans, E., Vandenberghe, A., and De Wachter, R.,** Collection of published 5S and 5.8S ribosomal RNA sequences, *Nucleic Acids Res.,* 11, r105, 1983.

118. **Nazar, R. N., Lo, A. C., and Wildeman, A. G.,** Effect of 2′-O-methylation on the structure of mammalian 5.8S rRNAs and the 5.8S-28S rRNA junction, *Nucleic Acids Res.,* 11, 5989, 1983.

119. **Tinoco, I., Jr., Borer, Ph. N., Dengler, B., Levine, M. D., Uhlenbeck, O. C., Crothers, D. M., and Gralla, J.,** Improved estimation of secondary structure in ribonucleic acids, *Nature (London) New Biol.,* 246, 40, 1973.

120. **Ninio, J.,** Prediction of pairing schemes in RNA molecules — loop contributions and energy of wobble and non-wobble pairs, *Biochimie,* 61, 1133, 1979.

121. **Nussinov, R. and Tinoco, I., Jr.,** Small changes in free energy assignments for unpaired bases do not affect predicted secondary structures in single stranded RNA, *Nucleic Acids Res.,* 10, 341, 1982.

122. **Dumas, J. P. and Ninio, J.,** Efficient algorithms for folding and comparing nucleic acid sequences, *Nucleic Acids Res.,* 10, 197, 1982.

123. **Salser, W.,** Globin mRNA sequences: analysis of base pairing and evolutionary implications, *Cold Spring Harbor Symp. Quant. Biol.,* 42, 985, 1977.

124. **Wildeman, A. G. and Nazar, R. N.,** Studies on the secondary structure of 5.8S rRNA from a thermophile, *Thermomyces lanuginosus, J. Biol. Chem.,* 256, 5675, 1981.

125. **Wildeman, A. G. and Nazar, R. N.,** Studies on the secondary structure of wheat 5.8S rRNA. Conformational changes in the A + U-rich stem during ribosome assembly, *Eur. J. Biochem.,* 121, 357, 1982.

126. **Walker, T. A., Johnson, K. D., Olsen, G. J., Peters, M. A., and Pace, N. R.,** Enzymatic and chemical structure mapping of mouse 28S ribosomal ribonucleic acid contacts in 5.8S ribosomal ribonucleic acid, *Biochemistry,* 21, 2320, 1982.

127. **Kelly, J. M. and Maden, B. E. H.,** Chemical modification studies and the secondary structure of HeLa cell 5.8S rRNA, *Nucleic Acids Res.,* 8, 4521, 1980.

128. **Toots, I., Metspalu, A., Villems, R., and Saarma, M.,** Location of single-stranded and double-stranded regions in rat liver 5S RNA and 5.8S RNA, *Nucleic Acids Res.,* 9, 5331, 1981.

129. **Eichler, D. C. and Eales, S. J.,** The effect of RNA secondary structure on the action of a nucleolar endoribonuclease, *J. Biol. Chem.,* 258, 10049, 1983.

130. **Luoma, G. A. and Marshall, A. G.,** Laser Raman evidence for new cloverleaf secondary structures for eukaryotic 5.8S RNA and prokaryotic 5S RNA, *Proc. Natl. Acad. Sci.U.S.A.,* 75, 4901, 1978.

131. **Burkey, K. O., Marshall, A. G., and Albcen, G. O.,** Determination of base pairing in ribonucleic acid by Fourier-transform infrared spectrometry: yeast ribosomal 5S ribonucleic acid, *Biochemistry,* 22, 4223, 1983.

132. **Stulz, J., Ackermann, Th., Appel, B., and Erdmann, V. A.,** Determination of base pairing in yeast 5S and 5.8S RNA by infrared spectroscopy, *Nucleic Acids Res.,* 9, 3851, 1981.

133. **Maruyama, S., Akazaki, S., Nitta, K., and Sugai, S.,** Equilibrium and kinetics of thermal unfolding of yeast 5.8S ribosomal RNA in aqueous salt solutions, *Int. J. Biol. Macromol.,* 5, 26, 1983.

134. **Kime, M. J. and Moore, P. B.,** Physical evidence for a domain structure in *Escherichia coli* 5S RNA, *FEBS Lett.,* 53, 199, 1983.

135. **Erdman, V. A.,** Structure and function of 5S and 5.8S RNA, *Progr. Nucleic Acids Res. Mol. Biol.,* 18, 45, 1976.

136. **Ursi, D., Vandenberghe, A., and De Wachter, R.,** Nucleotide sequences of the 5.8S rRNAs of a mollusc and a porifer, and considerations regarding the secondary structure of 5.8S rRNA and its interaction with 28S rRNA, *Nucleic Acids Res.,* 11, 8111, 1983.

137. **Boseley, P. G., Tuyns, A., and Birnsteil, M. L.,** Mapping of the *Xenopus laevis* 5.8S rRNA by restriction and DNA sequencing, *Nucleic Acids Res.,* 5, 1121, 1978.

138. **Peters, M. A., Walker, T. A., and Pace, N. R.,** Independent binding sites in mouse 5.8S ribosomal ribonucleic acid for 28S ribosomal ribonucleic acid, *Biochemistry,* 21, 2329, 1982.

139. **Kelly, J. M. and Cox, R. A.,** The nucleotide sequence at the 3'-end of *Neurospora crassa* 25S-rRNA and the location of a 5.8S-rRNA binding site, *Nucleic Acids Res.,* 9, 1111, 1981.

140. **Walker, Th. A., Endo, Y., Wheat, W. H., Wool, I. G., and Pace, N. R.,** Location of 5.8S rRNA contact sites in 28S rRNA and the effect of α-sarcin on the association of 5.8S rRNA with 28S rRNA, *J. Biol. Chem.,* 258, 333, 1983.

141. **Michot, B., Bachellerie, J.-P., and Raynal, F.,** Sequence and secondary structure of mouse 28S rRNA 5'-terminal domain. Organization of the 5.8S-28S rRNA complex, *Nucleic Acids Res.,* 10, 5273, 1982.

142. **Chan, Y.-L., Olvera, J., and Wool, I. G.,** The structure of rat 28S ribosomal ribonucleic acid inferred from the sequence of nucleotides in a gene, *Nucleic Acids Res.,* 11, 7819, 1983.

143. **Veldman, G. M., Klootwijk, J., DeRegt, V. C. H. F., Planta, R. J., Branlant, C., Krol, A., and Ebel, J.-P.,** The primary and secondary structure of yeast 26S rRNA, *Nucleic Acids Res.,* 9, 6935, 1981.

144. **Olsen, G. J. and Sogin, M. L.,** Nucleotide sequence of *Dictyostelium discoideum* 5.8S ribosomal ribonucleic acid: evolutionary and secondary structural implications, *Biochemistry,* 21, 2335, 1982.

145. **Nazar, R. N. and Wildeman, A. G.,** Altered features in the secondary structure of *Vicia faba* 5.8S rRNA, *Nucleic Acids Res.,* 9, 5345, 1981.

146. **Sitz, T. O., Banerjee, N., and Nazar, R. N.,** Effect of point mutations on 5.8S ribosomal ribonucleic acid secondary structure and the 5.8S-28S ribosomal ribonucleic junction, *Biochemistry,* 20, 4029, 1981.

147. **Sitz, T. O., Kuo, S.-C., and Nazar, R. N.,** Multimer forms of eukaryotic 5.8S ribosomal RNA, *Biochemistry,* 26, 5811, 1978.

148. **Speirs, J. and Birnsteil, M.,** Arrangement of the 5.8S RNA cistrons in the genome of *Xenopus laevis, J. Mol. Biol.,* 87, 237, 1974.

149. **Toots, I., Metspalu, A., Lind, A., Saarma, M., and Villems, R.,** Immobilized eukaryotic 5.8S RNA binds *Escherichia coli* and rat liver ribosomal proteins, *FEBS Lett.,* 104, 193, 1979.

150. **Todokoro, K., Ulbrich, N., Chan, Y.-L., and Wool, I. G.,** Characterization of the binding of rat liver ribosomal proteins L6, L8, L19, S9 and S13 to 5.8S ribosomal ribonucleic acid, *J. Biol. Chem.,* 256, 7207, 1981.

151. **Chan, Y.-L., Ulbrich, N., Ackerman, E. J., Todokoro, K., Slobin, L. I., Sater, B., Sigler, P. B., and Wool, I. G.,** The binding of transfer ribonucleic acids to 5S and 5.8S eukaryotic ribosomal ribonucleic acid-protein complexes, *J. Biol. Chem.,* 257, 2522, 1982.

152. **Lee, J. C., Henry, B., and Yeh, Y.-C.,** Binding of proteins from large ribosomal subunits to 5.8S rRNA of *Saccharomyces cerevisiae, J. Biol. Chem.,* 258, 854, 1983.

153. **Lo, A. C. and Nazar, R. N.,** Topography of 5.8S rRNA in rat liver ribosomes. Identification of diethyl pyrocarbonate-reactive sites, *J. Biol. Chem.,* 257, 3516, 1982.

154. **Liu W., Lo, A. C. and Nazar, R. N.,** Structure of the ribosome associated 5.8S ribosomal RNA, *J. Mol. Biol.,* 171, 217, 1983.

155. **Goodman, M.,** Decoding the pattern of protein evolution. *Progr. Biophys. Mol. Biol.*, 37, 105, 1981.
156. **Prager, E. M. and Wilson, A. C.,** Construction of phylogenetic trees for proteins and nucleic acids: empirical evaluation of alternative matrix methods. *J. Mol. Evol.*, 11, 129, 1978.
157. **Holmquist, R.,** The method of parsimony: an experimental test and theoretical analysis of the adequacy of molecular restoration studies. *J. Mol. Biol.*, 135, 939, 1979.
158. **Fitch, W. M.,** Estimating the total number of nucleotide substitutions since the common ancestor of a pair of homologous genes: comparison of several methods and three beta hemoglobin messenger RNAs. *J. Mol. Evol.*, 16, 153, 1980.
159. **Penny, D., Hendy, M. D., and Foulds, L. R.,** Techniques for the verification of minimal phylogenetic trees illustrated with ten mammalian hemoglobin sequences. *Biochem. J.*, 187, 65, 1980.
160. **Wagner, M.-J.,** The minimum number of mutations in an evolutionary network. *J. Theor. Biol.*, 91, 621, 1981.
161. **Tateno, Y., Nei, M., and Tajima, F.,** Accuracy of estimated phylogenetic trees from molecular data. I. Distantly related species. *J. Mol. Evol.*, 18, 387, 1982.
162. **Sankoff, D., Cedergren, R. J., and McKay, W.,** A strategy for sequence phylogeny research. *Nucleic Acids Res.*, 10, 421, 1982.
163. **Felsenstein, J.,** Numerical methods for inferring evolutionary trees. *Q. Rev. Biol.*, 57, 379, 1982.
164. **Klotz, L. C. and Blanken, R. L.,** A practical method for calculating evolutionary trees from sequence data. *J. Theor. Biol.*, 91, 261, 1981.
165. **Savicz-Ljubitzkaja, L. L. and Abramov, I. I.,** The geological annals of Bryophyta. *Rev. Bryol. Lichenol.*, 28, 330, 1959.
166. **Hueber, F. M.,** Hepaticites devonicus, a new fossil liverwort from the Devonian of New York. *Ann. Missouri Bot. Gard.*, 48, 125, 1961.
167. **Shlyakov, R. N.,** *The Hepaticae: Morphology, Phylogeny and classification,* Nauka, Leningrad, 1975.
168. **Ishchenko, T. A. and Shlyakov, R. N.,** Middle Devonian liverworts (Marchantiidae) from Podolia. *Paleontol. J.*, 13, 369, 1979.
169. **Schuster, R.,** *The Hepaticae and Anthocerotae of North America East of the Hundredth Meredian,* Columbia University Press, New York, 1966.
170. **Hinnebusch, A. G., Klotz, L. C., Blanken, R. L., and Loeblich, A. R., III,** An evaluation of the phylogenetic position of the Dinoflagellate *Crypthecodinium cohnii* based on 5S rRNA characterisation, *J. Mol. Evol.*, 17, 334, 1981.
171. **McCarroll, R., Olsen, G. J., Stahl, Y. D., Woese, C. R., and Sogin, M. L.,** Nucleotide sequence of the *Dictyostelium discoideum* small subunit ribosomal ribonucleic acid inferred from the gene sequence: evolutionary implications, *Biochemistry*, 22, 2858, 1983.
172. **Huysmans, E., Dams, E., Vandenberghe, A., and De Wachter, R.,** The nucleotide sequences of the 5S rRNA of four mushrooms and their use in studying the phylogenetic position of basidiomycetes among the eukaryotes, *Nucleic Acids Res.*, 11, 2871, 1983.
173. **Cedergren, R. J., Sankoff, D., La Rue, B., and Grosjean, H.,** The evolving tRNA molecule, *CRC Crit. Rev. Biochem.*, 11, 35, 1981.
174. **Cavalier-Smith, T.,** Eukaryotic kingdoms: seven or nine? *BioSystems*, 14, 461, 1981.
175. **Corliss, J. O.,** What are the taxonomic and evolutionary relationships of the Protozoa to the Protista? *Biosystems*, 14, 445, 1981.
176. **Rohdendorf, B. B. and Rasnitsyn, A. P., Eds.,** *Historical Development of Insects,* Nauka, Moscow, 1980.
177. **Kawata, Y. and Ishikawa, H.,** Nucleotide sequence and thermal property of 5S rRNA from the elder aphid, *Acyrthosiphon magnoliae, Nucleic Acids Res.*, 10, 1833, 1982.
178. **Xian-Rong, G., Nicoghosian, K., and Cedergren, R. J.,** 5S RNA sequence from the *Philosamia* silkworm: evidence for variable evolutionary rates in insect 5S RNA, *Nucleic Acids Res.*, 10, 5711, 1982.
179. **Gray, P. W. and Hallick, R. B.,** Isolation of *Euglena gracilis* chloroplast 5S ribosomal RNA and mapping the 5S rRNA gene on chloroplast DNA, *Biochemistry*, 18, 1820, 1979.
180. **Kumano, M., Tomioka, N., and Sugiura, M.,** The complete nucleotide sequence of a 23S rRNA gene from a blue-green alga *Anacystis nidulans, Gene,* 24, 219, 1983.
181. **Takaiwa, F., Kusuda, M., and Sugiura, M.,** The nucleotide sequence of chloroplast 4.5S rRNA from a fern *Dryopteris* acuminata, *Nucleic Acids Res.*, 10, 2257, 1982.
182. **Ohyama, K., Yamano, Y., Fukuzawa, H., Komano, T., and Yamagishi, H.,** Physical mapping of chloroplast DNA from liverwort *Marchantia polymorpha, Mol. Gen. Genet.,* 189, 1, 1983.
183. **Kumagai, I., Pieler, T., Subramanian, A. R., and Erdmann, V. A.,** Nucleotide sequence and secondary structure analysis of spinach chloroplast 4.5S RNA, *J. Biol. Chem.,* 257, 12924, 1982.
184. **Wildeman, A. G. and Nazar, R. N.,** Nucleotide sequence of wheat chloroplastid 4.5S ribonucleic acid. Sequence homologies in 4.5S RNA species, *J. Biol. Chem.,* 255, 11896, 1980.

185. **Keus, R. J. A., Roovers, D. J., Dekker, A. F., and Groot, G. S. P.,** The nucleotide sequence of the 4.5S and 5S rRNA genes and flanking regions from *Spirodela oligorhisa* chloroplasts, *Nucleic Acids Res.,* 11, 3405, 1983.

186. **Kumagai, I., Bartsch, M., Subramanian, A. R., and Erdmann, V. A.,** Chemical accessibility of the 4.5S RNA in spinach chloroplast ribosomes, *Nucleic Acids Res.,* 11, 961, 1983.

187. **Komarnitskii, N. A., Kudrjashov, A. V., and Uranov, A. A.,** *Plant Systematics,* Utchpedgiz, Moscow, 1962.

188. **Keus, R. J. A., Dekker, A. F., van Roon, M. A., and Groot, G. S. P.,** The nucleotide sequences of the regions flanking the genes coding for 23S, 16S and 4.5S ribosomal RNA of chloroplast DNA from *Spirodela oligorhisa, Nucleic Acids Res.,* 11, 6465, 1983.

189. **Brosius, J., Dull, T. J., and Noller, H. F.,** Complete nucleotide sequence of a 23S ribosomal RNA gene from *Escherichia coli, Proc. Natl. Acad. Sci. U.S.A.,* 77, 201, 1980.

190. **MacKay, R. M. and Doolittle, W. F.,** Nucleotide sequence of *Acanthamoeba castellanii* 5S and 5.8S ribosomal ribonucleic acids: phylogenetic and comparative structural analyses, *Nucleic Acids Res.,* 9, 3321, 1981.

191. **Schnare, M. N. and Gray, M. W.,** Nucleotide sequence of an exceptionally long 5.8S ribosomal RNA from *Crithidia fasciculata, Nucleic Acids Res.,* 10, 2085, 1982.

192. **Otsuka, T., Nomiyama, H., Sakaki, Y., and Takagi, Y.,** Nucleotide sequence of *Physarum polycephalum* 5.8S rRNA gene and its flanking regions, *Nucleic Acids Res.,* 10, 2379, 1982.

193. **Selker, E. and Yanofsky, C.,** Nucleotide sequence and conserved features of the 5.8S rRNA coding region of *Neurospora crassa, Nucleic Acids Res.,* 6, 2561, 1979.

194. **Rubin, G. M.,** The nucleotide sequence of *Saccharomyces cerevisiae* 5.8S ribosomal ribonucleic acid, *J. Biol. Chem.,* 248, 3860, 1973.

195. **Schaak, J., Mao Jen-i, and Söll, D.,** The 5.8S RNA gene sequence and the ribosomal repeat of *Schizosaccharomyces pombe. Nucleic Acids Res.,* 10, 2851, 1982.

196. **Rafalski, J. A., Wiewiórowski, M., and Söll, D.,** Organization of ribosomal DNA in yellow lupine (*Lupinus luteus*) and sequence of the 5.8S RNA gene, *FEBS Lett.,* 152, 241, 1983.

197. **Tanaka, Y., Dyer, T. A., and Brownlee, G. G.,** An improved direct RNA sequence method: its application to *Vicia faba* 5.8S ribosomal RNA, *Nucleic Acids Res.,* 8, 1259, 1980.

198. **MacKay, R. M., Spencer, D. F., Doolittle, W. F., and Gray, M. W.,** Nucleotide sequence of wheat-embryo cytosol 5S and 5.8S ribosomal ribonucleic acids, *Eur. J. Biochem.,* 112, 561, 1980.

199. **Nazar, R. N. and Roy, K. L.,** Nucleotide sequence of rainbow trout, (*Salmo gairdneri*) ribosomal 5.8S ribonucleic acid, *J. Biol. Chem.,* 253, 395, 1978.

200. **Khan, M. S. N. and Maden, B. E. H.** Nucleotide sequence relationships between vertebrate 5.8S ribosomal RNAs, *Nucleic Acids Res.,* 4, 2495, 1977.

201. **Ford, P. J. and Mathieson, T.,** The nucleotide sequences of 5.8S ribosomal RNA from *Xenopus laevis* and *Xenopus borealis, Eur. J. Biochem.,* 87, 199, 1978.

202. **Nazar, R. N. and Roy, K. L.,** The nucleotide sequence of turtle 5.8S rRNA, *FEBS Lett.,* 72, 111, 1976.

203. **Nazar, R. N., Sitz, T. O., and Busch, H.,** Sequence homologies in mammalian 5.8S ribosomal RNA, *Biochemistry,* 15, 505, 1976.

Chapter 7

MOLECULAR ANALYSIS OF PLANT DNA GENOMES: CONSERVED AND DIVERGED DNA SEQUENCES

A. S. Antonov

TABLE OF CONTENTS

I. INTRODUCTION

The discovery of the genetic role of DNA has set the stage for studying the structure and evolution of genomes as a means of improving and further elaborating the systematics and the theories of biological evolution. Originally, microorganisms were the target of this research; but since the early 1960s (and especially after the DNA hybridization technique had been developed), eukaryotic taxa were likewise taken up. Recently, genetic engineering and nucleic acid sequencing have opened up new opportunities in this field.

The pioneering studies of the DNAs of most different organisms have led to three basic conclusions. First, the chemical composition and fundamental principles of genetic material organization of all living matter reveal a similar pattern; this is essential for correct genome comparisons. Second, the rate of divergent evolution of DNA varies in different branches of the phylogenetic tree; e.g., if nuclear DNA is compared, it is much higher among Angiospermae classes than among Mammalia (a taxon of the same rank and of the same evolutionary age as the classes of Angiospermae, monocots, and dicots). Third, it is now obvious that the objectively evaluated degree of DNA similarity between organisms can be used to measure their phylogenetic relatedness. This conclusion also applies to nucleotide gene sequences.

Despite these breakthroughs an objective assessment of genotype similarities via DNA comparisons is still hampered by lack of basic information: the fundamental principles of genome organization and functioning have not yet been studied in full, especially in the case of eukaryotes. Thus far we do not know the functional role of most eukaryotic DNA; the current hypotheses appear to be insufficient.[1-5]

Molecular phylogenetic research has recently focused on comparing individual nucleic acid and protein sequences. This method, although not free from restrictions, compares functionally definite genome components to determine the rate and mode of the evolution of individual genes and of "auxiliary" DNA sequences. On this basis, hypotheses on the phylogenetic relatedness of the organisms may be suggested.

This may be a promising approach for systematics and phylogenetic studies because the evolution tempo of individual genome nucleotide sequences may be quite different. In other words, taxa of different degrees of phylogenetic relatedness may be compared via comparisons of genes differing in the rate of evolution. Until recently the different evolution rates of individual genes were thought to be determined largely by different selection pressure; now other mechanisms have been considered to explain this phenomenon.[6,7]

The new approach is useful for examining groups of organisms which are difficult to study by conventional systematic and phylogenetic techniques. Among higher eukaryotes, green plants are in this category. Although botanists have offered a multitude of plant systems, they can hardly be taken as natural. Our knowledge of plant evolution has quite a number of blank spots: even interrelations of the orders of angiosperms have not yet been specified, not to mention archegoniates. The genosystematic approach seems highly advisable for research into these "perennial" problems of botany.

Information gathered using the comparative approach should be evaluated in the light of the latest findings on the general patterns of plant genomes organization and functioning. Since the molecular structure of plant genomes is exceedingly labile, this instability must affect the pattern of individual gene evolution.

II. THE STRUCTURE AND EVOLUTION OF CONSERVED AND DIVERGED DNA SEQUENCES

We have not sufficient space here to examine all the results obtained in comparative studies of the evolution of nuclear DNA (nDNA) sequences, so we restrict the subject matter to their evolution in higher plants.

A. Some General Notes on the Structure and Evolution of Plant Genomes

Although plant species may differ significantly both in the quantity of nDNA in the haploid set of chromosomes[8.9] and in its composition,[10] their genome structural pattern is similar: plant genomes are formed by single copy (Sc) and repeated nucleotide sequences (Rs).[10-13] These operational notions[11] have no functional meaning. For instance, protein-coding genes in plant genomes may be represented by one or many copies. Nevertheless, the study of Sc and Rs (especially at the initial stage of plant DNA research) has proved to be highly useful for an understanding of the very general trends in plant genome evolution.

It was found, to begin with, that broad quantitative variations of Sc and Rs content in nDNA are typical of plants,[12-16] even of closely related species.[12,15,16] It followed from these observations that Rs families are rapidly being formed in plants, and early data on plant DNA hybridization proved that the divergent evolution of such sequences is also rapid.[17-20]

Different Sc and Rs migrate quickly within a plant genome; as a result, the Sc-Rs patterns differ even for phylogenically closely related species.[21,22] All these processes take place against the backdrop of ongoing quantitative nDNA changes, deletions, and amplifications. On the whole, the evolutionary transformation of plant genome is much more rapid than that in most of the higher eukaryote taxa studied.

One can form a general idea about the Sc and Rs change accumulation rate through the use of nDNA hybridization. Table 1 shows the values of DNA homology within Rs and Sc fractions for different phylogenetically related species. Similar results were obtained in Sc and Rs nDNA hybridization experiments with plants from many other taxa.[23-29] A statistical analysis made it possible to establish hiatus values for ΔTm and homologies for different-rank taxa of higher plants.[30] When these results are compared with similar data for vertebrates, it is easy to see the nonequivalency of taxa of the same rank in their systems, a significant factor to be taken into account for assessing the evolution tempos in eukaryotes.

Plant systematics have also been aided by the discovery of a clear-cut correlation between the degree of reproductive isolation of species within the genera of Angiospermae and the results of their Sc and Rs nDNA hybridization. If the degree of isolation is small and the species are able to form fertile hybrids in natural conditions (for instance, within the genus Achillea), then the Sc and Rs distinctions are not large.[29] When reproductive isolation increases (see the results of comparisons for Sc nDNA of the *Atriplex* species),[28] these differences are more pronounced.

Most studies of the hybridization of Sc and Rs of plant nDNA testify to the close accumulation rates of nucleotide substitutions in these fractions under speciation. As the phylogenetic distance between species increases, the ΔTm values for Sc and Rs go up. Hence, Rs comparisons may also be useful for assessing genome similarities, although contrary to certain theoretical premises and recommendations to work with Sc nDNA only.[31] Actually, however, these recommendations are at variance with the data obtained in the same laboratory in accordance with which the bulk of Sc are "fossil", deeply diverged Rs;[32] i.e., there is no qualitative difference between Sc and Rs.

The study of cloned individual Sc and Rs promises to provide an insight into their evolution. Plant speciation has been shown to be accompanied by formation of new Rs families, by a change in the number of copies in them, and by divergence of their primary structures.[33,34] Such cloned sequences may be useful as probes in phylogenetic research.

Until recently, we knew little about the causes of rapid Sc and Rs divergent changes in plant genomes; lately, however, attempts have been made to assess the role of individual factors of evolution in this process.

B. The Role of Polyploidy in Plant DNA Evolution

Polyploidy is one of the major factors of the microevolution of angiosperms, and hence it may underlie their more rapid nDNA divergence; the role of polyploidy in the evolution

Table 1
HOMOLOGIES IN Rs AND Sc DNA OF SOME APIACEAE SPECIES[30]

Plant species	Anthriscus glacialis				Prangos pabularia				Seseli nemorosum	
	Cot 1.0		Cot 10^2—10^4		Cot 1.0		Cot 10^2—10^4		Cot 140—10^4	
	1	2	1	2	1	2	1	2	1	2
Anthriscus glacialis Lipsky	0.0	100.0	0.0	100.0	10.7	30.6	6.5	33.8	6.5	35.5
Anthriscus ruprechtii Boiss.	3.8	79.0	—	—	13.6	35.9	—	—	—	—
Elaeosticta hirtula (Regel et Schmalh.) Kijukov. M. Pimen. et V. Tichomirov	7.7	53.3	—	—	10.7	46.5	—	—	—	—
Siella erecta (Huds.) M. Pimen.	9.1	54.6	—	—	13.0	47.5	—	—	—	—
Seseli libanotis (L.) Koch.	10.4	48.9	—	—	13.3	42.7	—	—	1.0	80.8
Seseli nemorosum (Korov.)	12.4	47.8	—	—	15.3	46.0	7.5	40.5	0.0	100.0
Seseli condensatum (L.) Reichnb.	—	—	—	—	—	—	5.1	42.7	2.2	86.7
Seseli mucronatum (Schrenk) M. Pimen. et Sdobn.	—	—	—	—	—	—	—	—	3.0	82.3
Pimpinella anthriscoides Boiss.	11.6	51.2	10.1	42.7	10.7	40.6	11.2	40.6	7.0	40.5
Ferula kokanica Regel et Schmalh.	8.9	46.0	9.7	40.7	11.5	41.0	12.8	32.3	11.8	29.9
Peucedanum latifolium (Bieb.)	9.1	42.6	10.2	—	12.3	49.5	7.9	31.6	12.5	30.2
Angelica komorovii (Schisch.) v. Tichomirov	12.2	48.5	8.0	35.2	13.4	46.7	11.6	33.5	10.8	47.1
Prangos pabularia Lindl.	8.7	43.9	9.9	40.6	0.0	100.0	0.0	100.0	8.4	39.6
Smyrniopsis aucheri Boiss.	10.3	43.4	10.1	35.0	6.4	52.2	6.4	62.3	9.0	50.3
Lecokia cretica DC	11.3	48.8	10.2	38.6	5.7	48.3	6.4	35.0	8.4	35.9
Laserpitium latifolium L.	8.8	57.5	—	—	10.7	37.2	—	—	7.5	38.8
Bupleurum aureum Fisch.	9.6	47.1	—	—	14.9	34.6	8.1	35.0	6.0	47.1
Conioselinum latifolium Rupr.	11.3	47.6	11.2	43.2	14.8	49.8	11.5	38.4	7.7	56.2
Paraligusticum discolor (Ledeb.) V. Tichomirov	11.2	53.6	—	—	11.9	51.0	10.8	43.9	8.9	36.4
Heracleum lehmannianum Bunge	12.6	44.5	—	—	13.0	35.8	9.6	25.1	6.9	39.7
Eryngium giganteum Bieb.	17.3	19.0	—	—	17.2	18.4	—	—	—	—

Labeled DNA of

1: Nucleotide substitutions, in %.
2: Homologies in DNA fractions, in %.

Table 2
HOMOLOGIES IN Rs AND Sc DNA OF SOME *SESELI*
SPECIES (APIACEAE)[27]

Plant species	Labeled DNA of					
	S. condensatum (2c)				*S. mucronatum* (2c)	
	Rs		Sc		Sc	
	a	b	a	b	a	b
Seseli condensatum (1)	0.0	100.0	0.0	100.0	3.5	76.0
Seseli condensatum (2)	1.0	72.5	0.5	88.0	2.5	86.5
Seseli mucronatum (3)	2.0	69.5	3.0	69.7	0.0	100.0
Seseli mucronatum (4)	3.5	63.5	8.5	77.5	4.0	90.7
Seseli nemorosum	—	—	3.5	77.6	4.0	88.0
Heracleum lehmanianum	—	—	9.5	45.9	6.0	47.0
Paraligusticum discolor	—	—	10.5	38.9	7.0	53.9
Peucedanum latifolium	—	—	12.5	30.0	7.0	56.9

1,2: Two different diploid populations.
3,4: Diploid and hexaploid populations.
a: Nucleotide substitutions, in %.
b: Homologies in DNA fractions, in %.

of other taxa of higher eukaryotes is less important. Up to 35% of the angiosperms are polyploids, and the proportion may be even higher for many rapidly evolving orders. Genome polyploidy increases the genetic variability of plant populations and intensifies the speciation process, yet nothing was known until recently about the intensity of nDNA changes following genome polyploidization.

Initially, the genera *Triticum* and *Aegilops* were taken as a model test object. Most of the cultivated wheats are polyploids; their genomes originate from the genomes of diploid wheats and aegilopses. Thus, interspecies nDNA comparisons seemed to be very promising.

Rs DNA hybridization showed that diploid wheats and aegilopses have more genome homologies than diploids and polyploids.[26] Similar results were also obtained for rapidly reassociating Rs nDNA of diploid and polyploid aegilopses.[25] Yet the cause of these distinctions was not completely evaluated since the relative role of natural and manmade selection remained unclear.

It would have been logical to proceed by studying natural diploid and polyploid plant populations and species. The genus *Seseli* (*Apiaceae*) was used for the purpose.[27] The most stable Rs DNA hybrids were obtained in hybridization experiments with DNA of plants from two different diploid *S. condensatum* populations. The thermostability was significantly lower for closely related species of the same genus, based on the tests with the DNAs of *S. condensatum* and of the diploid population *S. mucronatum* (ΔTm = 3°C). In concurrence with earlier observations,[25,26] the thermostability of DNA hybrid molecules obtained for the diploid population of *S. condensatum* and diploid or hexaploid *S. mucronatum* proved to be different (ΔTm = 2.0 and 3.5°C, respectively) (see Table 2). We suggested[27] that these distinctions might be due to a higher rate of accumulation of nucleotide substitutions in polyploid genome DNA. This hypothesis is supported by the results of investigations of gene expression in plant polyploids[35,36] and also by the data on rRNA evolution in animals: diploid and polyploid *Hyla* species.[37] As seen in Table 2, the same pattern applied for Sc fraction distinctions. The thermostability of hybrid DNA molecules formed in *S. condensatum*

Table 3
HYBRIDIZATION OF Rs AND Sc FRACTIONS OF DIPLOID *ACHILLEA SETACEA* DNA WITH "TOTAL" DNA OF SOME DIPLOID AND POLYPLOID ASTERACEAE SPECIES (Δ Tm VALUES = NUCLEOTIDE SUBSTITUTIONS, %)[29]

| | DNA fraction | | |
Plant species	Cot < 1	1—100	100—1000
1. *Achillea setacea* (2C)	0.0	0.0	0.0
2. *A. setacea* (4C)[a]	0.2	0.0	0.1
3. *A. setacea* (4C)[b]	0.1	0.1	0.1
4. *A. millefolium* (4C)[c]	0.5	0.3	0.3
5. *A. millefolium* (4C)[d]	0.6	0.3	0.4
6. *A. inundata* (6C)	0.8	0.6	0.7
7. *A. pannonica* (8C)	1.0	0.8	1.1
8. *A. nobilis* (2C)	1.1	1.0	1.2
9. *A. euxina* (4C)	0.9	0.8	1.5
10. *A. taurica* (2C)	1.5	1.4	1.7
11. *A. micrantha* (4C)	1.3	1.2	1.6
12. *A. micranthoides* (4C)	1.3	1.2	1.9
13. *A. birjuczensis* (4C)	0.9	0.8	1.2
14. *A. ochroleuca* (2C)	2.7	2.2	2.8
15. *Ptarmica borysthenica*	3.7	2.3	2.7
16. *Tanacetum odessanum*	2.5	1.9	2.2
17. *Anthemis* sp.	2.9	—	—

[a] Population from Kherson.
[b] Odessa region.
[c] Kiev region.
[d] Moscow region.

(2C) x *S. mucronatum* (6C) reaction was appreciably lower (ΔTm = 8.5°C) than that for molecules obtained in interspecific reactions (*S. condensatum* (2C) x *S. mucronatum* (2C) or *S. condensatum* (2C) x *S. nemorosum* (2C), ΔTm = 3.0 and 3.5°C, respectively).

Additional data were obtained in assays with Sc DNA of *S. mucronatum* (2C) (Table 2); the thermostability of DNA hybrids obtained in the experiment with *S. mucronatum* (2C) and *S. mucronatum* (6C) (ΔTm = 4.0°C) was close to that found in interspecies hybrids. The lowest thermostability (ΔTm = 7 to 19°C) was registered in intergeneric hybridization experiments.

Very similar regularities were revealed[29] in the experiment with diploid and polyploid milfoils (*Achillea*). Within the whiteflower milfoils section (species 1 to 7 in Table 3), a negative correlation was detected between the ploidy level and thermostability of DNA hybrid molecules. Although this genus is less diverged at the molecular level than are the genus *Seseli* and the majority of other plant genera studied previously, these two parameters reveal a clear-cut interdependence. The least similarity is exhibited by DNA of diploid *A. cetacea* and octaploid *A. pannonica*; in this case, thermostability is comparable with that of hybrid DNAs obtained in intersection comparisons.

The nature of polyploid species of *Seseli* and *Achillea* genera is still unknown. It is possible that at least some of them are allopolyploids and that the distinctions in ΔTm may be due to their hybrid origin. One cannot completely deny this possibility, yet available data suggest it is improbable. The DNA of diploid *Triticum boeoticum* is more similar to the diploid *Aegilops speltoides* or *A. squarrosa* than to the DNA of the allopolyploid wheats *T. durum* and *T. aestivum.*[26]

The thermostability of hybrid DNAs determined in tests with distantly related diploids is equal to (and sometimes even higher than) that for diploid-polyploids. It would have been lower had it been allopolyploid origin-dependent.

An alternative explanation may be that in the case of *S. mucronatum* diploid and hexaploid populations, we are actually dealing with sibling species. Plant sibling species have not been studied as deeply as those of animal due to some conceptual controversies between plant and animal taxonomists.[38] Plant DNA hybridization data may help to elaborate a new approach to this problem.

Summing up, we may conclude that polyploidy increases the nucleotide substitution rate in DNA evolution probably through a less pronounced selection pressure on the individual genes of multigene complexes of polyploid genomes. This evidence has to be taken into account when the phylograms of individual genes (and corresponding RNAs and proteins) are analyzed to reveal the phylogenetic relatedness of taxa. The mosaic pattern of polyploidy may have the most unpredictable effect on a gene evolution rate, and this may hamper assessment of phylogenetic distances and the topology of reconstructions.

C. The Evolution of Protein-Coding Sequences of Plant Genomes: Interspecies Comparisons

The DNA hybridization-revealed similarity of plant genomes does not always agree with botanists' conceptions of the phylogenetic relatedness of taxa. Data from these studies cannot yet be used to produce a fully substantiated correction of plant systems.

Although the higher plant genotypes are alike in complexity (i.e., formed by a similar number of genes), DNA hybridization reactions, particularly in the case of large "C-value" genomes, involve mainly those genome fractions whose functions have not been specified in full. Since transcriptionally active gene sequences in plant genomes comprise no more than a few percent of the entire nDNA,[28,39-42] estimates necessary for genome-genotype comparisons are only approximations. The situation is even more complicated because some temporarily nonexpressed nDNA sequences (pseudogenes, for instance) may be involved in genotype evolution. Moreover, the matrix function may not be the only nDNA function in eukaryotes; a part of nDNA may have skeletal functions[3] and be involved in the formation of supramolecular genotype structure and in chromosomal interactions.[5] The interdependence between a plant "nucleotype" and morphological characters has received special scrutiny. In view of DNA hybridization method restrictions,[30] nucleotide and amino acid sequence comparisons have become very popular.

The first comparisons of protein primary structures showed that the rate of evolution is protein-specific; the results for cytochromes, histones, fibrinopeptides, and some other animal proteins are well known. Since the first phylograms of animal kingdom based on these data dovetailed with zoologists' conceptions, the same approach was applied to other taxa. As soon as this had been done, the original euphoria vanished.

The results of the first comparisons of cytochrome *c* amino acid sequences caused doubts[43] about the prospects of this approach for the study of the plant phylogeny. Soon after, data were published on the structure of plastocyanines,[44,45] but the resulting conclusions were not widely accepted[46] (the point is that the phylogram of certain species does not accord with their taxonomic relations. Thus, *Phaseolus* and *Vigna* were separated from the seven other *Fabaceae* species studied in this work; *Prunus* and *Crataegus* of *Rosaceae* are far apart, and so forth). Similar inconsistencies mark another work of this laboratory: homologies in *Asteraceae* plastocyanines;[45] here, discrepancies are observed in the evaluation of phylogenetic kinship of Lactuceae species.

The merits and demerits of protein amino acid sequence methods were studied by means of computer modeling of the evolution processes,[47] and this made it possible to determine the real potencies of the two principal methods: the ancestor sequence and the matrix methods. A deliberate choice of protein for concrete phylogenetic objectives became a practical possibility; the ancestor sequence method was proven to be the best for closely related sequences. It follows from this analysis that the frequency of convergent evolutionary changes of protein structures is considerably lower than that of morphological structures. The conclusions of this work may also be useful for an analysis of the evolution of gene polynucleotide sequences.

As a rule, plant protein-coding genes have the same exon-intron structure as the genes of other eukaryotes.[48-50,57,71] There are exceptions; e.g., zein, lactin, and protease inhibitor genes lack introns.[54] Codon frequencies are close to those for protein-coding animal genes, with some exceptions (the thaumatine gene, for instance[55]).

Recently, comparative studies of plant gene nucleotide sequences opened new horizons in molecular phylogenetics. It appeared that the relatedness of very distant taxa may be evaluated. Thus, it was shown that the primary structure of one of the genes (SAc3) of the soya actin gene family has much in common even with animal actin genes. Previously it has been shown that actin amino acid sequences have a geat deal in common in such distantly related species as *Physarum*, yeast, and *Dictyostelium*.[56] The exons and introns of actin genes evolved at markedly different rates.[57] It is noteworthy that evolutionary conservative actin genes of plants accumulated nucleotide substitutions with higher rates than did actin genes of other eukaryotes. If we take the mean substitution accumulation rate for actin genes in animals and fungi to determine the divergency point of the main taxa of flowering plants, it appears to be several hundred million years away,[57] which in no way accords with paleobotanic evidence.[58] Previous studies of cytochrome *c* evolution rates led to a similar conclusion.[43] We regard the results for actin gene evolution rates as still another proof of the rapid evolution of plant genomes.[10]

The list of slowly evolving plant genes suitable for long-distant comparisons is increasing very fast. Judging by the related physical and chemical properties of plant and animal tubulin,[59] the genes of this protein have evolved slowly. Ferredoxin genes may be a suitable probe for distant phylogenetic comparisons as well; this follows from the results of comparative studies of amino acid sequences.[60] Complications may come because different ferredoxins function in diverse metabolic systems, and also because the evolution of ferredoxin genes included repeated duplications. Thus, instead of orthological, paralogical sequences may be erroneously compared. The pronounced relatedness of the primary structures of these proteins, present in pro- and eukaryote cells may indicate that they originate from the same ancestor sequence. Methods of comparisons, elaborated for animal globin genes, may help in this and other phylogenetic studies.

Since homologies were detected in amino acid sequences of the plastocyanins of phylogenetically distant species,[61] the genes of this protein, as well as those of other copper-containing "blue" proteins, may be suitable for the study of the distant evolutionary relationships of plant taxa.

Unfortunately, both amino acid sequences and corresponding histone gene nucleotide sequences in plants have not been studied in detail.[62] By analogy with animals, we may assume that this case involves a whole spectrum of change accumulation rates. It is known that plant gene histones include highly conserved genes (H4); on the other hand, the primary structures of histone H1 genes are rapidly evolving in all eukaryotes.

The crambin gene may be a suitable candidate for comparing distant plant taxa (crambin is a protein contained in the seeds of *Crambe abyssinica* (*Cruciferae*)). Primary structure-similar proteins, viscotoxin A3 (43% of homologies), and α_1-purothyonin (46% of homologies) were isolated from plants related to quite different orders of Angiospermae.[63] The nuclear gene of the small subunit of *RuBPCase* may be ranked among the evolutionary conserved; it exhibits 72% homology in pea and spinach.[64,65]

Valuable data were obtained by comparing evolution rates of glyceraldehyde-3-phosphate dehydrogenases of cytosol and chloroplasts. The protein-subunit genes of both enzymes are localized in the nucleus, but their evolution rates proved unequal. The structure of the cytosol enzyme is very conservative and the chloroplast enzyme evolved faster.[66] Consequently, the evolution rate of these two genes does not match that of the corresponding gene compartments; the nuclear plant genome is known to have evolved faster than the chloroplast genome.

The subunit genes of some plant storage proteins evolve relatively fast, therefore, comparison of the amino acid sequences of a vicilin subunit with the homological part of the phaseolin molecule has revealed 30% of homologies only;[67] similar results have been obtained for lectin cDNA of *Phaseolus vulgaris* (cv. Tendergreen) and *Pisum sativum*.[68]

Such molecular probes can well be used for analysis of both the family Fabaceae itself and its phylogenetic ties with other Angiospermae families. It may appear surprising, but even oat globuline and pea legumine reveal homologies.[69]

Trypsin inhibitor genes may be good for the study of the phylogenetic ties of individual taxa within Fabaceae as well. The amino acid sequences of the classical Kunitz trypsin inhibitor from soya and the WTI-I trypsin inhibitor from winged bean are only 50% homologous, i.e., the corresponding genes evolved at a very rapid rate.[70]

This list of differently evolving genes could be continued. However, it is obvious from what has been said above that even now one can select a cloned gene for a specific phylogenetic objective from among those which have been investigated (but taking into account some conditions, see the next section). The study of primary structures of individual RNAs (rRNA, for instance) opens up fresh possibilities. Since these results are considered by other authors in this book, they will not be discussed here.

D. Quickly and Slowly Evolving Gene Families in Plant Genomes

It is known that many plant proteins are coded by gene families. A detailed study of the nucleotide sequences of individual genes from such families is of particular significance for molecular phylogenetics. These families have proved to be heterogenous, e.g., the soya leghemoglobin gene family includes normal, pseudo, and truncated genes.[50,72] For the most part, gene families were formed as a result of repeated duplication-amplification events of the ancestor gene.[73-75] Subsequent substitution accumulation rates in individual genes of the family could have been different; at times, gene "subfamilies" were formed. For this reason, attempts to use the nucleotide sequence of a fortuitously cloned gene of a family for interspecific comparisons may lead to erroneous conclusions (a quite different situation emerges by comparison of rRNA sequences; here we deal with the "mean statistical sequence" reflecting the properties of the entire family).

The actin gene family[76] may be a good example. The nucleotide sequence of three genes of the family was determined — SAcI and SAc3 (soya), and MAcI (maize) — which are highly homologous on the whole (73 to 77%). Rapid changes at "silent" nucleotide residues of the genes were discovered. The rate was 1% for 0.7 to 1 million years, so the overall accumulation now is as much as 200 to 400% among plants and other eukaryotes (i.e., the changes occurred repeatedly in the same position).

The accumulation rate of amino acid changing substitutions was considerably lower. The differences among SAc1, SAc3, and MAcI is 8 to 11%. Significantly, interspecific distinctions between these plant genes from among different classes of *Angiospermae* are equal (!) to those between genes in a single family; within a single genome, an unexpected phenomenon compelled the authors to desist from comparing divergent processes of genes and plant species.[57] Yet this is not the only observation; it looks as if the evolution of genes of lupine 5.8S rRNA followed a similar pattern.[77] Pronounced differences were observed in two cloned 5.8S rRNA sequences. Paralogical 5S rRNA sequences were detected in a ribbon worm.[78] I am certain there are bound to be more observations like this in the future.

The genes of legume and grass storage proteins have been extensively studied. Proteins of two classes have been found in the seeds of most of the Leguminosae: legumines (II S) and vicilins (7S) with a subunit structure. Individual subunit types are coded by gene subfamilies, and the similarity of gene nucleotide sequences both between such subfamilies and within varies significantly.

Thus, comparison of the nucleotide sequences coding the α and α′-subunit of the complex 7S soya storage protein conglycin has made it possible to divide them into two groups.[79] The nucleotide sequences are nearly identical within each group, but the groups themselves differ by 6 to 7%. These differences are predominantly localized in the sequences, corresponding to COOH-terminal parts of the protein molecules. It is interesting that the adjacent 3′-noncoding sequences of the two subfamily genes are also highly homologous; complementary regions have been found in some other genes of soybeans as well. The evolutionary conservatism of these sequences may be due to the part they play either under gene expression or under stabilization of mRNA molecules. Analogous results have been obtained for the globin gene family in mammals.

Conglycin β-subunit-coding genes form another subfamily which differs to a far greater extent from genes of α and α′-subunits than among each other.[80] It has been demonstrated that the α, α′, and β-subunits are homologous only in a region adjacent to COOH-terminus. Comparison of the amino acid sequences of glycinine components also testified to a complex structure and evolution of the corresponding gene family.[81]

In soya species (the genus *Glycine*), the storage protein complex has undergone both qualitative and quantitative changes in the course of speciation. Its composition differs for annuals and perennials, although the seeds of all of these have 11S and 7S proteins. Broad interspecific intragenome gene comparisons can furnish much valuable information on the mechanisms and tempos of the evolution of plant multigene families.[81]

There is much evidence in literature on the gene structure of grass storage protein.[51-53,82,83] Since the analysis leads to about the same results as those for legumes, we shall not deal with that in this chapter.

III. CONCLUSION

The plant genome is a complex form with a very high evolutionary lability. The genome evolution rate was higher in plants than in the other groups of higher eukaryotes studied. The rate of evolution was influenced by a specific evolutionary factor pervasive in the plant kingdom — polyploidy.

The plant genome is formed by a spectrum of nucleotide sequences with different functional loads and is affected by different selection pressures. For this reason, the change accumulation rate varies considerably in different types of sequences in the course of evolution.

By using differently conserved nucleotide sequences as molecular probes, one can study the phylogenetic relatedness of any plant taxa, as well as the other taxa of pro- and eukaryotes. Proceeding from available evidence, we may infer that classical systematics and phylogenetics sometimes operate with erroneous conceptions concerning interrelations among many plant taxa; a revison of these conceptions is inevitable on the basis of the data obtained from comparative studies of plant genes.

New data on phylogenetic interrelatedness of plant taxa will undoubtedly contribute to the plant evolution theory.

REFERENCES

1. **Britten, R. J. and Davidson, E. H.,** Gene regulation for higher cells: a theory, *Science,* 165, 349, 1969; Repetitive and non-repetitive DNA sequences and a speculation on the origins of evolutionary novelty, *Q. Rev. Biol.,* 46, 111, 1971.
2. **Doolitle, W. F.,** Selfish DNA after fourteen months, in *Genome Evolution,* Dover, G. and Flavell, R., Eds., Academic Press, New York, 1982, 3.
3. **Cavalier-Smith, T.,** Nuclear volume control by nucleoskeletal DNA, selection for cell volume and cell growth rate, and the solution of the C-value paradox, *J. Cell. Sci.,* 34, 247, 1978.
4. **Davidson, E. H., Jacobs, H. T., and Britten, R. J.,** Very short repeats and coordinate induction of genes, *Nature (London),* 301, 468, 1983.
5. **Bennett, M. D.,** Nucleotypic basis of the spatial ordering of chromosomes in eucaryotes and the implications of the order for genome evolution and phenotypic variation, in *Genome Evolution,* Dover, G. A. and Flavell, R. B., Eds. Academic Press, London, New York, 1982, 239.
6. **Dover, G. A.,** Molecular drive: a cohesive mode of species evolution, *Nature (London),* 299, 111, 1982.
7. **Rose, M. R. and Doolittle, W. F.,** Molecular biological mechanisms of speciation, *Science,* 220, 157, 1983.
8. **Bennett, M. D. and Smith, J. B.,** Nuclear DNA amounts in angiosperms, *Philos. Trans. R. Soc. London Ser. B:,* 274, 227, 1976.
9. **Price, H. J.,** Evolution of DNA content in higher plants, *Bot. Rev.,* 42, 27, 1976.
10. **Antonov, A. S., Microschnichenko, G. P., and Slusarenko, A. G.,** Data on DNA primary structure in plant systematics, *Usp. Sovrem. Biol.* 74, 247, 1972 (in Russian).
11. **Britten, R. and Kohne, D.,** Repeated sequences in DNA, *Science,* 161, 529, 1968.
12. **Miroschnichenko, G. P., Antonov, A. S., and Valiejo-Roman, K. M.,** A study of reassociation of denatured, fragmented DNAs of some higher plants, *Dokl. Akad. Nauk SSSR,* 205, 1243, 1972 (in Russian).
13. **Flavell, R. B., Bennett, M. D., Smith, J. B., and Smith, D. B.,** Genome size and the proportion of repeated nucleotide sequences in plants, *Biochem. Genet.,* 12, 257, 1974.
14. **Ingle, J., Timmis, J. N., and Sinclair, J.,** The relationship between satellite deoxyribonucleic acid, ribosomal ribonucleic acid gene redundancy and genome size in plants, *Plant Physiol.,* 55, 496, 1975.
15. **Karavanov, A. and Jordansky, A.,** Genome structure of *Allium cepa* L. and *Allium fistulosum* L., *Mol. Biol.,* 7, 366, 1973 (in Russian).
16. **Miroshnichenko, G. P., Valiejo-Roman, K. M., and Antonov, A. S.,** DNA reassociation kinetics of some *Liliatae* species, *Dokl. Akad. Nauk SSSR,* 214, 1199, 1974 (in Russian).
17. **Bendich, A. J. and Bolton, E. T.** Relatedness among plants as measured by the DNA-agar technique, *Plant Physiol.,* 42, 959, 1967.
18. **Marinova, E. I., Antonov, A. S., and Belozersky, A. N.,** Homologies in DNA of some monocotyledonous plants, *Dokl. Akad. Nauk SSSR,* 184, 483, 1969 (in Russian).
19. **Bendich, A. and McCarthy, B. J.,** DNA comparisons among barley, oats, rye and wheat, *Genetics,* 65, 545, 1970.
20. **Slusarenko, A. G., Antonov, A. S., and Belozersky, A. N.,** Homological nucleotide sequences in DNA's of some *Liliatae* species, *Dokl. Akad. Nauk SSSR,* 209, 5, 1973 (in Russian).
21. **Murray, M. G., Cuellar, R. F., and Thompson, W. F.,** DNA sequence organization in the pea genome, *Biochemistry,* 17, 5781, 1978.
22. **Murray, M. G., Palmer, J. D., Cuellar, R. E., and Thompson, W. F.,** Deoxyribonucleic acid sequence organization in the mung bean genome, *Biochemistry,* 18, 525, 1979.
23. **Shnejer, V. S. and Antonov, A. S.,** Homologies in DNA of some species of *Iris* L., *Dokl. Akad. Nauk SSSR,* 222, 1975 (in Russian).
24. **Narayan, R. and Rees, H.,** Nuclear DNA divergence among *Lathyrus* species, *Chromosoma (Berlin),* 63, 101, 1977.
25. **Flavell, R., O'Dell, M., and Smith, D.,** Repeated sequence DNA comparisons between *Triticum* and *Aegilops* species, *Heredity,* 42, 309, 1979.
26. **Janeva, J. N. and Antonov, A. S.,** Homologies in repetitive DNA fractions of *Triticum* and *Aegilops* species, *Genetica,* 13, 578, 1977 (in Russian).
27. **Valiejo-Roman, K. M., Antonov, A. S., and Pimenov, M. G.,** Homologies in DNAs of some species from *Apioidea* subfamily, *Dokl. Akad. Nauk SSSR,* 245, 1021, 1979 (in Russian).
28. **Belford, H. S. and Thompson, W. F.,** Single copy DNA homologies in *Atriplex.* I. Cross reactivity estimates and the role of deletions in genome evolution, *Heredity,* 46, 91, 1981.
29. **Kashevarov, G. P. and Antonov, A. S.,** Analysis of phylogenetically closely related species from *Achillea* L. *(Asteraceae)* genus by means of DNA hybridization, *Bot. J.,* 67, 537, 1982 (in Russian).
30. **Valiejo-Roman, K. M., Antonov, A. S., and Kamaletdinova, M. A.,** An analysis of phylogeneitic interrelatedness of some *Umbelliferae* genera by means of DNA hybridization, *Dokl. Akad. Nauk. SSSR,* 262, 749, 1982.

31. **Belford, H. S. and Thompson, W. F.,** Single copy DNA homologies in *Atriplex.* II. Hybrid thermal stabilities and molecular phylogeny, *Heredity,* 46, 109, 1981.

32. **Murray, M. G., Peters, D. L., and Thompson, W. F.,** Ancient repeated sequences in the pea and mung bean genomes and a model for genome evolution, *J. Mol. Evol.,* 17, 31, 1981.

33. **Bedbrook, J. R., Jones, J., O'Dell, M., Thompson, R. D., and Flavell R. B.,** A molecular description of telomeric heterochromatin in *Secale* species, *Cell,* 19, 545, 1980.

34. **Appels, R., Dennis, E. S., Smyth, D. R., and Peacock, W. J.,** Two repeated DNA sequences from the heterochromatic regions of rye (*Secale cereale*) chromosomes, *Chromosoma (Berlin),* 84, 265, 1981.

35. **Garcia-Olmedo, F., Carbonero, P., Aragoncillo, C., and Salcedo, G.,** Loss of redundant gene expression after polyploidization in plants, *Experientia,* 34, 332, 1978.

36. **Wilson, H. D., Barber, S. C., and Walters, T.,** Loss of duplicate gene expression in tetraploid *Chenopodium, Biochem. Syst. Ecol.,* 11, 7, 1983.

37. **Toivonen, L. A., Crowe, D. T., Detrick, R. J., Klemann, S. W., and Vaughn, J. C.,** Ribosomal RNA gene number and sequence divergence in the diploid-tetraploid species pair of North American hylid tree frogs, *Biochem. Genet.,* 21, 299, 1983.

38. **Cronquist, A.,** Once again: what is a species? in *Beltsville Symp. in Agric. Res.,* Vol. 2, *Biosystematics in Agriculture,* 1978, 3.

39. **deVries, S. C., Springer, J., and Wessels, G. H.,** Sequence diversity of polysomal mRNAs in roots and shoots of etiolated and greened pea seedlings, *Planta,* 158, 42, 1983.

40. **Goldberg, R., Hoschek, G., Kamalay, J. C., and Timberlake, W. E.,** Sequence complexity of nuclear and polysomal RNA in leaves of the tobacco plant, *Cell,* 14, 123, 1978.

41. **Kiper, M., Bartels, D., Köchel, H.,** Gene number estimates in plant tissues and cells, *Plant Syst. Evol.,* 2(Suppl.), 129, 1979.

42. **Goldberg, R., Hoschek, G., Tam, S. H., Ditta, G. S., and Briedenbach, R. W.,** Abundance, diversity and regulation of mRNA sequence sets in soybean embryogenesis, and developmental regulation of cloned superabundant embryo mRNAs in soybean, *Dev. Biol.,* 83, 201, 218, 1981.

43. **Cronquist, A.,** The taxonomic significance of the structure of plant proteins: a classical taxonomist's view, *Brittonia,* 28, 1, 1976.

44. **Boulter, D., Peacock, D., Guise, A., Gleaves, J. T., and Estabrook, G.,** Relationship between the partial amino acid sequences of plastocyanin from members of ten families of flowering plants, *Phytochemistry,* 18, 603, 1979.

45. **Boulter, D.,** Present status of the use of amino acid sequence data in plant phylogenetic studies, in *Evolution of Protein Molecules,* Matsubara, H. and Yamanaka T., Eds., Japanese Scientific Society Press, Tokyo, 1979, 243.

46. **Cronquist, A.,** Chemistry in plant taxonomy: an assesment of where we stand, in *Chemosystematics: Principles and Practice,* Bisby, F. A., Ed. Academic Press, New York, 1979.

47. **Peacock, D. and Boulter, D.,** Use of amino acid sequence data in phylogeny and evaluation of methods using computer simulation, *J. Mol. Biol.,* 95, 513, 1975.

48. **Sheldon, E., Ferl, R., Fedoroff, N., and Hannoh, L. C.,** Isolation and analysis of a genomic clone encoding sucrose synthetase in maize: evidence for two introns in *Sh. Mol. Gen. Genet.,* 190, 421, 1983.

49. **Fischer, R. L. and Goldberg, R. B.,** Structure and flanking regions of soybean seed protein genes, *Cell,* 29, 651, 1982.

50. **Brisson, N. and Verma, D. P. S.,** Soybean leghemoglobin gene family. Normal, pseudo and truncated genes, *Proc. Natl. Acad. Sci. U.S.A.,* 79, 4055, 1982, see also *Nucleic Acids Res.,* 10, 689, 1982.

51. **Printer-Toro, J. A., Langridge, P., and Feix, G.,** Isolation and characterization of maize genes coding for zein proteins of the 21000 dalton size class, *Nucleic Acids Res.,* 10, 3845, 1982.

52. **Wienand, U. and Feix, G.,** Zein specific restriction enzyme fragments of maize DNA, *FEBS Lett.,* 116, 14, 1980.

53. **Pederson, K., Devereux, J., Wilson, D. R., Sheldon, E., and Larkins, B. A.,** Cloning and sequence analysis reveal structural variation among related zein genes in maize, *Cell,* 29, 1015, 1982.

54. **Messing, J., Geraghty, D., Heidecker, G., Hu, N.-T., Kride, J., and Rubenstein, I.,** Plant gene structure, in *Genetic Engineering of Plants,* Kosuge, T., Meredith, C. P., and Hollaender, A., Eds., Plenum Press, New York 1983, 211.

55. **Lycett, G. W., Delauney, A. J., and Groy, R. R. D.,** Are plant genes different? *FEBS Lett.,* 153, 43, 1983.

56. **Shah, D. M., Hightower, R. C., and Meagher, R. B.,** Complete nucleotide sequence of a soybean actin gene, *Proc. Natl. Acad. Sci. U.S.A.,* 79, 1022, 1982.

57. **Shah, D. M., Hightower, R. C., and Meagher, R. B.,** Genes encoding actin in higher plants: intron positions are highly conserved but the coding sequences are not, *J. Mol. Appl. Genet.,* 2, 111, 1983.

58. **Taylor, T. N.,** The origin of land plants: a paleobotanic perspective, *Taxon,* 31, 155, 1982.

59. **Yadav, N. S. and Filner, P.,** Tubulin from cultured tobacco cells: isolation and identification based on similarities to brain tubulin, *Planta,* 157, 46, 1983.

60. **Matsubara, H., Hase, T., Wakabayashi, S., and Wada, K.,** Gene duplications during evolution of chloroplast-type ferredoxins, in *Evolution of Protein Molecules,* Matsubara, H. and Jamanaka, T., Eds., Japanese Scientific Society Press, Tokyo, 1978, 290.

61. **Aitken, A.,** Plastocyanin and evolutionary relationship between chloroplasts and cyanobacteria, in *Evolution of Protein Molecules,* Matsubara, H. and Yamaneka, T., Eds., Japanese Scientific Society Press, Tokyo, 1978, 251.

62. **Thomas G. and Padayatty, J. D.,** Organization and bidirectional transcription of H2A, H2B and H4 histone genes in rice embryos, *Nature (London),* 306, 82, 1983.

63. **Teeter, M. M., Mazer, J. A., and L'Italien, J. J.,** Primary structure of the hydrophobic plant protein crambin, *Biochemistry,* 20, 5437, 1981.

64. **Bedbrook, J. P., Smith, S. M., and Ellis, R. J.,** Molecular cloning and sequencing of cDNA encoding the precursor of the small subunit of chloroplast ribulose-1,5-bisphosphate carboxylase, *Nature (London),* 287, 692, 1980.

65. **Berry-Lowe, S. L., McKnight, T. D., Shah, D. M., and Meagher, R. B.,** The nucleotide sequence, expression and evolution of one member of a multigene family encoding the small subunit of ribulose-1,5-bisphosphate carboxylase in soybean, *J. Mol. Appl. Genet.,* 1, 483, 1982.

66. **Cerff, R. and Kloppstech, K.,** Structural diversity and differential light control of mRNAs coding for angiosperm glyceraldehyde-3-phosphate dehydrogenase, *Proc. Natl. Acad. Sci. U.S.A.,* 79, 7624, 1982.

67. **Hirano, H., Gatehouse, J. A., and Boulter, D.,** The complete amino acid sequence of a subunit of the vicilin seed storage protein of pea *(Pisum sativum L.), FEBS Lett.,* 145, 99, 1982.

68. **Hoffman, L. M., Ma, Y., and Barker, R. F.,** Molecular cloning of *Phaseolus vulgaris* lectin mRNA and use of cDNA as a probe to estimate lectin transcript levels in various tissues, *Nucleic Acids Res.,* 10, 7819, 1982.

69. **Matlashewsky G. J. et al.,** Oat globulin and pea legumin are homologous proteins, in *Miami Winter Symposium,* Vol. 20, Ahmad, F. et al., Eds. Academic Press, New York, 1984.

70. **Yamamoto, M., Hara, S., and Ikenoka, T.,** Amino acid sequence of two trypsin inhibitors from winged bean seeds *(Psophocarpus tetragonolobus (L DC.), J. Biochem.,* 94, 849, 1983.

71. **Dennis, E. S. et al.,** Molecular analysis of the alcohol dehydrogenase (Adh 1) gene of maize, *Nucl. Acids Res.,* 12, 3983, 1984.

72. **Marcker, K. A., Bojsen, K., Jensen, E. Q., Paludan, K., and Wiborg, O.,** The structure and organization of the soybean leghemoglobine genes, in *Molecular genetics of the bacteria-plant Interaction,* Puhler, A., Ed., Springer-Verlag, Berlin, New York, 1983, 149.

73. **Pichersky, E. and Gottlieb, L. D.,** Evidence for duplication of the structural genes coding plastid and cytosolic isozymes of triose phosphate isomerase in diploid species of *Clarkia, Genetics,* 105, 421, 1983.

74. **Miflin, D. E. and Scandalios J. G.,** Genetic analysis of the two groups of duplicated genes coding for mitochondrial malate dehydrogenase in *Zea mays:* possible origin of *Mdh* genes by chromosome segment duplication, *Mol. Gen. Genet.,* 182, 211, 1981.

75. **Ellstrand, N. C., Lee J. M., and Foster, K. W.,** Alcohol dehydrogenase isozymes in grain sorghum *(Sorghum bicolor):* evidence for a gene duplication, *Biochem. Genet.,* 21, 147, 1983.

76. **Nagao, R. T., Shah, D. M., Eckcurode, V. K., and Meagher, R. B.,** Multigene family of actin-related sequences isolated from soybean genomic library, *DNA,* 1, 1, 1981.

77. **Rafalski, J. A., Wiewiorowski, M., and Söll, D.,** Organization of ribosomal DNA in yellow lupin *(Lupinus luteus),* and sequence of the 5,8S RNA gene, *FEBS Lett.,* 152, 241, 1983.

78. **Kumazaki, T., Hori, H., and Osawa, S.,** The nucleotide sequences of 5S rRNAs from two ribbon worms: *Emplectonema gracile* contains two 5S rRNA species differing considerably in their sequences, *Nucleic Acids Res.,* 11, 7141, 1983.

79. **Schuler, M. A., Schmitt, E. S., and Beachy, R. N.,** Closely related families of genes code for the α and α'-subunits of the soybean 7S storage protein complex, *Nucleic Acids Res.,* 10, 8225, 1982.

80. **Schuler, M. A., Ladin, B. P., Pollaco, J. C., Freyer, G., and Beachy, R. N.** Structural sequences are conserved in the genes coding for the α, α' and β-subunits of the soybean 7S storage protein, *Nucleic Acids Res.,* 10, 8245, 1982.

81. **Staswick, P. E., Broue, P., and Nielsen, N. C.,** Glycinin composition of several perennial species related to soybean, *Plant Physiol.,* 72, 1114, 1983.

82. **Spena, A., Viotti, A., and Pirrota, V.,** Two adjacent genomic zein sequences: structure, organization and tissue-specific restriction pattern, *J. Mol. Biol.,* 169, 799, 1983.

83. **Forde, J., Forde, B. G., Fry, R. P., Kreis, M., Shewry, P. R., and Miflin, B. J.,** Identification of barley and wheat cDNA clones related to the high-M_2 polypeptides of wheat gluten, *FEBS Lett.,* 162, 360, 1983.

Chapter 8

A CRITICAL REVIEW OF SOME TERMINOLOGIES USED FOR ADDITIONAL DNA IN PLANT CHROMOSOMES

Arun Kumar Sharma

TABLE OF CONTENTS

I. INTRODUCTION

In recent years due to marked development of physical and chemical methods of the study of chromosome architecture, numerous new terminologies have been introduced in the literature. In the eukaryotic systems, the chromosomes are visualized as giant complex molecules of DNA composed of genes of variable length. Refinements in ultrastructural techniques[1] have led to the resolution of chromosomes into fibrils 20 to 30 Å in diameter, folded several times to give the ultimate thickness of 100 Å. Cytologically, it is a continuous deoxyribonucleoprotein fiber having alternating condensed and uncondensed segments. Pulse labeling, as well as high resolution autoradiography, has revealed that chromosomes are made up of numerous replicons which undergo simultaneous replication during reproduction. The application of X-ray diffraction analysis has shown the chromosome to be composed of a bead-like structure, each bead being designated as a *nucleosome*. Five histone fractions are found in the nucleosomes. Four of these, namely, H-2a, H2b, H-3, and H-4 form an octamer, H-1 being associated as a linker. A DNA segment of approximately 200 bp is coiled around each nucleosome. The DNA wrapped around the octamer of histones makes the diameter of the spherical structure to be 100 Å, thus agreeing with the earlier demonstration of the same diameter of the DNA fiber. Thus, the proteins entering into the chromosome architecture of the nucleosomes are also repeated units, whose composition may be variable in certain cases.

The discovery of repeated DNA sequences in plants assisted considerably the interpretation of chromosome structure in terms of function and evolution. The enormity of the problem can be judged from the very fact that in several plant species, 70 to 75% of DNA is repetitive. Additional elements in plant chromosomes include the repeated sequences and amplified copies. Various authors have attributed different functions to the repeated sequences and several terms have also been applied. Moreover, if the concept of additional genetic elements in the chromosomes is accepted, then both phylogenetic and ontogenetic increases are to be taken into account. A critical assessment of several terminologies (glossaries) currently being used for additional DNA sequences has been the subject matter of this chapter. Most of the references are taken from different eukaryotic systems with special reference to plant chromosomes.

II. INCREASE IN DNA

The importance of additional DNA during development and differentiation has been recognized.[2] Endomitotic replication of chromonema has been recorded during differentiation. This has been attributed to the need for additional protein synthesis, whereas some consider this method of replication as a mechanism for the supply of fresh strands for continued transcription when the original strand is no longer operative.[3-6] The entire process is under genetic control and the need for such replication is entirely dependent on the genetic constitution of the species determining the period during which the genes may continue to transcribe without undergoing replication. Several cases have been recorded from this laboratory where such amplification of DNA has been shown to be associated with differentiation.[7,8] The amplified sequences need not necessarily involve the entire genome and therefore variable contents of DNA may characterize the different organs of individuals.[8-10]

Nagl[2] has suggested that plants normally possess a mechanism for phylogenetic increase in DNA as exemplified by the presence of polyploidy, generative polyploidy, and repeated sequences. However, an increase in DNA may involve multiple copies of the same or introduction of new information contents. Polyploidy, on the other hand, merely involves addition of back-up copies. Phylogenetic increase does not affect constancy of the amount of DNA in different cells. In addition to earlier works (see Sharma[5]), in later years ontogenetic increase of DNA has been reported in several organisms. Sekerka[11] reported a change in DNA content of interkinetic nuclei of the epicotyl of *Vicia faba* during differentiation. Such amplification during root development of *Allium cepa* has also been noted.[12] In *Arachis hypogea* a variation from 2C to 8C DNA was recorded in various tissues, the minimum being in root and shoot apices and leaf tissues (Sharma[5]).

Such high DNA values have been correlated with protein synthesizing capacity. In the scutellum of *Triticum durum*, a difference in DNA content has been recorded, associated with different histone-DNA ratios, in different tissues following aging. Such repeats may originate out of tandem or lateral duplication and unequal crossing-over. Species in which the mechanism of phylogenetic increase is not operative resort to amplification of DNA during ontogeny. This issue, however, needs to be thoroughly investigated.

The significance of high frequency repeats has not yet been fully established. The increase in copies of existing sequences may form the basis for the generally accepted existence of families of repeated sequences, provided however that such multiple copies remain long enough to become a family of repeated sequences. It would imply that *Xenopus* ribosomal genes may form a family. However, evidence for such a mechanism has yet to be obtained.

Several functions have been attributed to these genes, including those of regulation, maintenance of chromosome structure, control of crossing-over, and differentiation of chromosome segments. Such repeats have also been claimed to play an important role in serving as a reservoir of loci for the accumulation of mutation or even as padding to keep the chromatin in the folded state.

III. C-VALUE PARADOX

The repeated sequences have given rise to a paradoxical situation with regard to the genomic content of different species. In most eukaryotic systems, the amount of DNA in the genome, otherwise known as *C-value*, is much in excess of the total number of structural genes as already mentioned in the case of human cells. This has led to the situation termed as *C-value paradox*. It is indeed very difficult to correlate the degree of differentiation with the amount of DNA in an organism. The best examples are the lilies and amphibians where the range in amount of DNA is 20 to 100 pg, as compared to 2 to 3 pg in mammals and 7 pg in the human system.[13] Evidently, the repeated sequences are involved with genes which do not code for structural proteins but which lead to variability of DNA values in a different hierarchy of organization. The redundancy is suggested in view of the absence of information content. The C-value paradox may not hold to the same extent for all members of a species. The extent of variability in C-values at the intraspecific level, so far noted in certain organisms, is not fully known.[14-16] Even in the human system, quantitative variations of the genome have been recorded.[17,18] A correct interpretation of the significance of C-value will have to await an analysis of its variability in natural populations at the intraspecific level.

IV. SATELLITE DNA

Satellite DNA (sat-DNA), with high homogenous repeats, has been located in several organisms. In the pea, four fractions of rRNA were observed to hybridize with the main band.[19] In *Drosophila viridis* sat-DNAs are very specific in location and are rich in A-T sequences. They are consistently located on the sides of the nuclei nearest to the vitelline membrane. Highly repetitive sat-DNA sequences have been found in Cucurbitaceous species. The restriction pattern suggests an internal Hind III sequence of repeats with 380 bp in *Cucumis melo*. In *Cucumis sativus*, on the other hand, excision results in repeated units of 180 bp. A certain amount of homology between the satellites of the two species has been recorded, together with the properties of amplification and dispersion. Sat-DNAs have also been traced through *in situ* hybridization in human acrocentrics, especially on the short arm. Some of them exhibit some heterogeneity in their DNA content. In this connection, the intensity of fluoresecence has not been considered a proper criterion for detecting homogeneity of satellites.[18] A satellite is historically a CsCl-density satellite. In this case there is no density difference and a satellite is not observed on CsCl (as in the green monkey), but a reassociation or restriction enzyme is given for a family of repeats whose members are not exact copies of each other.

V. OTHER REPEATS

In addition to highly homogenous very short repeats, *moderate* and *minor* repeated sequences form a significant part of repeated DNA in biological systems.[20] In general, moderate and minor repeats remain interspersed between nonrepeated sequences. Repeats of diverse sequences have been recorded in different organisms, including *Drosophila*[21] and man.[22] Though highly repeated sequences often remain associated with heterochromatin, their association with other repeated sequences is also not ruled out. High frequency repeats have been observed in telomeric heterochromatin.[23] Heterozygosity of the repeated DNA is found to be associated with heteromorphicity in heterochromatin, especially in out-breeders.[24,25] Long repeated DNA sequences have been located in maize, as well as shorter sites which are 150 nucleotides long.[26] The heterochromatic knob in maize also has a very high content of repeated sequences.[27] In finger millets nearly 40 to 50% of repeated DNA is interspersed with 18% nonrepeats.[28]

In *Scilla autumnalis* repeated sequences have been clearly demonstrated in B-chromosomes. In *Secale cereale* and *S. montana,* the same complement of repeated sequences is found in both. The respective amounts of 630 and 610 bp and distribution of 480 bp families show substantial differences.[24] In rye, on the other hand, each simple subrepeat is interspersed by unrelated small subrepeats. Even *in vitro* growth of some *Drosophila* cells leads to addition of several repeated sequences.[29] This is an example of conservatism and dispersion but simultaneously each taxonomic unit remains distinct.

Though usually moderate and minor repeats remain interspersed, in a few cases the repeats are not necessarily interspersed with nonrepeats. In Syrian hamsters, short repetitive sequences are organized in scramble-tandem clusters[30] rather than individually interspersed with nonrepetitive regions. In rice genomes, such sequence interspersion has been noted in higher $C_o t$ values. At lower $C_o t$ values, however, DNA sequences have been interspersed within the repetitive fraction. All these facts clearly indicate that minor and moderate repeats, which are undoubtedly amplified and dispersed, may sometimes not be associated with unique sequences, but generally interspersion with the latter is recorded.[30,31]

A. Intervening Sequences

The most widely distributed additional DNA sequences in the eukaryotic genes are the *intervening sequences* or *introns* between coding elements. Such introns may be located at the terminal or initiation points or at intercalary positions.[31-33] The intervening sequences are transcribed but excised before translation. There is a high degree of homology between the intervening sequences of the two species. In *Drosophila melanogaster* the amplified dispersed copies belong to two categories; in one the sequences are related to each other and in the other they are not related.[34,35] However, such amplified intron-related sequences occur elsewhere in the genome as well,[36] and these have been suggested to be insertion elements.

B. Transposons

The idea of transposable (mobile) elements was first suggested by McClintock,[37] who visualized transposition of insertion sequences in maize. These sequences have a high degree of adjacent repeats, as in *Drosophila* and yeast. These are comparable to jumping genes (transposons). In interspecific hybrids of *Drosophila,* such transposition of mobile genetic elements has also been recorded. *In situ* hybridization has led to the insertion of a small mdg element (jumping element) of *Drosophila viridis* to the 5th chromosome of *D. littoralis*.[38] This is a case of artificial transposition between different chromosomes and four such mobile dispersed genetic elements have been recorded for a specific family of repeats. There may even be 35 dispersed copies in a family of repeated sequences such as the Ty-1 gene in *Saccharomyces cereviscae,* which constitute about 2% of the genome. Tandem clusters of Ty-1 genes have also been located and culturing flies for 1 month has led to a detectable shift of their location in 2 strains.[39] The transposable elements in yeast are quite remarkable in the sense that their movement is spontaneous and not activated by mutagens. In *Drosophila melanogaster* several families of such dispersed genes have been located, out of which copia are 5 kb long with direct repeats of 300 bp. The 412 sequences are each 7.3 kb with direct repeats of 500 bp.[40] In contrast to Ty-1 of yeast which has a repetition of 258 bp presenting 100 copies of the gene, in *Drosophila* dispersed, amplified, and mobile elements have also been noted in 297 and 225 bp sequences, but these are not as well defined. In view of the fact that interrelationships have been noted between transposable elements, a detailed study of their occurrence in several other dipterans has been suggested.[41] Transposable elements have also been located in the human system.[42]

C. Spacers

Amplified sequences have been recorded as *spacers* in rDNA of *Xenopus,* in *Drosophila,* and in other organisms.[13,43,44] The spacer sequences have also been noted to be heterogenous and located in 5-histone gene clusters in mammals and other organisms.[45] In *Xenopus borealis* 5-H genes are contained in clusters, about 80 bp apart with spacers of variable length. Recently, a new class of human interspersed repeated sequences different from the Abr family has been recorded. A nontranscribed spacer group (rDNA-NTS) of the mouse ribosomal gene, and utilized for screening a human gene library. It is a 250-bp segment located between human 5 and β-globin genes, which is mostly a tandem block of 17 TG dinucleotides. It is remarkable that homology of these spacer repeated sequences has been noted among *Xenopus,* pigeon, slime mold, and yeast DNAs. This homology in a wide spectrum of organisms indicates their highly conserved nature. Amplification and dispersion of such spacer sequences have been clearly demonstrated. In certain cases, the heterogeneity in size of rDNA repeating units is found to be due to the difference in length of the NTS regions.[46] These differences have been interpreted as reflecting the simple insertions into the NTS region of the major "short" repeat. Evidently such insertions may also indicate mobility of such sequences.

D. Nucleotypic DNA

In order to find a suitable explanation for the C-value paradox, the term *nucleotypic* DNA was coined.[47-49] This type of DNA is highly amplified and repeated in nature and is dispersed in its location in the genome. The word *nucleotypic* was used to account for its action related to properties of the nucleus, such as volume and duration of mitosis. A more detailed discussion is given later while dealing with the function of repeated sequences.

E. Palindromes

Palindromes or inverted repeats have been recorded at initiation and termination points as well as at other specific loci,[50,51] and their ultrastructural and biochemical natures have been worked out. Besides lower organisms,[52] genomes of several eukaryotes, such as mammals, amphibia, insects, and plants have been seen to possess inverted repeats.[53-55]

F. Selfish DNA

The terminology adopted for the amplified sequences is often unusual. *Selfish DNA* is applied to the repeated sequences which exist because of their capacity for duplication in a congenial cellular environment.[56] No evolutionary function is visualized. This form of DNA may often be harmful to the phenotype, like the segregation-distortion locus in *Drosophila*. However, large portions of DNA in eukaryotic genes are of this type. The genes included are not only amplified and regulated to carry out the vital activities of the cell, but their existence is also entirely dependent on their capacity to survive in the cellular environment.

The selfish DNAs have been categorized differently by various authors and termed accordingly. It is suggested[56] that selfish DNAs are sequence-dependent and should be distinguished from those that are sequence-independent; these are referred to as *ignorant DNA*. The latter possesses the properties of dispersion and amplification with selfish DNA. The sharing of similar sequences, such as 5S genes in different chromosomes, is a property of ignorant DNA, whereas copia and Ty-I (transposons) are selfish in nature. Selfish DNA sequences, having the properties of mobility and capacity of transfer between different chromosomes, have been designated as *parasitic* or *symbiotic DNA*.[57] The term *incidental DNA* has been applied to the amplified selfish DNA sequences, taking into account their mode of origin.[58] It has been suggested that the pressure of mutation often leads to amplified sequences incidental to the mutation process, which may provide a steady pool of potential gene resources.

Some of the duplicated functional genes often become nonfunctional following mutation. Such sequences have been referred to as *pseudogenes* or *dead sequences*.[59] These have been noted in different mammalian systems adjacent to the globin genes. The transcription of a pseudogene is responsible for the origin of human leukocyte interferon.[60] In view of the importance of these sequences in certain cellular functions, the term pseudo or dead genes is inappropriate.

G. Dynamic DNA

Excluding the unique sequences present in one or a few copies which code for enzyme proteins, all other DNA sequences have several common properties. All the sequences so far mentioned show more or less the common properties of *amplification, dispersion*, and *mobility*. The term *dynamic DNA* was thus applied to cover all the terms mentioned so far.[9,61] Introns have been compared with transposons because of the common property of mobility which leads to their capacity for dispersion. In fact, selfish DNA includes introns and therefore all mobile sequences with the property of dispersion. Spacer sequences, as noted in 5S genes, are considered to be ignorant and are amplified, dispersed, and possibly mobile. All three properties have been noted in copia and Ty-I-sequence-dependent transposons. Parasitic and symbiotic DNAs are also amplified, dispersed, and are capable of movement. Incidental DNA, however, assumes that the origin of such amplified sequences is incidental to mutation. Nucleotypic DNA is also repeated, dispersed, and may have the property of movement. In general, amplification and dispersion are common to all types of DNA, whereas mobility has been demonstrated in some and not observed in others. The application of the term dynamic DNA takes into account all the properties attributed to such DNA sequences, which do not necessarily code for structural proteins, but have the capacity of amplification, dispersion, and mobility. Accessory chromosomes, as the evidence presented thus far shows, contain a high degree of repeated sequences. The extent to which these chromosomes represent the cytological embodiment of dynamic sequences has yet to be ascertained. Since the repeated sequences may later be converted into unique genes through mutations, these definitions are semantic in nature.

The term dynamic DNA, proposed to embrace all such amplified sequences having the capacity of amplification, dispersion, and mobility, describes the functions of repeats in biological systems.[62] It exerts a dynamic influence on several nonspecific and vital functions of the cell, including nuclear behavior, cell volume, and chromosome size. Dynamic DNA has a distinctive role in messenger processing, reshuffling of exons, and maintenance of integrity of chromosome structure by providing padding at respective loci. Notwithstanding, the fact that evolution is not anticipatory, multiple copies are to be regarded as a natural mechanism for a steady supply of potential genetic diversity. Absolute functional redundancy or triviality, whether at a cellular or an organismic level, can hardly be reconciled with adaptations against the rigors of selection. The mobility and dispersion at multiple sites may be strategies adopted by these amplified sequences to promote genetic diversity and as a measure against complete elimination in evolution.

H. Fluid Genome

Although many essential aspects of the eukaryotic genome are stable, the potential for variation is now believed to be enormous. Dawid[63] has recently summarized this as "it has become more difficult to put our fingers on the aspect of the genome that is stable. Split genes and gene reshuffling supply a possible source of new and useful proteins. The movable repeats supply a great potentiality of regulatory rearrangements which could lead to new structures. These two possibilities taken together change by orders of magnitude the potentialities for useful organized novelty. These are probably only the first set of identifiable events of genomic variation that the new methods have identified."

VI. FUNCTIONS OF INTERSPERSED REPEATS

Various functions have been attributed to interspersed repeats.[64] Their role in repair synthesis has been demonstrated in plant systems. Moderate repeats in *Lilium* have been shown to undergo specific repair synthesis during pachytene, through conservation of such DNA sequences termed as pDNA (pachytene DNA). It has been suggested that for families with high thermostability the lack of internal divergence is evidence for fairly recent introduction into a moderately repeated DNA class. pDNA sequences as a whole represent evolutionary ancient families, the products of strong selective pressure for an indispensible meiotic function. The heterochromatin in rye shows rearrangements where each subrepeat is interspersed by unrelated nonsubrepeats. The importance of such repeated sequences in the regulation of chromosome structure is indicated in their involvement in folding during pairing[65] as well as in differentiation of chromosome structure. Their presence at different loci in chromosomes in different strains of *Drosophila* may indicate a functional role.[66,67] Similarly, the increase in amplified sequences in cultured cells of *Drosophila* is also signficant.[29]

The importance of repeated sequences, especially in gene conversion and expression, has been demonstrated in fission yeast.[68] Exchanges between repeated genes, leading to intergenic conversion and reappearance of suppressor active alleles, have become a powerful tool for genome exchange. The maintenance of sequence homogeneity of repeats is facilitated by such conversions.[69] In Asian and Caucasian human systems, genetic exchanges occur within large repeated gene clusters of the α-globin region.[70] The best example for the control of repeats in the expression of nonrepeats is provided in *Saccharomyces purpuratus* where RNA hybridization has been noted preferentially with nonrepetitive sequences linked with repeats.[13]

In different organisms, sequences coding for histone, tRNA, and rRNA are all repeats of a different kind which can be transcribed. All five genes coding for sea urchin histone are repeated sequences having variable efficiencies of transcription.[71]

An interesting case of gene expression is recorded in the oocyte nuclei of *Xenopus* where injection of L-22 repeat sequences allows expression of the histone gene of the sea urchin.[72,73] Various other functions have been attributed to moderate repeats, including roles in evolution,[74] adaptive radiation,[75] and as a reservoir of new sequences.[76] Sharma[4,5] interpreted such sequences as loci for the accumulation of mutations.

Inverted repeats or palindromes, in view of their occurrence in clusters at specific loci, have been assigned certain functions.[77] The term *fold back* or *snapback* DNA has been used and involvement in the formation of micronuclear DNA in ciliates has been suggested. Polymorphisms in inverted repeats are common and may have an evolutionary importance. Several functions have been attributed to palindromes. Their role in DNA replication at chromosome end has been suggested by Cavalier-Smith[78] and Heumanns.[79] Hartman et al.[80] have ascribed more than one function to these sequences.

Palindromic and repetitive sequences are intensely replicated under specified conditions.[81] The initiation of replication involves certain parts of comparatively long palindromes which are identical or very similar in the nucleotide sequences. Synchrony of replicon activation can be induced under specific conditions. Another extreme view has been taken by Deininger and Schmidt[82] who attribute no function to palindromes. In general, the role of such sequences in specific protein synthesis has been visualized at different levels.[83] They may serve as recognition and functional systems at the DNA and RNA levels involving deletion and translocation of the genetic material.[52] In messenger processing and protein synthesis, their roles involve different functions, including the recognition of cleavage sites, termination of transcription, and binding of regulatory proteins.[84] Cavalier-Smith[77] suggested a role in attachment of chromosomes to each other, implying possibly information transfer. Bassi et al.[55] noted a gradient of interspersion of palindromes in the genome, with their gradual increases in higher organisms. In the maintenance of chromosome orientation in interphase and nuclear structure, the significance of such sequences has been emphasized. All these data in relation to palindromes may suggest their multiple functions, and the preservation of such specific sequences at distinct loci may indicate a selective adaptation.

A. Location-Specific Functions

The location of repeated sequences in the introns has been clearly demonstrated. Such intervening sequences in multiple copies are present in the primary transcript following transcription, but are spliced off before translation. Their role in the processing of the messenger, its transport and its translation is signified by their localization at the intercalary, terminal, and initiation points.[31,32] Their specific activity in the rearrangement of functional exons, leading to the synthesis of new transcripts, has been demonstrated by recombination with introns in hen lysozymes.[85] In the human globin gene, the expressed sequences contain intervening repeats involved in intergenic conversion.[86] In fact, the intervening sequences with high degree repeats may play a very significant role in the synthesis of new translatable transcripts and variable structural proteins. Splicing followed by rejoining of different exons may lead to variable messengers if alternate sequences are introduced in a different order. The information content of different allied antibodies may thus be stored in a single gene sequence, which has varying exon combinations following the excision of introns. The importance of intervening segments with repeated sequences assumes added significance in terms of accelerating intragenic recombinations.

The location of repeats in transposons is difficult to reconcile with any concept involving no apparent function.[88] The mobility itself permits dispersion leaving aside accelerating accumulation of certain segments of specific loci. It is likely that such mobile sequences aid in the promotion of genetic diversity. The survival of sequences is also influenced by transfer to an environment where they will be tolerated.

The presence of repeated DNA in spacer sequences has been studied extensively in different organisms.[43,89] Such sequences often form heterogenous clusters[13] and their function is indicated in all the five histone gene clusters of mammals and other organisms.[45] In *Xenopus borealis* the clusters contain 5S genes, 80 bp apart, separated by spacers of variable length.

In vivo experiments have indicated that initiation and termination of transcription are facilitated through such sequences. However, the presence of detectable dissimilar 5S gene clusters in species of *Xenopus* may suggest that common control is exerted only by a few sequences. In mouse, NTS fragments contain 13 tandem copies of 13 bp subrepeating units. It has been postulated that regions of inverted repeats as well as large poly-T tracks may be related to a high level of rRNA synthesis.

In general, these repeated sequences with dynamic functions do not code for structural proteins, but they do play a role in the maintenance and functioning of structural sequences. Similarly, genes for nonspecific functions in cells are subject to physiological influences. The properties of amplification, dispersion, and mobility confer a certain amount of flexibility and a wide functional range and may be subject to physiological and extracellular influences. Therefore, these sequences, which are often heterogenous in nature as revealed by different restriction sites, exhibit complexity in structure and flexibility in behavior — the two features acquired during evolution.

Accessory chromosomes in plants, as the evidence so far indicates, may contain a high proportion of repeated DNA, perhaps as the cytological embodiment of repeated sequences. The properties of amplification and dispersion are inherent and mobility can be assumed in view of the dispersive property. There has been considerable debate with regard to the function of the accessory chromosomes. Significant correlation between soil type, climate, and accessory chromosomes has been recorded in different species of *Festuca, Phleum, and Centaurea*.[87] Adaptability of B-chromosomes in temperate and alpine climates has been clearly demonstrated in *Allium stracheyi* and species of *Arisaema*.[10,88-90] The effects of crossover are noted in interspecific hybrids of *Aegilops, Lolium, Secale*, and some insects.[24,91,92] The accessory chromosomes certainly confer a buffering effect on the adaptability of a species and a threshold point over which a negative influence may be recorded.

ACKNOWLEDGMENT

The author is thankful to Professor S. K. Dutta for kindly going through the manuscript and suggesting valuable modifications.

REFERENCES

1. **Sharma, A. K. and Sharma, A.,** *Chromosome Techniques — Theory and Practice,* 3rd ed., Butterworths, London, 1980.
2. **Nagl, W.,** Molecular and structural aspects of the endomitotic chromosome cycle in angiosperms, in *Chromosomes Today,* Darlington, C. D. and Lewis, K. R., Eds., Oliver & Boyd, London, 1972, 3, 17.
3. **Evans, L. S. and van't Hof, J.,** Is polyploidy necessary for tissue differentiation in higher plants?, *Am. J. Bot.,* 62, 1060, 1975.
4. **Sharma, A. K.,** A new look at chromosome and its evolution, *Proc. Indian Natl. Sci. Acad.,* 42B, 12, 1976.
5. **Sharma, A. K.,** Change in chromosome concept, *Proc. Indian Acad. Sci.,* 87B, 161, 1978.
6. **Sen, S.,** Differentiated nuclei and elucidation of chromosomal control of differentiation, *Nucleus,* 17, 40, 1974.
7. **Sharma, A. K. and Mookerjea, A.,** Induction of division in cells — a study of the causal factors involved, *Bull. Bot. Soc. G.C. Bose Mem.,* 824, 1954.
8. **Banerjee, M. and Sharma, A. K.,** Variation in DNA content, *Experientia,* 35, 42, 1979.
9. **Sharma, A. K.,** Additional genetic materials in chromosomes, in *Proceedings of the 2nd Chromosome Conference at Kew,* Brandham, P. E. and Bennett, M. D., Eds., George Allen & Unwin, London, 1983.
10. **Sau, H., Sharma, A. K., and Choudhuri, R. K.,** DNA, RNA and protein content of isolated nuclei from different plant organs, *Indian J. Exp. Biol.,* 18, 1519, 1980.

11. **Sekerka, V.**, Changes in DNA content of interkinetic nuclei of epicotyl cells of *Vicia faba* L during the process of differentiation, *Biologia*, 36, 741, 1981.

12. **Cremonini, R., Ioro, M. L., and Duranti, M.**, Differentiation of metaxylem cell line in the root of *Allium cepa*. II. Changes in nucleotide sequence redundancy, *Protoplasma*, 108, 1, 1981.

13. **Lewin, B.**, *Gene Expression — Eukaryotic Chromosomes*, Wiley Interscience, New York, 1980.

14. **Kurnitt, D. M.**, Satellite DNA and heterochromatin variants: the case of unequal mitotic crossover, *Hum. Genet.*, 47, 169, 1979.

15. **Patton, J. L. and Sherwood, S. W.**, Genome evolution in pocket gophers (genus *Thomomyces*). I., *Chromosoma (Berlin)*, 85, 149, 1982.

16. **Sherwood, S. W. and Patton, J. L.**, Genome evolution in pocket gophers (genus *Thomomyces*). II., *Chromosoma (Berlin)*, 85, 163, 1982.

17. **Bostock, C. J., Gosden, J. R., and Mitchell, A. R.** Localization of a male-specific DNA fragment to a sub-region of human Y-chromosome, *Nature (London)*, 272, 324, 1978.

18. **Gosden, J. R., Lawrie, S. S., and Gosden, C. M.**, Satellite DNA sequences in human acrocentric chromosomes. Informations from translocations and heteromorphisms, *Am. J. Hum. Genet.*, 33, 243, 1981.

19. **Wall, L. V. M., and Bryant, J. A.**, Isolation and preliminary characterization of cryptic satellite DNA in pea, *Phytochemistry*, 20, 1767, 1981.

20. **Davidson, E. H., Jacobs, H. T., and Britten, R. J.**, Eukaryotic gene expression of very short repeats and coordinate induction of genes, *Nature (London)*, 301, 468, 1983.

21. **Bruttlag, D. and Peacock, W. J.**, Sequences of the 1.672 g/cm³ satellite DNA of *Drosophila melanogaster*, *J. Mol. Biol.*, 135, 565, 1979.

22. **Cooke, H. J. and Hindley, J.**, Cloning of human satellite. III. Different components are on different chromosomes, *Nucleic Acids Res.*, 6, 3177, 1979.

23. **Appels, R., Driscoll, C., and Peacock, W. J.**, Heterochromatin and highly repeated DNA sequences in Rye *(Secale cereale)*, *Chromosoma (Berlin)*, 70, 67, 1978.

24. **Jones, J. D. G. and Flavell, R. B.**, The structure amount and chromosomal localization of defined DNA sequences in species of the genus *Secale*, *Chromosoma (Berlin)*, 86, 613, 1982.

25. **Giraldez, R., Cermemo, M. C., and Orellana, J.**, Comparison of C-banding pattern in the chromosomes of inbred lines and open pollinated varieties of rye, *Z. Pflanzenzuch*, 83, 40, 1979.

26. **Lobov, V. P.**, Repeated sequences in maize DNA, *Fiziol. Biochim. Kult. Rast.*, 13, 477, 1981.

27. **Rhoades, M. M., Peacock, W. J., Dennis, E. S., and Prior, A. J.**, Highly repeated DNA sequence limited to knob heterochromatin in maize, *Proc. Natl. Acad. Sci. U.S.A.*, 78, 4490, 1981.

28. **Gupta, V. S. and Ranjekar, P. K.**, DNA sequence organisation in finger millet, *J. Biosci.*, 3, 417, 1981.

29. **Potter, S. S., Brorein, W. J., Dunsmuir, P., and Rubin, G. M.**, Transposition of elements of the 412, copia and 297 dispersed repeated gene families in *Drosophila*, *Cell*, 17, 415, 1979.

30. **Moyzis, D. K., Bonnet, J., Li, D. W., and Ts'o, P.O.P.**, An alternative view of mammalian DNA sequence organisation, *J. Mol. Biol.*, 53, 871, 1981.

31. **Crick, F.**, Split genes and RNA splicing, *Science*, 204, 264, 1979.

32. **Darnell, J. E.**, Implications of RNA-RNA splicing in evolution of eukaryotic cells, *Science*, 202, 1257, 1978.

33. **Sogin, H. L., Pace, B., and Pace, N. R.**, Partial purification and properties of a ribosomal RNA maturation endonuclease from *Bacillus subtilis*, *J. Biol. Chem.*, 252, 1350, 1977.

34. **Glover, D. M.**, Cloned segment of *Drosophila melanogaster* rDNA containing new types of sequence insertion, *Proc. Natl. Acad. Sci. U.S.A.*, 74, 4932, 1977.

35. **Wallaver, P. K. and Dawid, I. B.**, Ribosomal DNA in *Drosophila melanogaster*. II. Heteroduplex mapping of cloned and uncloned rDNA, *J. Mol. Biol.*, 126, 769, 1978.

36. **Dawid, I. B. and Botchun, P.**, Sequences homologous to ribosomal insertions occur in the *Drosophila* genome outside the nuclear organizer, *Proc. Natl. Acad. Sci. U.S.A.*, 74, 4233, 1977.

37. **McClintock, B.**, Chromosome organisation and genic expression, *Cold Spring Harbor Symp. Quant. Biol.*, 16, 13, 1952.

38. **Evans, M. B., Yeninolopov, G. H., Peunova, N. I., and Ityin, Y.**, Transposition of mobile genetic elements in the interspecific hybrids in *Drosophila*, *Chromosoma (Berlin)*, 85, 375, 1982.

39. **Cameron, J. R., Loh, E. Y., and Davis, R. W.**, Evidence of transposition of dispersed repetitive DNA families in yeast, *Cell*, 16, 739, 1979.

40. **Strobel, S. W., Dunsmuir, P., and Rubin, G. M.**, Polymorphism in the chromosomal location elements of the 412, copia and 297 dispersed repeated gene families in *Drosophila*, *Cell*, 17, 429, 1979.

41. **Green, M. M.**, Transposable elements in *Drosophila* and other Diptera, *Annu. Rev. Genet.*, 14, 104, 1980.

42. **Calabretta, B., Robertson, D. L., Barrera-Saldona, H. A., Lambrou, T. P., and Saunders, G. F.**, Genome instability in a region of human DNA enriched in Alu repeat sequences, *Nature (London)*, 216, 219, 1983.

43. **Jacq, B., Jourdan, R., and Jordan, B. R.**, Structure and processing of precursor 5S RNA in *Drosophila melanogaster*, *J. Mol. Biol.*, 177, 785, 1979.

44. **Fedorof, N. V.,** On spacers, *Cell,* 16, 697, 1979.
45. **Cohn, R. H. and Kedes, L. H.,** Non-allelic histone gene clusters of individual sea urchins *(Lytechinus pictus)* polarity and gene organisation, *Cell,* 18, 843, 1979.
46. **Waldron, J., Dansmuir, P., and Bedbrook, J.,** Characterization of rDNA repeat unit in Mitchell *Petunia* genome, *Plant Mol. Biol.,* 2, 57, 1983.
47. **Evans, G. M. and Rees, H.,** Mitotic cycles in dicotyledons and monocotyledons, *Nature (London),* 233, 350, 1971.
48. **Bennet, M. C.,** Nuclear DNA content and minimum generation time in herbaceous plants, *Proc. R. Soc. Lond Ser. B:,* 181, 109, 1972.
49. **Price, H. J.,** Evolution of DNA contents in higher plants, *Bot. Rev.,* 42, 27, 1976.
50. **Bostock, C. J.,** The organisation of DNA sequences in chromosomes, in *Cell Biology,* Goldstein, L. and Prescott, D. M., Eds., Academic Press, New York, 1980.
51. **Flavell, R. B.,** Molecular changes in chromosomal DNA organisation and origins of phenotypic variation, in *Chromosomes Today,* Bennett, M. D., Bobrow, M., and Hewitt, G., Eds., George Allen & Unwin, London, 1981, 42.
52. **Klein, H. L. and Welch, S. K.,** Inverted repeated sequences in yeast nuclear DNA, *Nucleic Acids Res.,* 8, 4651, 1980.
53. **Deumling, B.,** Localization of fold back DNA sequences in the nuclei and chromosomes of *Scilla, Secale* and Mouse, *Nucleic Acids Res.,* 5, 3589, 1978.
54. **Stack, S. M. and Comings, D. E.,** The chromosomes and DNA of *Allium cepa, Chromosoma (Berlin),* 70, 161, 1979.
55. **Bassi, P., Cremonini, R., and Cionini, P. G.,** Cytological localization of inverted repeated DNA sequences in *Vicia faba, Chromosoma (Berlin),* 85, 453, 1982.
56. **Orgel, L. E. and Crick, F. H. C.,** Selfish DNA — the ultimate parasite, *Nature (London),* 284, 604, 1980.
57. **Dover, G. and Doolittle, W. F.,** Modes of genome evolution, *Nature (London),* 288, 646, 1980.
58. **Jain, H. K.,** Incidental DNA, *Nature (London),* 288, 647, 1980.
59. **Proudfoot, N.,** Pseudogenes, *Nature (London),* 286, 840, 1980.
60. **Dawid, I. B., Long, E. O., Di Novera, P. P., and Pardue, M. L.,** Ribosomal insertion-like elements in *Drosophila melanogaster* are interspersed with mobile sequences, *Cell,* 25, 399, 1981.
61. **Sharma, A. K.,** Additional genetic elements in chromosomes, *Nucleus,* 21, 113, 1978.
62. **Sharma, A. K.,** DNA repeats and their terminology, *Nucleus,* 24, 87, 1981.
63. **Dawid, I.,** Genomic change and morphological evolution: group report, in *Evolution and Development,* Bonner, J. T., Ed., Springer-Verlag, Basel, 1982, 19.
64. **Davidson, E. H. and Britten, R. J.,** Regulation of gene expression: possible role of repetitive sequences, *Science,* 204, 1052, 1979.
65. **John, B. and Miklos, C. L. G.,** Functional aspects of satellite DNA and heterochromatin, *Int. Rev. Cytol.,* 58, 114, 1979.
66. **Beauchamp, R. S., Mitchell, A. R., Buckland, R. A., and Bostock, C. J.,** Specific arrangements of human satellite III DNA sequences in human chromosomes, *Chromosoma,* 71, 153, 1979.
67. **Young, M. W.,** Middle repetitive DNA: a fluid component of the *Drosophila* genome, *Proc. Natl. Acad. Sci. U.S.A.,* 76, 6274, 1979.
68. **Egel, R.,** Intergenic conversion and reiterated genes, *Nature (London),* 290, 20, 1981.
69. **Klein, H. L. and Petes, T. D.,** Intrachromosomal gene conversion in yeast, *Nature (London),* 289, 144, 1981.
70. **Liebhader, S. A., Gossens, M., and Kan, Y. W.,** Homology and concerted evolution at the 1 and 2 loci of human globin, *Nature (London),* 290, 26, 1981.
71. **Henstschel, C. H. and Birnsteil, M. U.,** The organisation and expression of histone gene families, *Cell,* 25, 301, 1981.
72. **Grosschedl, R. and Birnsteil, M. L.,** Identification of regulatory sequences in the prelude sequences of H2A histone gene by the study of specific deletion mutants *in vivo, Proc. Natl. Acad. Sci. U.S.A.,* 77, 1432, 1980.
73. **Probst, E., Kressmann, A., and Birnsteil, M. L.,** Expression of sea urchin histone genes in the oocyte of *Xenopus laevis, J. Mol. Biol.,* 135, 705, 1979.
74. **Bachmann, K., Goin, O. B., and Goin, C. J.,** Nuclear DNA amounts in vertebrates, *Brookhaven Symp. Biol.,* 23, 419, 1972.
75. **Stebbins, G. L.,** Ecological distribution centers of adaptive radiation in angiosperms, in *Taxonomy, Phytogeographs and Evolution,* Valentine, D. H., Ed., Academic Press, New York, 1972, 7.
76. **Hinegardnar, R.,** Evolution of genome size, in *Molecular Evolution,* Ayala, F. J., Ed., Sinauer Associated, Sunderland, Mass., 1976, 179.
77. **Cavalier-Smith, T.,** How selfish is DNA? *Nature (London),* 285, 617, 1980.

78. **Cavalier-Smith, T.,** Long palindromes in eukaryotic DNA, *Nature (London),* 262, 255, 1976.
79. **Heumanns, J. M.,** A model of replication of the ends of linear chromosomes, *Nucleic Acids Res.,* 3, 3167, 1976.
80. **Hartman, N., Bell, A. J., and McLanchlan, A.,** Organisation of inverted repeat sequences in hamster cell nuclear DNA, *Biochim. Biophys. Acta,* 564, 372, 1979.
81. **Borschsenius, S. N., Merk Ina, N. A., Romanov, G. A., and Vanyshin, B. F.,** Palindromic and repetitive sequences in initiation sites of DNA replication in *Tetrahymena, Mol. Biol.,* 15, 816, 1981.
82. **Deininger, P. L. and Schmidt, C. W.,** An electron microscope study of the DNA sequence organisation of the human genome, *J. Mol. Biol.,* 106, 773, 1976.
83. **Gailit, J. O., and Fredrickson, D. W.,** Possible palindromic DNA, *J. Theor. Biol.,* 88, 241, 1981.
84. **Jelinek, W.,** Specific nucleotide sequences in HeLa cell inverted repeated DNA. Enrichment for sequences found in double stranded regions of heterogenous nuclear RNA, *J. Mol. Biol.,* 115, 591, 1977.
85. **Artymiuk, P. J., Blake, C. C. F., and Dippel, A. E.,** Genes pieced together — exons delineate homologous structures of diverged lysozymes, *Nature (London),* 290, 287, 1981.
86. **Slighton, J. L., Blechl, A. E., and Smithies, O.,** Human fetal γ^G and γ^A globin genes: complete nucleotide sequences suggest that DNA can be exchanged between these duplicated genes, *Cell,* 21, 627, 1980.
87. **Müntzing, A.,** Accessory chromosomes, *Ann. Rev. Genet.,* 8, 243, 1977.
88. **Sharma, A. K.,** Genetic diversity of some monocotyledonous crops and their wild relatives in the Eastern Himalayan Region, Workshop Conf. Tropical Plant Res. SE Asia, New Delhi, 1982.
89. **Sharma, A. K. and Aiyangar, H. R.,** Occurrence of B chromosomes in diploid *Allium stracheyii* and their elimination, *Chromosoma,* 12, 310, 1961.
90. **Sharma, A. K.,** Chromosomes and distribution of Monocotyledons in the Eastern Himalayas, in *Tropical Botany,* Larsen, K. and Holm-Nilsen, L. B., Eds., Academic Press, New York, 1979, 327.
91. **Jones, R. N.,** B chromosome system in flowering plant and animal species, *Int. Rev. Cytol.,* 40, 1, 1975.
92. **John, B.,** The role of chromosome change in the evolution of orthopteroid insects, in *Chromosomes in Evolution of Eukaryotic Groups,* Vol. 1, Sharma, A. K. and Sharma, A., Eds., CRC Press, Boca Raton, Fla., 1983, 1.

INDEX

O

Oats *(Avena sativa)*
  gene pools of, 23
  haploid DNA content for, 26
  phylogenetic relationships of, 72
  repeated DNA sequences of, 26, 29, 34, 36
  sequence organization pattern in, 29
Oenothera, 71
Oryza, 6
Osmunda cinnamomea (cinnamon fern), 64, 65
Osteichtyes, rDNA units in, 90

P

Palindromes, description of, 189
Papilionoieae, evolution of, 72
Parasitic DNA, 190
Parsimony, principle of, 67—68
pDNA (pachytene DNA), 191
Pea *(Pisum sativum)*, see also *Pisum*, 74
Pearl millet, see Millet
Petunia hybrida (petunia), 73
Petunia parodii, 72
Phalaris
  interspecific variation in DNA content of, 5, 12
  variation in DNA content of, 7
Phaseolus
  interspecific variation in DNA content of, 6, 12
  phylogenetic relationships of, 177
Phaseolus vulgaris (dwarf bean)
  phylogenetic relationships of, 72
  4.5S rRNA from, 158
Philosamia, 5.8S rRNAs of, 150, 151
Phylogenetic probes, IVS, 117
Phylogenetic trees, 67—68
  construction of, 155
  "present-day ancestor" method of building, 156
Phylogenies
  of basidiomycetes, 48
  for *Brassica*, 68
  of fungi, 47
  molecular approaches to derivation of
    hybridization, 108
    hybrid melting point (Tm) analysis, 108
    restriction enzyme analyses, 107—108
    sequence analyses, 111
  plant vs. animal, 138
Physarum, 157
Physarum polycephalum
  extra chromosomal rDNA of, 84
  gene duplication in, 50
Picea, 6
Pinus, 7
Pisum
  chloroplast DNA relationships in, 71
  phylogenetic studies in, 68
Pisum sativum (pea), 74
Plant leaf, "universal model" for, 153, 154
Plants, higher

genomes of
  evolution of protein-coding sequences, 177—179
  evolving gene families in, 179—180
  formation of, 180
  structure and evolution of, 173
  role of polyploidy in DNA evolution of, 173—177
  5.8S rRNA sequences for, 155
  sequenced 5.8S rRNAs for, 145
Plasmodium lophurae, 143
Point mutations, 72
Polymorphisms
  fragment length, 115
  restriction enzyme site, 115
Polyploidy
  DNA content and, 38
  DNA diminution in, 10
  generative, 186
  of Gramineae, 22
  in higher plant evolution, 10—11
  in plant DNA evolution, 173—177
  significance of, 180
Porifera, sequenced 5.8S rRNAs for, 145
Prokaryotes, rDNA units in, 85
Promoter sequences, for chloroplast gene transcription, 66
Protein-coding sequences, of plant genomes, 177—179
Protein synthesis, chloroplast, 66
Protozoa
  rDNA units in, 86, 142
  sequenced 5.8S rRNAs for, 145
Protozoa, ciliated, restriction enzyme analysis of, 118
Prunus, 177
Pseudogenes
  description, 190
  formation, 75
Pulsatilla, 5

R

Radish *(Raphanus sativa)*, 69
Ranunculus, interspecific variation in DNA content of, 5
Raphanus sativa (radish), 69
Rattus, 151
Rattus norvegicus (rat), 91
rDNA
  extrachromosomal vs. chromosomal, 101
  molecular analysis of, 104—107
rDNA genes, electron microscopic visualization of, 93
rDNA locus
  evolutionary change at
    differentiation at species level and above, 115—119
    individual and population variation, 111—115
  evolutionary trends at, 82—93

Printed in the United States
by Baker & Taylor Publisher Services